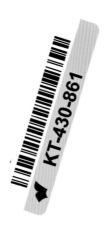

Pearce's Surgical Companion

Essential notes for postgraduate exams

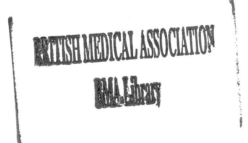
Oliver Pearce

tfm Publishing Limited, Castle Hill Barns, Harley, Nr Shrewsbury, SY5 6LX, UK.

Tel: +44 (0)1952 510061; Fax: +44 (0)1952 510192

E-mail: nikki@tfmpublishing.com; Web site: www.tfmpublishing.com

Design & Typesetting:	Nikki Bramhill BSc Hons, Dip Law, Solicitor
First Edition:	© May 2009
Illustrations:	Nicki Averill, Nicki Averill Design and Illustration
Front cover images:	© 1999 Image 100 Ltd.
	© Comstock Inc., www.comstock.com

ISBN: 978 1 903378 48 9

Printed by Gutenberg Press Ltd., Gudja Road, Tarxien, PLA 19, Malta.

Tel: +356 21897037; Fax: +356 21800069.

Contents

Contents

Preface

The inspiration for this book came from undertaking my own postgraduate surgical exams, specifically the MRCS in the UK, in 2001. It cannot escape the notice of candidates that the list of textbooks one needs to read is long, and large sections of each book are simply not aimed towards passing these exams, but rather they are aimed very much at their own specialist subject; there felt like a lot of redundancy in reading them.

Why then, shouldn't there be a single book aimed at the level of postgraduate surgical exams, containing much of the information needed in a user friendly format? Well, if there wasn't such a book out there, why not write it? The answer, it would seem, is because it is an enormous undertaking. It is a difficult niche to fill and after all, who out there really has the breadth of knowledge to write such a book? The only individuals who encompass that knowledge (however transiently) are those poor souls actually taking the exam. Thus, the time to write it is immediately post-exam. There will of course be subjects too specialised for inclusion in this book, which by its very nature is focused on the level of knowledge you must acquire to enter the ranks of specialist surgical training.

This book was written whilst I was a Specialist Registrar in Orthopaedic Surgery in the Oxford region. I have a great personal interest in medical education. I am a Clinical Tutor at the Nuffield Orthopaedic Centre, Oxford, and a College Tutor for the graduate-entry medical degree at Worcester College, Oxford, for the Clinical Surgery course. I have edited a number of orthopaedic chapters in the new edition of the Surgical Trainee Education Program (STEP) course, a series of modules which forms the syllabus of the UK surgical exam, the Membership of the Royal College of Surgeons (MRCS). I also sit, as National Trainee Representative, on the Royal College of Surgeons Committee, the Faculty Steering Group, with the brief of training consultants on how to train the trainees of the future in the Intercollegiate Surgical Curriculum Project (ISCP). I am also a reviewer for the *Journal of Bone and Joint Surgery* (British edition).

When I'm not writing or teaching, I quite enjoy running, cycling and swimming, competing in regular triathlons and runs around the region. I enjoy reading books other people have written too!

I sincerely hope you benefit from everything this book has to offer; it has been a labour of love for the last six years of my life.

Oliver Pearce MBBS FRCS
April 2009

Acknowledgements

I would like to extend a special thank you to all the following consultants, experts in their fields, who kindly gave their time to ensure the information contained in each chapter is contemporary, correct and clearly set out.

Mr. S. Aiono MSc FRCS FRACS Consultant General Surgeon, Wanganui Hospital, New Zealand. *General surgery and vascular surgery sections.*

Mr. C. Aldren MA MB BS FRCS FRCS(ORL) Consultant ENT Surgeon, Wexham Park Hospital, Slough, UK. *ENT sections.*

Mr. A. Andrade FRCS MSc Consultant Orthopaedic Surgeon, Royal Berkshire Hospital, Reading, UK. *Orthopaedic chapters.*

Dr. M. Bradley BSc MB BS MRCP FRCR Consultant Neuroradiologist, Frenchay Hospital, North Bristol NHS Trust, Bristol, UK. *Head injury and neurology sections.*

Dr. I. Decamps MD Consultant Anaesthetist (Practicien Hospitalier), University Hospital St. Marguerite, Marseille, France. *Physiology chapter.*

Mr. A. Gandhe BSc FRCS Fellow in Hip and Knee Arthroplasty, Royal Berkshire Hospital, Reading, UK. *For his expert help with illustrations.*

Mr B. Harrison MB BS MS FRCS(Eng) Consultant Endocrine Surgeon, Royal Hallamshire Hospital, Sheffield, UK. *Endocrine sections.*

Dr. A. Helaine Doctor of Medicine, Assistant Chef de Clinique, Anaesthetics and Intensive Care Medicine, University Hospital St. Marguerite, Marseille, France. *Physiology chapter.*

Dr. R. Jack FRCA Consultant Anaesthetist and Medical Director, Wexham Park Hospital, Slough, UK. *Physiology chapter.*

Dr. A. Lessing MBChB (Hon) MSc FRCP FRCPI FRCPath DTM&H Consultant Physician & Clinical Director Infectious Diseases, Heatherwood and Wexham Park Hospitals NHS Foundation Trust, HCAI Evaluation Group, South Central Strategic Health Authority, Slough, UK. *Microbiology section.*

Mr. H. Motiwala MS FRCSUrol Consultant Urological Surgeon, Clinical Lead (Urology) and Programme Director (London Deanery), Wexham Park Hospital, Slough, UK. *Urology and renal sections.*

Mr. S. Pearce MRCS Specialist Registrar in Orthopaedics, South East London region, UK. A thank you for his overall input in the organization of this textbook. As someone who was going through the exam at the time of writing, his comments, and individual contributions to chapters were instrumental to the book. Especially useful were his identification of glaring omissions that needed further attention. He has provided a fresh perspective that brought new life to this textbook.

Mr. R. Ragoowansi MB MSc FRCS (Plast) Consultant Plastic & Hand Surgeon, Barts and the London NHS Trust, London, UK. *Burns section.*

Mr. A.R. Rao MS DNB MSc FRCSEd Specialist Registrar and Honorary Research Fellow in Urology, Wexham Park Hospital, Slough, UK. *Urology and renal sections.*

Dr. H. Sharif MB ChB FRCPath Consultant Histopathologist, Wexham Park Hospital, Slough, UK. *Histology and pathology sections.*

Mr. A. Sierakowski BSc (Hons) MB BS MRCS Clinical Fellow in General Surgery, Lister Hospital, Stevenage, UK. *Breast and vascular surgery sections.*

And, of course, to my dear wife, Lina, who has been the very ideal of support throughout the creation of this book and without whom I could never have actually finished.

Bibliography

Basic Pathology (Kumar Cotran and Robbins).

Colour Atlas of Human Anatomy (McMinn, Abrahams, Hutchings and Marks).

Last's Anatomy (Last).

Principles of Physiology (Berne and Levy).

Clinical Surgery in General (Kirk, Mansfield and Cochrane).

The New Aird's Companion in Surgical Studies (Burnand and Young).

Clinical Anatomy (Ellis).

Concise Medical Dictionary (Oxford reference).

Contemporary Operative Surgery (Adrian Marston).

General Surgical Operations (Kirk).

An Introduction to Human Anatomy (Green and Silver).

An Introduction to the Signs and Symptoms of Surgical Disease (Browse).

Apley's System of Orthopaedics and Fractures (Apley).

Miller's Review of Orthopaedics (Miller).

And, of course, the STEP Course, 1996 edition.

Abbreviations

AAA Abdominal aortic aneurysm
ABG Arterial blood gas
ABPI Ankle Brachial Pressure Index
ACDF Anterior cervical disc fusion
ACh Acetylcholine
ACJ Acromioclavicular joint
ACL Anterior cruciate ligament
ACTH Adrenocorticotrophic hormone
ACV Assist control ventilation
ADH Antidiuretic hormone
ADP Adenosine diphospate
Adr Adrenaline
AF Atrial fibrillation
AIN Anterior interosseous nerve
Alb Albumin
ALP Alkaline phosphatase
ANA Antinuclear antibody
ANP Atrial natriuretic peptide
ANS Autonomic nervous system
AP Action potential
APACHE Acute Physiolgy And Chronic Health Evaluation
APC Antigen-presenting cell
APL Abductor pollicis longus
APS Acute physiology score
APTR Activated partial thromboplastin ratio
APTT Activated partial thromboplastin time
ARDS Acute respiratory distress syndrome
ASA American Society of Anaesthesiologists
ASIS Anterior superior iliac spine
AST Aspartate transaminase
ATFL Anterior talofibular ligament
ATLS® Advanced Trauma Life Support®
ATP Adenosine triphosphate
AV Atrioventricular
AVN Avascular necrosis
AXR Abdominal X-ray
BCC Basal cell carcinoma
BCG Bacille Calmette-Guerin
BKA Below-knee amputation
BOO Bladder outflow obstruction
BP Blood pressure
BPH Benign prostatic hypertrophy
BSE Bovine spongiform encephalopathy
CA Carbonic anhydrase
CABG Coronary artery bypass graft

CAH Congenital adrenal hyperplasia
CBD Common bile duct
CBT Cognitive behavioural therapy
CC Costal cartilage
CCF Congestive cardiac failure
CCK Cholecystokinin
CEA Carcino-embryonic antigen
CF Cystic fibrosis
Ch Choline
CIS Carcinoma in situ
CISC Clean intermittent self-catheterisation
CK Creatine kinase (CK MB = The isoenzyme fraction of CK of the MB type. M = Muscle, B = Brain, therefore there are 3 different combinations of isoenzymes possible, CK MM, CK MB or CK BB).
CMCJ Carpometacarpal joint
CMV Cytomegalovirus
CNS Central nervous system
CO Cardiac output
COAD Chronic obstructive airways disease
COPD Chronic obstructive pulmonary disease
CPAP Continuous positive airway pressure
CPM Continuous passive movement
CRF Chronic renal failure
CRH Corticotrophin releasing hormone
CRP C-reactive protein
CRPS Chronic regional pain syndrome
CS Clotting screen
CSF Cerebrospinal fluid
CTS Carpal tunnel syndrome
CVA Cerebrovascular accident
CVP Central venous pressure
CVS Cardiovascular system
CXR Chest X-ray
D1 First part of the duodenum
DCIS Ductal carcinoma in situ
DCS Dynamic condylar screw
DDAVP Desmopressin (1-desamino-8-d-arginine-vasopressin)
DHEA Dihydroepiandrosterone
DHS Dynamic hip screw
DIC Disseminated intravascular coagulation
DIPJ Distal interphalangeal joint
DMSA 99mTc dimercaptosuccinic acid scan
2,3 DPG 2,3 Diphosphoglycerine

DRE Digital rectal examination
DUSS Distal urethral striated sphincter
DVT Deep vein thrombosis
DXT Radiotherapy
EBV Epstein-Barr virus
ECF Extracellular fluid
ECG Electrocardiogram
EMG Electromyography
EMLA Eutectic mixture of local anaesthetics
EO Ethylene oxide
EPB Extensor pollicis brevis
EPL Extensor pollicis longus
ERCP Endoscopic retrograde cholangiopancreatography
ESR Erythrocyte sedimentation rate
ET Endotracheal
EUA Examination under anaesthetic
FAP Familial adenomatous polyposis
FBC Full blood count
FDP Flexor digitorum profundus
FDS Flexor digitorum superficialis
FESS Functional endoscopic sinus surgery
FEV Forced expiratory volume
FFP Fresh frozen plasma
FHx Family history
FMTC Familial medullary thyroid cancer
FNA Fine needle aspiration
FOB Faecal occult blood
FPB Flexor pollicis brevis
FPL Flexor pollicis longus
FRC Functional residual capacity
FSH Follicular stimulating hormone
FVC Forced vital capacity
GA General anaesthesia
GABA Gamma-aminobutyric acid
GammaGT Gamma glutamyl transpeptidase
GB Gallbladder
GCS Glasgow Coma Scale
GFR Glomerular filtration rate
GHIH Growth hormone inhibitory hormone
GHJ Glenohumeral joint
GHRH Growth hormone releasing hormone
GIP Gastro-inhibitory peptide
GIT Gastrointestinal tract
Glu Glucose
GnRH Gonadotrophin releasing hormone
G+S Group and save
GT Greater trochanter
GTN Glyceryl trinitrate
H Hydrogen
Hb Haemoglobin
HCG Human chorionic gonadotrophin
Hct Haematocrit
HGH Human growth hormone

HIT Heparin-induced thrombocytopaenia
HLA Human leucocyte antigen
HPT Hyperparathyroidism
HPV Human papilloma virus
HR Heart rate
5-HT 5-Hydroxytryptamine (also known as serotonin)
HTLV1 Human type leukocyte virus type 1
IADSA Intra-arterial digital subtraction angiogram
ICP Intracranial pressure
ICS Intercostal space
IFN Interferon
IJV Internal jugular vein
IL Interleukin
IMA Inferior mesenteric artery
INR International normalised ratio
IPJ Interphalangeal joint
ITP Idiopathic thrombocytopaenic purpurae
IVC Inferior vena cava
IVDSA Intravenous digital subtraction angiogram
IVU Intravenous urethrogram
K Potassium
KUB Kidney, urethra, bladder
LA Local anaesthetic
LAD Left anterior descending
LCIS Lobular carcinoma in situ
LCL Lateral cruciate ligament
LDH Lactate dehydrogenase
LFT Liver function test
LH Luteinising hormone
LISS Less invasive stabilisation system
LMP Last menstrual period
LMWH Low-molecular-weight heparin
LN Lymph node
LT Leukotriene
LTN Long thoracic nerve
LUTS Lower urinary tract symptoms
LVF Left ventricular failure
MALT Mucosa-associated lymphoid tissue
MAP Mean arterial pressure
MCL Medial cruciate ligament
MCPJ Metacarpophalangeal joint
MC+S Microscopy, culture and sensitivity
MCV Mean cellular volume
MEN Multiple endocrine neoplasia
MHC Major histocompatabilty complex
MI Myocardial infarction
MIBG Meta-iodobenzylguanidine
MLC Mixed lymphocyte culture
MM Malignant melanoma
MNG Multi-nodular goitre
MODS Multiple organ dysfunction syndrome
MOF Multi-organ failure
MRA Magnetic resonance angiography

MRSA Methicillin-resistant *Staphylococcus aureus*
MSH Melanocyte stimulating hormone
MSU Mid-stream urine
MTC Medullary thyroid cancer
MTPJ Metatarsophalangeal joint
MUA Manipulation under anaesthetic
Na Sodium
NAC Non-albicans Candida
NBM Nil by mouth (also known as NPO, nil per orum)
NdYAG Neodynium yttrium argon
NCS Nerve conduction studies
NG Nasogastric
NHL Non-Hodgkin's lymphoma
NO Nitrous oxide
NOF Neck of femur
NSAID Non-steroidal anti-inflammatory drug
OA Osteoarthritis
OCP Oral contraceptive pill
OGD Oesophago-gastroduodenoscopy
OH Chemical symbolism for hydroxide, i.e. oxygen and hydrogen (OH)
ORIF Open reduction and internal fixation
PAC Pulmonary artery catheter
PAF Paroxysmal atrial fibrillation
PAM Post-amputation mobility
PAN Polyarteritis nodosum
PCL Posterior cruciate ligament
PCNL Percutaneous nephrolithotomy
PDS Polydiaxalone (type of suture material, a polymer)
PE Pulmonary embolism
PEEP Positive end expiratory pressure
PG Prostaglandin
PIH Prolactin inhibitory hormone
PIN Posterior interosseous nerve
PIPJ Proximal interphalangeal joint
PNS Peripheral nervous system
POP Plaster of Paris
PPI Proton pump inhibitor
PR Per rectum
PRH Prolactin releasing hormone
PSA Prostate-specific antigen
PTC Percutaneous transhepatic cholangiography
PTFE Polytetrafluoroethylene
PTH Parathyroid hormone
PTHrP Parathyroid hormone-related peptide
PV Per vaginum
PVR Peripheral vascular resistance
QOL Quality of life
RA Rheumatoid arthritis
RBC Red blood cell
RC Residual capacity
RIF Right iliac fossa
RLN Recurrent laryngeal nerve
RR Respiratory rate

RSD Reflex sympathetic dystrophy
RTA Road traffic accident
RUQ Right upper quadrant
RV Residual volume
SA Sino-atrial
SBE Subacute bacterial endocarditis
SCC Squamous cell carcinoma
SCIDS Severe combined immunodeficiency syndrome
SCIWORA Spinal cord injury without radiological abnormality
SCM Sternocleidomastoid
SF Saphenofemoral
SIMV Synchronised intermittent mandatory ventilation
SIRS Systemic inflammatory response syndrome
SLE Systemic lupus erythematosus
SMA Superior mesenteric artery
SSI Surgical site infection
SUFE Slipped upper femoral epiphysis
SV Stroke volume
SVC Superior vena cava
SVR Systemic vascular resistance
TAO Thyroid-associated ophthalmopathy
TB Tuberculosis
TBSA Total body surface area
TCC Transitional cell carcinoma
TEDS Thrombo-embolic deterrent stockings
TFL Tensor fascia lata
TFT Thyroid function tests
TIA Transient ischaemic attack
TIPS Transjugular intrahepatic portosytemic shunt
TLC Total lung capacity
TLC-RC Total lung capacity-residual capacity
TMJ Temperomandibular joint
TNF Tumour necrosis factor
TPA Tissue plasminogen activator
TRH Thyrotrophin releasing hormone
TRUS Transrectal ultrasound
TSH Thyroid stimulating hormone
TUNA Transurethral needle ablation
TURBT Transurethral resection of bladder tumour
TURP Transurethral resection of the prostate
TV Tidal volume
UC Ulcerative colitis
U&E Urea and electrolytes
URTI Upper respiratory tract infection
USS Ultrasound scanning
UTI Urinary tract infection
VAU Vein, artery, ureter
VCMG Video cystometrogram
VF Ventricular fibrillation
VMA Vanillimandelic acid
WCC White cell count
XGP Xanthogranulomatous pyelonephritis

Section 1

Applied basic sciences

Chapter 1

Pathology and practice of surgery

Basic pathological terminology

This is a brief introduction to a few basic terms of pathology. More definitions relating to pathology will arise throughout the book. Definitions are an important basic premise from which to build more complex concepts within a particular subject.

Terminology

Aetiology
The 'cause' of a disease.

Pathogenesis
The 'mechanism(s)' by which a disease occurs.

Cellular adaptive responses
- Atrophy: partial or complete wasting, from the Greek 'trophy' meaning growth, and the prefix 'a' meaning absence of.
- Hypertrophy: increase in size of cells.
- Hyperplasia: increase in number of cells.
- Metaplasia: reversible change of one mature tissue cell type, for another mature tissue cell type.
- Necrosis: cell death (not dependent on an energy-using process), usually from ischaemic causes.
- Apoptosis: a cell death reaction (dependent on an energy-using process), which is pre-programmed as part of the normal cell life cycle. It can also be induced by toxins (e.g. free radicals), micro-organisms or some inflammatory mediators (e.g. interferon).

Note
- Apoptosis stems from the etymological root to 'fall away'.
- Cell injury can be classified into 'reversible' and 'irreversible' cell injury.

Ischaemia
Supply of blood inadequate for a tissue/organ's metabolic need.

Infarction
Death of tissue following acute ischaemia where irreparable damage has occurred.

True gangrene
Necrosis with putrefaction.

Dry gangrene (mummification)
Dessication of necrosed tissues usually secondary to chronic ischaemia. Tissues appear black because of deposits of iron sulphide from degraded haemoglobin. There is a dry, shrivelled area with an inflammatory zone at the junction of living and dead tissue (line of demarcation).

Wet gangrene

Saprophytic infection and putrefaction of tissues. Progressive infection exacerbates ischaemia, spreading gangrene and necessitating more proximal amputation.

Gas gangrene

Spreading tissue necrosis when Clostridia spores gain access to the wound (most commonly *Clostridium perfringens*) in which there is extensive soft tissue or muscle injury. Clostridium produces gas and powerful toxins which cause further tissue damage and spreads infection.

Meleney's gangrene

May occur at the site of abdominal surgery. It is caused by a combination of aerobic and anaerobic bacteria forming a cellulitis followed by gangrene.

Fournier's gangrene

Spontaneous onset of rapidly progressing gangrene of the scrotum in otherwise healthy men. It is caused by synergism of faecal bacteria and anaerobes (similar aetiology to Meleney's).

Necrotising fasciitis

Rapidly spreading necrosis through fascial planes often with normal looking overlying skin in the early stages. Later, the skin is deprived of blood supply and becomes painful, red and, finally, necrotic. The patient is then severely ill with fever and toxaemia. It is caused by mixed flora including Streptococcus, Staphylococcus, gram-negatives and anaerobes.

Transudate

An imbalance of hydrostatic and oncotic pressures resulting in a fluid of low protein content (<30g/L) crossing an intact endothelial surface.

Causes:

- Increased hydrostatic pressure (congestive cardiac failure [CCF], sodium/fluid retention, venous thrombosis).
- Decreased oncotic pressure (hepatic failure, malnutrition, nephrotic syndrome).
- Decreased lymphatic drainage (irradiation, lymphadenectomy).

Exudate

Inflammatory process resulting in a fluid of high protein content (>30g/L) crossing a damaged endothelium.

Causes:

- Serous (malignant ascites).
- Haemorrhagic (peritonitis).
- Purulent (*Escherichia coli* peritonitis).
- Fibrinous (pericarditis).
- Pseudomembranous colitis (*Clostridium difficile*).

Fistula

An abnormal communication between two epithelialised surfaces lined by chronic granulation tissue. Fistulae can be congenital or acquired (inflammatory causes, neoplastic causes, traumatic causes, infective causes). They can also be classified according to output: low <200ml in 24 hours, moderate 200-500ml in 24 hours, high >500ml in 24 hours.

Granuloma

Histologically, an apparently expansile mass of macrophages. Immunologically, a collection of activated macrophages surrounded by lymphocytes.

Causes:

- Indigestible organisms (e.g. TB).
- Foreign bodies.
- Crohn's disease.
- Idiopathic.

Abscess

A localised collection of pus, surrounded and walled off by damaged and inflamed tissue.

Pus

Fluid at the site of an established infection, containing dead white blood cells, both living and dead bacteria, and fragments of dead tissue.

Acute inflammation

This is defined as the immediate and early response to injury:

- Vascular changes, vasodilation and increased permeability, results in an exudate of protein-rich fluid, 'tissue oedema'.

- Leukocytes (mainly neutrophils) adhere and migrate to, then through, the vessel wall, to the site of the injury (they follow a chemotactic gradient).
- Phagocytosis of the offending agent then follows.
- During phagocytosis, there is release of toxic metabolites and proteases that can damage surrounding tissue.

Note

— Galen's mnemonic for acute inflammatory characteristics is Rubor, Calor, Dolor, Tumour, and Functio laesa.

— Vasoactive mediators in the above reaction are: histamine, 5-Hydroxytryptamine (5-HT), lysosomal enzymes, prostaglandins (PGs), leukotrienes (LTs), paroxysmal atrial fibrillation, nitrous oxide (NO), cytokines.

— Another system that kicks in at the stimulus of tissue injury is the coagulation cascade as well as the complement cascade.

The possible outcomes of acute inflammation are:

- Complete resolution.
- Scarring of affected tissue (in tissue incapable of regeneration).
- Abscess formation.
- Chronic inflammation.

Chronic inflammation

This is defined as inflammation of a prolonged duration (days to years), during which inflammation and tissue healing are proceeding simultaneously. It is characterised by the following:

- Infiltration of mononuclear cells. These are different from the cells seen in acute inflammation (neutrophils), as they are made up of lymphocytes, macrophages and plasma cells.
- Tissue destruction secondary to the effects of the inflammatory cells.
- New vessel formation, fibroblast proliferation and fibrosis.

Note

— An important definition to realise is that neutrophils are polymorphonucleocytes, and that macrophages are a type of monocyte. Both, however, are capable of phagocytosis.

Functions of the lymphatic system are:

- To drain the fluid from acute inflammation.
- To present antigen to the T- and B-cell systems located in more central lymph nodes for the purpose of the immune response. This is usually a good thing, but it can have a downside. When the lymphatic ducts become a pathway for spread of the infection, this is termed lymphangitis, or when the infection reaches the lymph nodes, this is termed lymphadenitis.

The systemic effects of inflammation are:

- Pyrexia.
- Leukocytosis.
- Raised erythrocyte sedimentation rate (ESR)/C-reactive protein (CRP).

Microbiology

Important definitions

- Gram stain: a technique named after Dr HC Gram, differentiating bacteria into two large groups, based on the properties of their cell wall, i.e. gram-positive, staining blue, or gram-negative, staining pink. The test is NOT a substitute for culture, and clinical application depends on whether the site is normally sterile, or not.
- Gram-positive organisms: a characteristic of gram-positive organisms is the ability to make exotoxins, which are proteins and enzymes that damage host cells. Examples are Staphylococci, Streptococci and Clostridia.
- Gram-negative organisms: a characteristic of gram-negative organisms is the production of endotoxins in their cell membranes, which have a clinical effect on death of the cell, stimulating macrophages to release inflammatory cytokines

with a toxic effect. Examples are *Escherichia coli*, Pseudomonas, Salmonellae.

- Cocci are spherical.
- Bacilli are rod-shaped.
- Aerobes need O_2 to grow.
- Anaerobes need an O_2-free environment to grow.
- Facultative anaerobes are aerobes that are capable of growing in O_2-free conditions.

Microflora

Staphylococci

A basic coagulase test rapidly differentiates between *Staphylococcus aureus* (SAU) (+) and the species of the coagulase-negative Staphylococci (CNS or CoNS) (-) which includes *S. epidermidis*, *S. haemolyticus* and many others.

Streptococci

The first differentiation is made based on haemolysis of red cells contained in the horse blood agar plate. Alpha-haemolysis (greenish colonies) denotes the *S. viridans* group, including the oral Streptococci (long coccal chains on microscopy), the faecal Streptococci (now named Enterococci) (short chains or diploccocal) and *S. pneumoniae* (short chains or diplococcal). Beta-haemolysis refers to complete lysis of the horse red cells resulting in complete clearing of the agar. These beta-haemolytic Streptococci are grouped as Group A, Group B, Group C, Group G, etc., and many species exist. A third group of Streptococci does not result in any haemolysis on the plate.

Rationale for antibiotic prophylaxis

It is essential to know about typical commensals of body surfaces and cavities. A commensal is an organism that forms part of the normal microbial flora of a body surface or cavity. Commensals are important because they can become infective organisms under certain circumstances. For example, *Staphylococcus aureus* is a skin (and nasal cavity) commensal organism, and when the skin is breached (i.e. cut) these organisms have the potential to cause wound infection.

Antibiotic prophylaxis is an essential concept to grasp; the administration of antibiotics to prevent infection by bacteria. Thus, it is important to know the appropriate antibiotic for prophylaxis. The choice of antibiotic is based on the recognised commensals that cause infection in the region of the intended surgery.

Prophylactic antibiotics are best given on induction of anaesthesia via the intravenous route, which achieves the maximal dose at time of surgery. There is no evidence in favour of giving more than one dose. The main aim of prophylaxis is to prevent postoperative wound infection.

Conventionally, surgical principles would suggest that antimicrobial prophylaxis is not required for 'clean' surgery. However, the case mix and comorbidities, and technical demands of the procedure, support the use of prophylaxis in selected clean procedures, e.g. joint replacement surgery.

Transmission of infection can be either via an exogenous or endogenous route. It should be emphasised at this point that endogenous organisms form the overwhelming majority of transmitted infections. Hand washing is a highly important preventative measure by hospital staff.

Surgical site infections

Surgical site infections (SSIs) can be either superficial or deep.

Superficial surgical site infections

This is infection of the incision site (see the classification of wound types [clean/dirty] on p12 for the incidence of superficial SSIs, although this is a guide only, as other factors affect the potential for wound infection, e.g. diabetes, chest infection [coughing on the wound], immune deficiency, etc). The consequences of superficial SSIs are less serious than for deep SSIs. The common causative organisms of superficial SSIs are *Staphylococcus aureus* or Streptococci. Antibiotics suitable for these organisms are flucloxacillin and benzyl penicillin.

Deep surgical site infections

This refers to infection of surgical implants (e.g. orthopaedic or vascular) or deep abdominal sepsis.

Orthopaedic implants are susceptible to coagulase-negative Staphylococci or alpha-haemolytic Streptococci.

Vascular grafts (e.g. Dacron aortic graft) are susceptible to *Staphylococcus aureus* or coagulase-negative Staphylococi. A special case occurs when there is an aorto-enteric fistula; this allows infection by gram-positive Staphylococci, Enterococci, and gram-negatives such as Pseudomonas and Bacteroides (i.e. polymicrobial infection).

An important point on deep SSIs is that they are highly resistant to antibiotic treatment, so much so that removing the prosthesis and inserting a replacement is the only alternative to long-term antibiosis (which more often than not only controls the infection rather than eradicating it).

Classification of antibiotics

Antibiotics are for the most part (95%) cell wall agents. Other groups can simply be summarised as the ribosomal group and others. For completeness, an antifungal section has been included.

Cell wall agents

It is worth emphasising that these represent 95% of all antibiotics used in clinical practice. Cell wall agents are divided into two basic subtypes, the beta lactams and the glycopeptides.

Beta lactams
Penicillins
Two examples are benzyl penicillin (anti-streptococcal activity) and flucloxacillin (anti-staphylococcal activity).

Note

—   Beta-lactamase inhibitor combinations are Augmentin (amoxycillin and clavulinic acid), and Tazocin (tazobactam). These are antibiotics where the major weakness of penicillins (the development of beta-lactamase by bacteria, which confers resistance to the antibiotic) has been compensated for.

Cephalosporins
Cefuroxime and cefotaxime have gram-positive and gram-negative cover, but no pseudomonal cover. Ceftazidime has gram-positive, gram-negative and anti-pseudomonal cover. It is not in general use due to side effect concerns, most notably infection with *Clostridium difficile*.

Glycopeptides
Vancomycin
Used in invasive MRSA infections intravenously. Levels need to be monitored twice a week (pre-dose, also known as 'trough' levels).

Ribosomal group (aminoglycosides)
These provide excellent gram-negative cover. They only require a once daily dose at 5mg/kg.

Their use for more than 72 hours is rarely needed. Examples of aminoglycosides are gentamicin, amikacin and doxycycline (which have good oral broad spectrum cover).

Others
Trimethoprim
Given orally, it is a useful anti-urinary tract infection agent.

Ciprofloxacin
Given orally, it is again a useful anti-urinary tract infection agent.

Rifampicin
For specialised use only. NEVER for monotherapy use; this is to prevent resistance.

Antifungals
These are used in invasive fungal infections such as intravenous line infections or intra-abdominal infections.

The 'azoles', e.g. fluconazole
Used to be first choice for *Candida albicans*. It is now less reliable as some types of *C. albicans* have become resistant.

The 'polyenes', e.g. amphotericin
Used commonly intravenously in the lipid complex formulation known as Abelcet. This version is particularly useful if the patient's serum creatinine is greater than 130µmol/L, as (unlike amphotericin) it is renal-sparing. Amphotericins tend to be replaced by echocandins, i.e. caspofungin, for non-*albicans* *Candida* (NAC) resistant to fluconazole (for example, NAC IV line or blood stream infection) or refractory invasive aspergillosis.

Sterilisation techniques

Sterilisation is the process of killing all micro-organisms:

- Steam under pressure: kills micro-organisms on the surface of instruments (3-15 minutes, depending on temperature).
- Hot air: temperature 160°C for two hours, therefore it is inefficient.
- Ethylene oxide (EO): mainly an industrial process for single-use instruments.
- Low temperature steam and formaldehyde: only requires a temperature of 73°C, so it is therefore useful for heat-sensitive instruments.
- Irradiation: industrial technique using gamma irradiation.

Disinfection is the process of reducing the number of micro-organisms.

- Low temperature steam.
- Boiling water.
- Formaldehyde.
- Glutaraldehyde.

Note

- Endoscopes are decontaminated by chemical means, due to the delicate nature of the instruments.

The immune system

The level of detail you need to know about this subject is limited, but you should be aware of the following basic principles.

Humoral immunity

This is the release of chemicals (cytokines) by immune cells in response to an immunogenic stimulus. Examples of cells implicated in humoral immunity are T cells, CD4 and CD8 cells. The cytokines released by them promote local inflammation.

Antigen presentation

An antigen is simply a molecule that stimulates an immune reaction. Antigen can be recognised by two possible mechanisms: either 'free' (B cells recognise free antigen) or, 'membrane-bound', i.e. phagocytosed foreign proteins are broken down into fragments which are presented on the cell's surface (T cells recognise membrane-bound antigen).

T cells

T cells are made in the thymus gland, hence the 'T'. The two types of T cell that you should be aware of are the CD4 (helper) cell, and the CD8 (killer) cell. Both recognise antigen presented on cell membranes. The difference between them is as follows:

- CD4 cells recognise antigen in association with Class II histocompatibility molecules on the surface of macrophages that have phagocytosed foreign material. They release cytokines as a result, a form of humoral immunity.
- CD8 cells recognise antigen in association with Class I histocompatibility molecules. This occurs when cells have synthesised 'non-self' (e.g. viral) proteins, not as for CD4, when a macrophage has actively phagocytosed foreign material. The CD8 cell then releases toxins to lyse or apoptose the infected cell(s).

B cells

B cells are made in the bone marrow, hence the 'B'. B cells recognise non-membrane-bound antigen, i.e. 'free'. They release immunoglobulins as a form of humoral immunity. Examples of immunoglobulins are IgA, IgM, IgG, IgD and IgE.

Immunoglobulins are antibodies; they are capable of acting in an antigen-presenting role on foreign material, as opsonins, and as an activator of the complement cascade.

Note

- B and T cell co-operation is often seen. Presentation of antigen to a T cell results in T cell stimulation of B cell monoclonal proliferation, i.e. high numbers of B cells with identical IgM molecules on their surface specifically targeted at the antigen that set off the process.

Macrophages

Macrophages are phagocytic and are able to present antigen to T cells, by Class II histocompatibility molecules. They contain toxic granules which lyse engulfed material.

Natural killer cells

Natural killer cells are a type of lymphocyte, but have neither T or B receptors. They are responsible for lysis of tumour cells and virally infected cells without prior sensitisation.

The immune response requires uptake and processing of antigen by an antigen-presenting cell (e.g. macrophage), expression on its surface, then clonal selection of T and B cells to proliferate and mature.

Immunoglobulins

Immunoglobulin is another word for antibody. There are five different types of immunoglobulins, each having a separate function as follows:

- IgG. Memory function, after previous infection, which mounts a strong and rapid response.
- IgA. Involved in mucosal defence, particularly in the gastro-intestinal tract where it lines the tract and detects antigen before or as it is being absorbed from the gut into the circulation, thus triggering an early response.
- IgM. Responsible for a rapid response to detected foreign material. Performs this via a mechanism using the major histocompatibility complex which is capable of recognising 'non-self' genetic (or other) material.
- IgE. Stimulates release of histamine from mast cells.
- IgD. Amplifies some of the above reactions.

Complement cascade

Complement is always referred to as C, followed by a number that represents the position of the complement molecule in its cascade, e.g. C3 or C5.

There are two different cascades:

- Classical (antigen-antibody stimulated).
- Alternative (antigen on surface of foreign molecule stimulated).

The functions of the complement cascade are:

- Opsonisation. Opsonin is Greek for 'relish'; it means that when complement has attached itself to a molecule, it is recognised and stimulates an attack by inflammatory cells.
- Membrane attack, directly.
- Speeding up the acute inflammatory response.

Summary

The mounting of an immune response requires the uptake and processing of antigen by an antigen-presenting cell (APC) (e.g. macrophage) and the expression of the antigen (or part of it) on the surface membrane of this cell.

This is followed by the clonal selection of B and T cells to proliferate and mature. The signals for this are cytokines from the T cells to more T cells and B cells. T and B cells alike are formed specifically for the immune response required.

Immune deficiency

Immune deficiency can be congenital or acquired.

Congenital immune deficiency

- IgA deficiency (recurrent sinusitis, chest infection, diarrhoea).
- Agammaglobulinaemia (Bruton's disease). Recurrent upper and lower respiratory infection, presenting after the age of 6/12 as maternal IgG has run out.
- Severe combined immunodeficiency (SCID) infections from any type of pathogen (viral, bacterial, fungal, protozoal).

- Problems with cell-mediated and humoral immunity of unknown cause.
- DiGeorge's syndrome (thymic hypoplasia). Decreased T cell synthesis which therefore results in increased infection from a virus, fungi and protozoa.

Treatment

Bone marrow transplant or gene therapy. In the special case of DiGeorge's syndrome, this can be treated with a thymic cell transplant.

Acquired immune deficiency

This is far more common than congenital immune deficiency.

- Malnutrition (reduced protein absorption).
- Liver disease (reduced protein synthesis).
- Protein-losing renal disease (increased protein loss).
- Drugs (immunosuppressive, e.g. azathioprine, steroids, methotrexate).
- Hodgkin's lymphoma.
- AIDS.
- Splenectomy (results in an increased risk of pneumococcal septicaemia).

Alternative categorisation of immune deficiency

Cellular immune dysfunction

Reduced macrophage (monocyte of bone marrow origin/B cell) levels and reduced T helper cell levels, which are needed for the activation of B cells. This results in increased:

- Bacterial (intracellular) infections, e.g. Listeria, Legionella, Salmonella, TB.
- Viral infections, e.g. Herpes family (simplex *Varicella zoster*)/cytomegalovirus (CMV).
- Fungal infections, e.g. *Cryptococcus neoformans*, *Toxoplasmosis gondii*, *Pneumocystis carinii*, Cryptosporidia.
- Helminthic infections, e.g. *Strongyloides stercoralis*.

Humoral immune dysfunction

A deficiency of immunoglobulins, e.g. IgA deficiency, SCIDS, Bruton's disease, resulting in recurrent *Streptococcus pneumoniae*, *Neisseria gonorrhoeae*, *Haemophilus influenzae*, *Neisseria meningitidis* infections.

Hypersensitivity reactions

These are disorders related to immune-mediated-tissue-damaging reactions.

Type I (anaphylactic)

IgE is released upon re-exposure to an antigen (contact, ingestion, inhalation, etc). This results in the release of histamine and complement cascade activation (C3 release) from mast cells and/or basophils. The result of these vasoactive mediators being released can be either local (e.g. urticaria or bronchospasm), or systemic (e.g. in severe cases, profound hypotension/shock).

Type II (antibody-mediated)

Antibodies react to antigenic components in cells, e.g. RBCs in transfusion reactions, or Rh +ve blood contamination in Rh -ve mother forming antibodies which cross the placental barrier and attack fetal RBCs, or auto-immune haemolytic anaemia.

Type III (immune complex-mediated)

Characterised by the formation of antibody/antigen complexes which travel in the circulation, depositing themselves favourably in the joints, kidneys, serosa, and heart, where they cause a vasculitic, necrotic reaction which determines the pattern of disease, e.g. systemic lupus erythematosus (SLE), rheumatoid arthritis, glomerulonephritis.

Note

- A localised Type III reaction can occur, called the Arthus reaction, e.g. injection of antigen which forms a localised inflammatory focus. A similar mechanism is behind 'farmer's lung' where a Type III reaction occurs in response to fungal growth in hay, causing respiratory symptoms.

Type IV (delayed hypersensitivity, cell-mediated)

T lymphocytes respond directly to stimuli in the form of mycobacteria, fungi, as well as other stimuli. They are responsible for T helper cell activation with its associated inflammatory reaction.

Specifically, lymphocytes metamorphose to epithelioid-type cells with a collar of lymphocytes (this is a granuloma); giant cells are also characteristically present.

An example of a Type IV reaction is the TB test (Heaf or Mantoux), where tuberculin is injected into the skin, in someone already sensitised to TB, i.e. previously had TB or BCG (Bacille Calmette-Guerin) immunisation. There is a granulomatous reaction which resolves after 2-7 days.

Note

- Broadly, T cells originate in the thymus, B cells originate in the bone marrow.

Mechanisms in the normal individual to protect against auto-immune (hypersensitive) reactions

Clonal deletion
Clonal deletion is the process of sifting out T cells that would (inappropriately) react against self-antigen, before they are released into the circulation. This is done by apoptosis.

Clonal anergy
B cells that react to self-antigens in the absence of co-stimulatory factors (i.e. those on antigen-presenting cells) cause a negative reaction which prevents the B cell from reacting to this antigen (even in the presence of APCs, next time).

Peripheral suppression
T suppressor cells are found to suppress peripheral activity of T cells at a local level.

Acute inflammatory response

A useful way of remembering the components of the inflammatory reaction is Galen's list of effects of inflammation: Rubor (redness), Calor (heat), Dolor (pain), Tumour (swelling) and Functio laesa (loss of function).

Tissue/cellular damage leads to microvascular dilatation, mainly at the arteriolar level, thus resulting in increased blood flow, hence 'Rubor' and 'Calor'. This is followed by an increase in the permeability of the microvasculature and thus, an exudation of protein-rich extravascular fluid, hence 'Tumour'. Leukocytes attach to the vessel walls (margination), then travel across them to the site of tissue damage (this is done by chemotaxis, the process of following a chemical gradient; in this case of complement, tumour necrosis factor [TNF] or interleukin-8 [IL8]). These leukocytes 'sensitise' nociceptors, hence 'Dolor'. They phagocytose the necrotic tissue and infective organisms by recognising complement and IgG opsonising their surface. Inside the leukocyte O_2-free radicals, H_2O_2, and Cl-free radicals are used to kill the ingested material.

Note

- Leaks of these toxic chemicals are responsible for damage to adjacent structures. This can become pathological, e.g. in rheumatoid arthritis, gout, etc.

The last of Galen's five cardinal signs of acute inflammation is 'Functio laesa' ('lack of function' due to the aforementioned reactions).

Note

- The complement cascade is the activation of C3 by the 'classic' (i.e. by exposure to the Ag-Ab complex, usually IgG or IgM) or 'alternative' pathway (direct activation by exposure to microbial surface polysaccharides).

Risk of wound infection (surgical site infection [SSI])

Classification of wound type

I Clean

Incision, uninfected skin, no hollow viscus. There is a 1.5% risk of wound infection.

II Clean contaminated

Incision breaches hollow viscus (non-colon) but contamination is minimal and controlled. There is a <8% risk of wound infection.

III Contaminated

Incision breaches hollow viscus and becomes contaminated (also includes open fracture and bite wounds). There is a 12% risk of wound infection.

IV Dirty

Wound in the presence of pus, or perforation, or a four-hour post-traumatic wound. There is a 25% risk of wound infection.

Note

—   The above classification should be learned as it is frequently asked in exams, e.g. what is the risk of wound infection post-excision of a gangrenous appendix?

Note

—   SSIs are a function of both surgical site integrity (see below) and host factors (various scores, i.e. ASA, APACHE II, etc).

Wound healing

Objectives of wound healing

♦   To restore the tensile strength of tissue.
♦   To cover areas exposed by the wound.

Healing by primary intention

The wound edges have good approximation, with no requirement for an epithelial covering.

Healing by secondary intention

Poor wound edge approximation, requiring epithelial cover; the edges cannot be brought together with sutures. Within hours of a wound forming, fibrin and fibronectin are released which act as glue to keep the wound edges together. This is followed by epidermal cell migration if not too large a defect exists. Epidermal cell proliferation begins if too much epidermis is damaged.

In the dermis, a mild acute inflammatory reaction begins within hours of the wound, resulting in:

♦   Removal of inflammatory exudate and debris.
♦   Restoration of tensile strength.
♦   Ingrowth of new blood vessels.

An acute inflammatory cell is the macrophage, which releases inflammatory mediators and ingests foreign material, resulting in release of growth promoting factors. A combination of richly vascularised gel, inflammatory cells and collagen-producing fibroblasts is known as granulation tissue. Wound contraction is produced by the action of myofibroblasts. Wound strength, when healed, is provided by collagen.

The steps of wound healing

♦   Coagulative. The clot forms at the wound site, which stops the bleeding and shields the wound from any further contamination.
♦   Inflammatory. Macrophages migrate to the wound site and engulf foreign material.
♦   Synthetic. Fibrocartilage is made from collagen precursor cells and fibroblasts to close the wound.
♦   Remodelling. A dynamic process by which the disorganised cartilage is re-aligned to resist the forces upon it in the wound.
♦   Maturation. The inflammatory nature of the scar decreases with time, going from pink to skin coloured.
♦   Epithelialisation. The process by which skin cells can migrate across small distances, covering the defect with skin.

Note

—   The scar formed will only have a maximum of 80% of tensile strength of skin.

Inhibitory factors of wound healing

The following is a useful list to remember, as it is frequently asked in viva exams.

Local

◆ Infection.
◆ Ischaemia.
◆ Foreign body.
◆ Haematoma.
◆ Malignancy.
◆ Denervation.
◆ Excess mobility, e.g. over a joint.

Systemic

◆ Poor nutrition.
◆ Vitamin A and C deficiency.
◆ Protein deficiency.
◆ Zinc and magnesium deficiency.
◆ Diabetes.
◆ Uraemia.
◆ Jaundice.
◆ Steroids.
◆ Immunosuppressants.
◆ Chemotherapeutic agents.
◆ Malignant disease.
◆ Irradiation.
◆ Increasing age.

The body's response to injury

Sympathetic

There is increased cardiac and cerebral blood flow, decreased blood flow to other organs, increased protein breakdown to glucose and increased glucose storage as glycogen.

Acute phase response

Chemical mediators known to influence the complex series of steps in the acute phase response to trauma or antigen, resulting in local inflammation, include cytokines, IL and TNF. There are many others, but these are the main ones to remember.

Endocrine

This includes the release of adrenocorticotrophic hormone (ACTH), cortisol, aldosterone, vasopressin, insulin, glucagon, thyroxine, heat shock proteins, 5-HT, histamine, growth hormone, and endogenous opioids.

Summary of results of body's response to injury

◆ Hypovolaemia. Impaired excretion of H_2O and Na^+, thus conserving body water.
◆ Pyrexia. A change in metabolic rate, i.e. initially a low metabolic rate conserving energy, then a high metabolic rate favouring tissue repair.
◆ Lipolysis. Fat stores are used for rapid energy.
◆ Carbohydrates. Glycogen stores only last 24 hours, then gluconeogenesis takes over through the stimulus of cortisol and glucagons, resulting in glucose formation.
◆ Albumin. Blood levels fall due to increased vessel permeability and, hence, loss into the soft tissues.
◆ Sodium. Falls due to an antidiuretic hormone (ADH)-mediated renal reabsorption of water, i.e. a dilutional effect.
◆ Acid-base. A variable response: either alkalosis, due to sodium reabsorption (in the renal tubule where it is swapped for either a potassium or a hydrogen ion); or, acidosis, due to anaerobic tissue perfusion when it is hypoperfused (in the shocked state).
◆ Impaired immune response.

Hypercoagulability

An increased coagulable state is good for stopping bleeding (a short-term benefit), but there are also down sides, in that it also results in an increased risk of deep vein thrombosis (DVT) or disseminated intravascular coagulation (DIC).

Acute respiratory distress syndrome (ARDS) and/or multiple organ dysfunction syndrome (MODS)

Severe injury can result in an inflammatory reaction in the lung parenchyma, resulting in pulmonary oedema; this is termed acute respiratory distress syndrome (ARDS). ARDS is effectively a single organ failure, but severe injury can progress onto multiple organ dysfunction syndrome (MODS), where other organ systems fail, especially renal, cardiac and cerebral.

Neoplasia

Neoplasia means 'new growth' (loss of responsiveness to normal growth controls).

Adenoma

A benign epithelial growth involving glandular patterns.

Papilloma

A benign epithelial growth producing 'finger-like fronds'.

Polyp

A mass whose surface projects over the level of the mucosa. It is usually benign, but some malignant tumours are polypoid. The most significant thing to know about polyps is that some of them are pre-malignant, e.g. colonic polyps.

Note

- Polyps are classified into: tubular, villous, tubulovillous, inflammatory, hamartomatous, metaplastic or benign vs malignant (and pre-malignant).

Cystadenoma

A hollow cystic mass commonly seen in ovarian tumours.

Carcinoma

A malignant tumour of epithelial origin.

Sarcoma

A malignant tumour of mesenchymal origin.

Teratoma

A tumour arising from totipotent stem cells, i.e. all three cell lines.

Hamartoma

A tumour-like malformation composed of haphazard arrangement of different amounts of tissue normally found at that site. It has no tendency to grow, other than under normal growth controls of the body.

Characteristics of tumours

Differentiation and anaplasia

Benign lesions are well differentiated. Malignant lesions are poorly differentiated or anaplastic.

Note

- Dysplasia is disorderly but non-neoplastic proliferation (loss of uniformity of individual cells, and of their architectural orientation).
- Pleomorphism is the variation in size and shape.
- Carcinoma *in situ* is marked dysplasia through the entire thickness of the epithelium, but no invasion.

Rate of growth

A characteristic of malignant tumours is rapid growth and, conversely, slow growth for benign tumours.

Local invasiveness

Only present if the tumour is malignant.

Metastatic spread

Only present if malignant.

Modalities of spread of tumours

- Seeding within body cavities.
- Lymphatic.
- Haematogenous.
- Transcoelomic, e.g. metastases to the peritoneal cavity.

Note

- Carcinomas tend towards lymphatic spread, and sarcomas to haematogenous spread.

Tumour staging

Staging is an attempt to quantify the extent of spread. The most common tumour staging system type is the TNM system: T1-4 (tumour size), N1-3 (number of nodes), M0 or 1 (presence or absence of metastases).

Tumour grading

Grading systems use cytologic differentiation to estimate the 'aggressiveness' of the tumour, usually Grades I-IV. Parameters used to decide the grade of a tumour are: differentiation, mitoses, nuclei and variation.

Epidemiology

Epidemiology is the study of the relationship between the environment and disease process.

Examples of epidemiological factors in neoplasia are:

♦ Heredity, e.g. a tumour with autosomal dominant inheritance.

Note

– Retinoblastomas show an increased risk of a second neoplasia, which is an osteogenic sarcoma.

♦ Environmental carcinogens, e.g. smoking, alcohol, asbestos, sunlight exposure.
♦ Age.
♦ Sex.

Paraneoplastic syndromes

Paraneoplastic syndromes are symptom complexes in cancer patients, unexplained by local or distal spread of tumour. They are caused by secretion of hormones from the tissue of origin, e.g. hypercalcaemia, Cushing's (ACTH), high parathyroid hormone-related peptide (PTHrP).

Tumour progression

Tumour cells can acquire greater malignant potential with time; this is known as tumour progression. Cells cease being monoclonal and become more heterogenous.

Another weapon in the armoury of the tumour is angiogenesis: as the tumour grows in size it requires a greater blood supply which it achieves by stimulating new vessel growth.

Carcinogenesis

Genetic damage is needed for carcinogenesis (the process of cause and effect of tumours).

Agents that are known to be carcinogenic:

♦ Radiation.
♦ Chemicals.
♦ Oncogenes.
♦ Viruses, e.g. HTLV1, HPV, EBV, Hep B.

Note

– The multi-hit theory states that numerous mutations may be needed before carcinogenesis occurs.

Clonal evolution

Clonal evolution describes the theory of one cell undergoing the appropriate mutations which then divides repeatedly forming the bulk of the tumour, i.e. the tumour is made up of clones of the original cell initially but later tumour progression creates a more heterogenous cohort of cells.

Mechanisms of action of carcinogens

♦ Activation of oncogenes.
♦ Inhibition of tumour suppressor genes.
♦ Inhibition of mutator gene oncogene and its corresponding oncoproteins are a normal component of cellular proliferation. It is only when they are over-expressed due to a mutation that they stimulate uncontrolled cell replication.

Note

– Oncogenes are dominant; it only takes one mutational event to contribute to neoplasia.

Tumour suppressor gene

Part of the multi-hit theory of carcinogenesis is that the tumour suppressor gene's activity is normally that of down-regulating cellular proliferation when activated. However, a mutation in the suppressor gene removes this protective mechanism from carcinogenesis.

Note

- Tumour suppressor genes are recessive, i.e. more than one mutation is needed to promote carcinogenesis.

A simple way of thinking of the roles of tumour suppressor genes and oncogenes is by the use of a car analogy: oncogenes represent the accelerator; tumour suppressor genes represent the brakes, i.e. too much accelerating (oncogene activation) or loss of brakes (tumour supressor gene loss) results in disorderly, malignant, cell proliferation.

Features of malignant tumours

- Mitoses (increased in number and abnormal).
- Increased nuclear to cytoplasmic ratio.
- Pleomorphism (variance of size and shape).
- Hyperchromatism (increased nuclear staining).
- Necrosis.
- Haemorrhage.
- Infiltrative borders.

Chemotherapy

Adjuvant chemotherapy

Chemotherapeutic agents used in combination with surgery for improved survival.

Neoadjuvant chemotherapy

Chemotherapeutic agents used prior to surgery to achieve improved local control.

Aim of chemotherapy

The aim of chemotherapy is to selectively kill tumour cells whilst sparing normal tissues.

Note

- The cell cycle must be understood before understanding the classification of cytotoxic agents.

A cell is normally to be found in the G0 phase.

The cell cycle

A cell undergoes replication by passing through the following phases:

- G1 (protein and RNA synthesis).
- S (DNA synthesis).
- G2 (RNA synthesis).
- M (mitosis).

The growth fraction (the proportion of the whole of the tumour cells that are involved in growth) of a tumour is important in how sensitive it will be to chemotherapy.

Note

- As a tumour increases in size its growth fraction falls.

It is known that at 37% of its maximum size, a tumour's growth fraction will be at its highest.

Pharmacology of cytotoxic drugs

Alkylating agents, e.g. cyclophosphamide

These add an alkyl group (R-CH-) covalently to proteins and nucleic acids.

Antimetabolites, e.g. azathioprine or mercaptopurine

Due to their similarity to metabolites in key chemical reactions, these competitively inhibit cell replication. Antitumour antibiotics bind to DNA and intercalate between the base pairs.

Plant alkaloids, e.g. vincristine

These contain mitotic spindle poisons which bind to tubulin, which is the protein of cellular microtubules.

Biological agents, e.g. tamoxifen

These use biological reagents to act as tumour suppressors. For example, hormonal therapy is useful in hormone-sensitive tumours, e.g. tamoxifen in breast cancer, or oestrogens in prostate cancer.

Combination chemotherapy

Used for the circumvention of resistance.

Modes of administration

- Intravenous.
- Intramuscular.
- Per orum.
- Intrathecal.

Note

- Implanted pumps can be used to administer chemotherapy, e.g. deliver chemotherapy directly into the portal vein in liver metastases of colorectal disease.

Complications of chemotherapy

Acute toxicity
- Bone marrow.
- Gastrointestinal.
- Alopecia.

Long-term toxicity
- Carcinogenesis.
- Gonadal damage.

Bladder
- Fibrosis.
- Haematuria.

Radiotherapy (DXT)

Radiotherapy is the therapeutic use of ionising radiation for the treatment of malignant disease, using gamma rays and beta particles.

Modes of administation

- Direct implantation, e.g. iridium needles into a tongue carcinoma.
- Inserted into a cavity, e.g. caesium beads in carcinoma of the cervix.

Note

- The above are forms of brachytherapy (implantation of source of radiation into the anatomical locale of the tumour).

- Systemic administration, e.g. iodine^{131} for cancer of the thyroid.
- External beam radiotherapy.

Mechanism of action of radiotherapy

High energy X-rays interact with body tissues to cause ionisation and release electrons of high kinetic energy. The electrons cause damage to adjacent molecules, including DNA, via an oxygen-dependent mechanism. This prevents further mitosis.

Note

- The size of tumour and radiosensitivity of tumour type are important factors in their response to DXT.

Adjuvant radiotherapy can be used pre-operatively or postoperatively to achieve improved local control Examples of factors improved by this method are:

- Spread of tumour cells beyond the resection margins.
- Spilled tumour cells at the time of surgery.
- Lymph node metastases.

Fractionation

Fractionation is the subdivision of total dose intended for treatment into fractions. The purpose is to allow tissues to recover between doses, and for necrotic areas in the centre of the tumour to become oxygenated; this allows for a better response to the treatment.

Side effects of radiotherapy

Skin
- Inflammation and desquamation.

Gastrointestinal
- Nausea and vomiting.
- Bleeding.
- Oesophagitis.
- Abdominal pain.
- Fibrosis causing stricture.

Bone marrow
- Bone marrow suppression.

Gonadal
- Infertility.

Lymph tissue
- Lymphoedema.

Malignant melanoma

Malignant melanoma is a tumour of melanocytes of the skin.

Types of malignant melanoma

Types of malignant melanoma are: superficial spreading; nodular; lentigo maligna (melanoma *in situ*, arises in Hutchinson's lentigo, on the face in the elderly); and acral lentiginous melanoma (found on hands or feet, often misdiagnosed as subungual haematoma).

Pathological classification (Breslow's thickness or Clark's level)

Breslow's thickness is thought to be a better indicator of prognosis:

- <0.76mm (incidence of metastases = 0%. 7-year survival is 100%).
- <1.5mm (metastases 8%. 7-year survival is 88%).
- 1.5-4mm (metastases 15%. 7-year survival is 61%).
- >4mm (metastases 72%. 7-year survival is 32%).

Clark's level:

- Confined to epidermis.
- Invasion of the papillary dermis.
- Invasion up to the level of the sub-papillary vessels but not into the reticular dermis.
- Invasion of the reticular dermis.
- Invasion of subcutaneous fat.

Note

— Clark's level cannot be used in polypoid melanomas, but Breslow's thickness is justified.

Useful prognostic factors

- Women have a better prognosis than men.
- Age is a poor prognostic factor.
- Anatomical site. There is a better prognosis if the lesion is on the lower limb; a worse prognosis if it is on the trunk and head. Nodular melanomas have a worse prognosis than a superficial spread, usually because of increased depth.
- Lentigo maligna (melanoma *in situ*) has a better prognosis than invasive malignant melanoma.

Risk factors

- Sunlight.
- Severe burns as a child.
- Fair skin and living near the equator.
- Legs in women.
- Trunks in men.

Clinical signs and symptoms indicating malignant change

- Change in size.
- Change in shape.
- Change in thickness.
- Change in colour.
- Sensation of itching.
- Bleeding.
- Ulceration.
- Halo (surrounding rim of hypo-pigmentation).
- Satellite nodules.
- Lymphadenopathy (indicating distant spread).

Blood and blood products

Blood

Responsible for transport of O_2, nutrients, waste products, cells involved in humoral and cellular immunity, and hormones.

Constituents of blood

Red blood cells
Transport of O_2 and CO_2.

White blood cells

Neutrophil polymorphs (macrophages)
Responsible for phagocytosis and breakdown of micro-organisms.

Lymphocytes
Responsible for humoral immunity, i.e. mature into plasma cells and memory cells, which can release immunoglobulins (production of antibody in response to antigen exposure). T lymphocytes are responsible for cell-mediated immunity, i.e. include T helper, T suppressor, and T killer cells, which release ILs and interferon alpha and gamma.

Platelets
Formed from megakaryocytes. Their functions include adhesion, activation of the clotting cascade, secretion, aggregation and contraction. They are able to secrete serotonin, adrenalin, adenosine diphosphate (ADP), prostaglandins and thromboxane.

Plasma
A transport medium for the above cells which allows transport of coagulation factors, fibrinolytic precursors, nutrients between the gastrointestinal tract (GIT) and liver, and waste products for metabolism and excretion in the liver and kidney.

Note

- The presence of anaemia on blood testing is not necessarily a reason for immediate blood transfusion; the cause should be looked into first and treated. If the patient still needs a transfusion when the cause is known, then it can be given.

Blood transfusion complications

This is a frequent question in viva exams, and should be learnt in a list format. You should be able to expand a little on each item on the list, if asked.

Immediate

- Circulatory overload (too much fluid given for the patient to cope with). Furosemide can be administered to prevent this.
- Hyperkalaemia (damaged cells in the blood bag, e.g. if not stored at a cool enough temperature potassium is released).
- Hypothermia (giving blood whilst still cold).
- Hypocalcaemia (citrate, which is used as an anticoagulant in the blood bag, binds to the free calcium in the patient's blood, lowering its level).
- Acidosis (similar reason as for hyperkalaemia; acidotic contents in the bag if cellular damage present, e.g. due to storage at an insufficiently low temperature).
- Haemolytic reaction (usually due to ABO incompatibility). Fever, discomfort, headache, vomiting, oliguria, haemoglobinuria are seen, which can result in acute renal failure. The mechanism of this is complement activation, targeting haemolysis of foreign cells. This can result in DIC.

Delayed

- Delayed haemolysis.
- Iron overload, e.g. in sicklers who require multiple transfusions. Treatment is by desferrioxamine administration.
- Blood-borne infection (e.g. HIV, hepatitis A, B, C, CMV, HTLV1, syphilis).

Note

- The above relate mainly to reactions against RBCs. However, reactions to WBCs (febrile reactions, pulmonary infiltrates), platelets (post-transfusion purpurae) or plasma (urticaria, and rarely, anaphylaxis) can develop.
- Transfusion of one unit of platelets raises the platelet count by approximately 40.

Massive transfusion

This is an important definition to remember: transfusion of greater than the individual's circulating volume within 24 hours.

Possible complications

- Cardiac abnormalities, e.g. ventricular extrasystoles, ventricular fibrillation (VF), arrest (secondary to low temperature, low calcium, high potassium).
- Acidosis.
- Failure of haemostasis, e.g. bleeding from wounds and puncture sites (secondary to low concentrations of coagulation factors in transfused blood).
- Adult respiratory distress syndrome (ARDS). A syndrome presenting clinically with dyspnoea and hypoxia. It results from an increase in pulmonary compliance, i.e. a restrictive deficit. The pathology at the base of this syndrome is pulmonary arteriolar thrombosis and localised DIC, resulting in leakage of fluid across the microvasculature into the lung parenchyma. Aggregates of leukocytes and macrophage appear in the parenchyma.

Treatment of blood transfusion ARDS

Stop transfusion and give IV steroids.

Note

- With every 10U of blood given, 1U of platelets is needed.
- FFP is plasma frozen within six hours of collection to <30°C. It contains coagulation factors; therefore, it is used in DIC in combination with platelets.

Fresh frozen plasma (FFP) - indications for IV administration

- Warfarin reversal (immediate).
- DIC.
- Massive transfusion.
- Idiopathic thrombocytopaenic purpurae (ITP).
- Coronary artery bypass graft (CABG).
- Bleeding associated with severe liver disease.
- Coagulation factor deficiency where a specific factor is missing.

Note

- If, when transfusing blood, platelets, or FFP, Rhesus D +ve blood is given to a Rh -ve female of childbearing age, they should be given Anti D 250U, with each unit of blood product transfused.

Platelets - indications for IV administration

- Severe burns.
- Hypoproteinaemia of liver or renal disease.
- Massive transfusion.
- Post-liver resection.
- Gram-negative septicaemia.

Clotting cascade

There are two main clotting pathways that form the clotting cascade: the intrinsic and extrinsic pathways (Figure 1.1). The aim of the pathways is to form a blood clot. This is an aggregate of fibrin threads that adhere to each other and the surrounding cells (e.g. of the vessel wall) trapping red, white and platelet cells together in one large mass. This clot is intended to plug breaches in vessel walls, and hence arrest bleeding.

The clot is the first stage towards thrombus formation. Thrombus is defined as a solid mass formed in living circulation from the components of a streaming circulation.

The intrinsic pathway is so called because it occurs in response to the exposure of blood to negatively charged molecules belonging to the body (i.e. intrinsic), but that are not normally part of the lining of the vessel. For example, 'raw' collagen exposed when a vessel wall is damaged.

The extrinsic pathway is so called because it occurs in response to exposure of blood to negatively

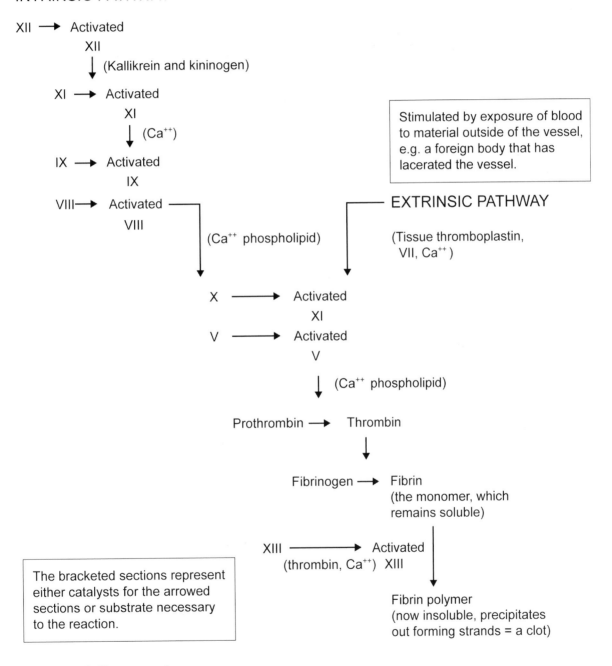

Figure 1.1. The clotting cascade.

charged surfaces that are not found in vessels, but outside of them, e.g. a sharp foreign body that has lacerated the vessel.

Both intrinsic and extrinsic pathways stimulate the final common part of the pathway leading to formation of an insoluble polymer of fibrin from its soluble monomer form. The insoluble polymer precipitates out of blood locally, forming threads as previously described.

The individual steps in both cascades require catalysis by various means, most important of which is the calcium ion.

Interference with these pathways results in anticoagulation.

Warfarin interferes with the synthesis of vitamin K-dependent clotting factors (VII, IX and X). Thus, the effect of warfarin takes a number of days to become clinically apparent, as one must wait for the already present vitamin K-dependent factors to be depleted before anticoagulation sets in.

Heparin and related low-molecular-weight heparins (LMWHs) act by binding to antithrombin III, a chemical present in normal blood, whose activity is greatly stimulated by heparin in a rapid reaction. Antithrombin III inhibits activation of thrombin and factor Xa. Thus, the effect of heparin is effectively instantaneous.

A separate issue to the clotting cascade is why does clotting not continue permanently, once initiated? The answer lies in a chemical called plasmin. It is proteolytic, and its action is to fibrinolyse (literally to break up fibrin) the clot. Plasminogen, which is a normal constituent of blood, is activated to plasmin by cells in tissues adjacent to the clot, thus preventing its excessive spread through the vascular system.

Just as anticoagulants can prevent clot formation, a group of drugs known as fibrinolytics can be used as clot busters. They are particularly useful in coronary artery clots, i.e. in acute myocardial infarction. Examples of fibrinolytics are streptokinase and tissue plasminogen activator (tPA).

Disorders of coagulation

Inherited

von Willebrand's disease
Deficiency of a factor responsible for platelet coagulation function. It is autosomal dominant and therefore affects both sexes equally. Treatment is by desmopressin (DDAVP).

Haemophilia (Factor VIII deficiency)
Sex-linked recessive and therefore usually affects males. Treatment is by Factor VIII concentrate.

Acquired

- Drugs, e.g. warfarin, aspirin, NSAIDs.
- Liver disease (decreased synthesis of clotting factors).
- Sepsis (DIC).
- Other (auto-immune, vasculitis, hypersplenism).

Note

- You should be familiar with 'Virchow's triad'. These are three factors that predispose to thrombosis (most commonly seen clinically, as deep venous thrombosis):
  1. Damage to the vessel wall.
  2. Decrease in blood flow rate (stasis).
  3. Increased coagulability of blood.

Deep venous thrombosis (DVT)

Risk factors for DVT

- Previous DVT.
- Pelvic tumour.
- Obesity.
- Oral contraceptive pill (OCP).
- Clotting abnormality.
- Smoking.
- Cancer.
- Immobility.
- Abdominopelvic surgery.
- Any prolonged surgery.
- Increasing age.

Differential diagnosis of DVT

◆ Ruptured Baker's cyst.
◆ Osteoarthritis (OA) of the knee.
◆ Ruptured popliteal aneurysm.
◆ Knee haemarthrosis.
◆ Cellulitis.
◆ Ruptured tendo achilles.
◆ Osteosarcoma.
◆ Lymphoedema.
◆ Ischaemic limb.
◆ Muscle strain.

DVT prophylaxis options

◆ Graduated stockings (thrombo-embolic deterrent stockings [TEDS]).

Note

– The term graduated refers to the fact that as the stocking becomes more proximal, the actual pressure that it exerts decreases gradually.

◆ Pneumatic calf compression devices.
◆ Intravenous heparin infusion.
◆ Subcutaneous heparin.

Note

– Dextran 70, antiplatelet agents and electrical calf stimulation can also be used, but these all have lower efficacy. Dextran 70 is a special case in that it is effective in pulmonary embolism (PE) prophylaxis but not in DVT prophylaxis.

Note

– Even with ideal prophylaxis, 5-20% of patients suffer DVT (depending on the type of surgery), and up to 0.2% suffer a fatal PE.

DVT treatment

Treatment is with an IV heparin infusion, using the activated partial thromboplastin time (APTT) to monitor the degree of anticoagulation (although this is of unproven accuracy) or subcutaneous LMWH, whilst starting warfarin therapy (for six months), obviously stopping the heparin when the international normalised ratio (INR) is high enough (usually considered to be >2).

Note

– The heparin infusion has been superseded by the advent of LMWHs (e.g. Fragmin), which can be used for treatment while waiting for the INR to rise above 2. The advantages are that you need only give one daily dose and do not need to check the APTT as with the heparin infusion.
– Sometimes an inferior vena cava (IVC) filter is indicated for prevention of PE in a patient with DVT, e.g. recent haemorrhagic cerebro-vascular accident (CVA), acute bleeding duodenal ulcer, etc., as anticoagulation is contraindicated in these patients. Another indication is recurrent PE, despite adequate anticoagulation.

The relevance of DVT in clinical practice

DVT can lead to breaking off of the clot within the venous system which then flows back to the heart and passes through the right heart into the pulmonary circulation (where the vascular diameter reduces again down to capillary level). Thus, the clot lodges in the pulmonary circulation, obstructing flow to a section of lung. This is termed a pulmonary embolism (PE).

Definition of embolus
Abnormal mass of undissolved material which passes in the blood from one part of the circulation.

Definition of embolism
When an embolus impacts in a vessel too small to allow it to pass obstructing the flow of blood.

Types of embolism
Thrombus, gas, fat, tumour, amniotic fluid, foreign body, and therapeutic.

The acute management of PE is with oxygen to maintain saturations if necessary. For DVT, the patient will require a prolonged course of warfarin, after treating with heparin, until the warfarin has raised the INR to greater than 2.

Massive PE can be rapidly fatal. But there is a minority of cases in which a massive PE is lodged in one of the pulmonary arteries, and the patient is able to survive on high-flow oxygen long enough for the clot to either be thrombolysed with interventional radiology assistance, or surgically removed via a thoracotomy, obviously requiring the immediate assistance of an experienced cardiothoracic surgeon.

Disseminated intravascular coagulation (DIC)

DIC is the inappropriate, excessive activation and consumption of coagulation factors. It is not a primary condition; it is always secondary to something (see below).

Note

— DIC can be acute or chronic.

Acute DIC

Acute DIC can be secondary to sepsis, post-partum haemorrhage, post-massive transfusion, an acute abdomen, shock, and acute liver failure. It presents as sudden and significant bleeding from wounds and puncture sites, urinary and genital tracts.

Chronic DIC

This is seen in disseminated malignancy and presents as recurrent thrombotic events, such as DVTs.

Management of DIC

- Find the cause.
- Treat the cause.

- Blood tests (full blood count [FBC], clotting screen [CS]). Fibrinogen degradation products (FDPs) are instrumental in diagnosis.
- Support coagulation (platelets, cryoprecipitate, FFP).

Hepatitis

The pathological definition is hepatocyte necrosis with inflammatory cell infiltration.

Signs and symptoms

- 2-6 weeks incubation.
- Prodrome:
  - anorexia;
  - nausea;
  - joint pain;
  - fever.
- Jaundice (first clinically apparent in the sclerae, but as the bilirubin level rises, the skin becomes more visibly jaundiced), tender hepatomegaly, splenomegaly, adenopathy.

Differential diagnosis

Acute
- Drug reaction, reaction to toxins, acute alcoholic hepatitis.
- Infectious mononucleosis.
- Leptospirosis (Weil's disease, a spirochaete from ingestion of water containing rat faeces or urine contamination).
- Syphilis.
- Q fever, yellow fever.

Chronic
- Chronic alcoholic hepatitis, drug reaction.
- Chronic auto-immune hepatitis.
- Wilson's disease (a congenital enzyme deficiency [of caeruloplasmin] resulting in a build up of copper in the liver, causing jaundice and cirrhosis).

Hepatitis A

This is the most common type of hepatitis (20-40% of all cases). It has a faecal-oral spread or may be contracted from infected food (shellfish)/water. Usually this is a self-limiting disease, therefore treatment is for the most part supportive and advice is given to avoid alcohol.

Hepatitis B

Contracted by the intravenous route or sexual transmission. It is self-limiting and therefore requires supportive therapy and no alcohol (interferon [IFN] can be used). Five percent may lead to fulminant liver failure or chronic hepatitis. It is a blood-borne virus with an incubation of six weeks to six months. Five to ten percent of patients develop a carrier status. Three viral antigens are present in the virus particle itself:

- HbsAg - surface antigen.
- HbcAg - core antigen.
- HbeAg - e antigen.

When acutely infected:

- HbsAg - present in patient's serum.
- HbeAg - present in patient's serum.
- HbcAg - present in the liver and anti-HbcAg in patient's serum.

After infection:

- Anti-HbsAg - present in patient's serum.
- Anti-HbcAg - present in patient's serum.
- Anti-HbeAg - present in patient's serum.

A carrier, by definition, has HbsAg persisting for over six months.

Hepatitis C

This is contracted by the intravenous route or sexual transmission. It used to be a major cause of post-transfusion hepatitis before screening. Approximately 50% develop chronic infection. Treatment is with interferon alpha.

Note

- Infective hepatitis is a notifiable disease.
- Hep D is activated in the presence of Hep B.

Bone

Bone is a dense connective tissue, containing cells and fibres in a calcified matrix, and is highly vascular. Cortical bone contains channels for blood flow, called canaliculi (small), Haversian canals (larger), and Volkman's canals (run at right angles to Haversian, as anastomoses); medullary bone contains nutrient arteries.

Types of bone

- Cortical (hard, dense, resembles ivory).
- Cancellous (trabecular structure, designed to resist force normally applied to it).

Marrow

Marrow is stored in the bony medulla. It is red in childhood, for haematopoiesis, gradually becoming more yellow in adulthood, as fat infiltrates it.

Periosteum

A thick fibrous tissue on the outer surface of bone, it is vascular, well innervated (very sensitive), and is not present at articulating surfaces of synovial joints.

Bone development

The formation of bone takes place by two different basic mechanisms, replacement of a cartilage bone-precursor-cartilage model (endochondral) and of a bone-precursor-fibrous model (intramembranous). Bone is not formed *de novo*, it always replaces tissue:

- Endochondral ossification. Pre-existing hyaline cartilage is replaced by bone, e.g. ossification centres in young bone.
- Intramembranous ossification. Osteoblasts lay down bone in fibrous tissue (no cartilaginous precursor).

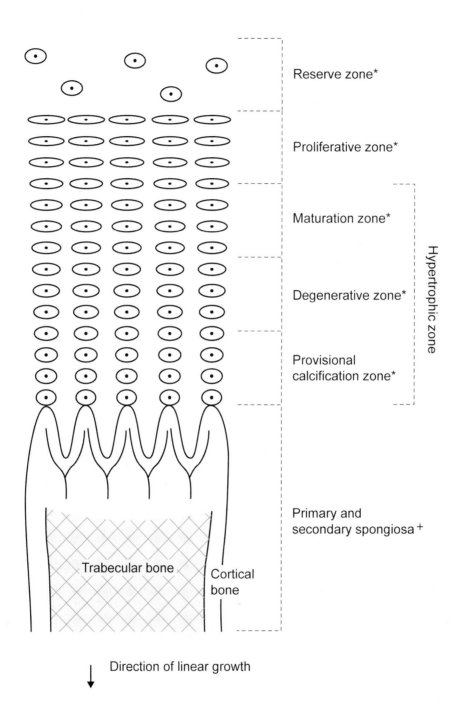

Figure 1.2. Long bone growth.
* Chondroctyes, which form cartilage.
+ At this stage the chondrocytes die and the cells that are involved in actual bone formation are osteoblasts.

Sesamoid bone

- Made of bone, cartilage, or a combination of the two.
- Largest sesamoid bone in the body is the patella.
- Sesamoid bones are usually found in tendons.
- One example of a sesamoid bone that is NOT associated with tendon is the fabella, which is in the muscular belly of gastrocnemius lateral head (commonly seen on knee X-rays).

Joints

Fibrous

A joint formed by bone, fibrocartilage, bone. It features little movement, e.g. skull sutures, or syndesmosis.

Cartilaginous
Primary

A joint formed by bone, hyaline cartilage, bone. It features little movement, e.g. first rib with manubrium, or (all) costal cartilages.

Secondary

A joint formed by bone, hyaline cartilage, fibrocartilage, hyaline cartilage, bone. It features as midline structures, e.g. pubic symphysis, manubrium sterni or intervertebral discs.

Synovial

Synovial joints have six main characteristics: a capsule, synovial secreting cells, a degree of movement, bone ends covered in hyaline cartilage, enclose a joint cavity, and are reinforced by ligaments.

Typical synovial joints

The contents are bone, hyaline cartilage, joint capsule, hyaline cartilage, bone, e.g. limb joints.

Atypical synovial joints

The contents are bone, fibrocartilage, joint capsule, fibrocartilage, bone, e.g. temperomandibular joint (TMJ), second rib to sternum, manubrioclavicular and sternoclavicular joints.

Note

- Joint capsules are technically ligaments and, as such, count as one of the ligamentous supports of the joint.
- The viscocity of the synovium changes with the speed of movement (thinner in faster movements, and vice versa).

Long bone growth

Longitudinal growth in long bones takes place at the growth plate in skeletally immature bones. This is a form of enchondral ossification, i.e. bone replaces a cartilage model.

The growth plate is divided into different zones or layers as follows (Figure 1.2):

- Epiphysis - the 'end' section of the bone (proximal or distal).
- Reserve zone - cells here store lipids, glycogen and proteoglycans for use in bone growth.
- Proliferative zone - horizontal rows of cells (chondrocytes, i.e. cells that go on to form cartilage [not bone]) divide and progress linearly along the axis of the bone, stacking themselves one on top of the other.
- Hypertrophic zone - subdivided into three layers:
  - maturation;
  - degeneration;
  - provisional calcification.

The chondrocytes die at this stage releasing calcium that was stored. Primary and secondary spongiosa - osteoblasts and osteoclasts - are responsible, between them, for weaving and remodelling new bone at this level from the calcium released from the dead chondrocytes.

Note

- The important point, if a little semantic, is that cartilage is replaced by bone, not converted into bone. The chondrocytes actually die in enchondral ossification.

Bone healing

Stages of bone healing

Fracture
Involves tearing of blood vessels, therefore resulting in haemorrhage (raises the periosteum).

Release of inflammatory mediators
Increases oedema and hence periosteal elevation, resulting in a fusiform swelling.

Bone necrosis
In areas where blood supply has been cut off, macrophages enter the fracture site and begin bone demolition, then granulation (granulation tissue extends up and down the bone for quite a distance).

Callus formation
Periosteum cells on the inner surface proliferate and lay down woven bone which is an unmineralised cartilage matrix, that is then ossified and remodelled by osteoblast and osteoclast activity.

Note

– Callus is the product of calcified woven bone, prior to remodelling to normal bony architecture.

Healing across the fracture gap
Healing is either by primary ossification or the gap is closed by fibrous tissue; only later by calcified bone.

Remodelling
The co-ordinated resorption and bone formation mediated by osteoblasts and osteoclasts in response to the forces across it, is known as Wolff's law. This process gradually re-forms the bone back to its original shape and structure.

Note

– Failure of the above is termed non-union.

Atherosclerosis

A condition affecting medium-sized arteries, characterised by atherosclerotic plaques consisting of a necrotic core rich in cholesterol and other lipids, surrounded by smooth muscle cells and fibrous tisue. It predisposes to ischaemic heart disease, CVAs and aortic aneurysm formation, all of which have considerable associated morbidity and mortality.

Risk factors for atherosclerosis

Constitutional
(i.e. about which you can do nothing).
- Age (begins in childhood, symptomatic from the 4th/5th decade onwards.
- Sex (male, until women become post-menopausal, and their risk catches up).
- Family history (first degree relative).

Acquired
(i.e. about which you can do something).
- Hypertension.
- Hyperlipidaemia.
- Smoking.
- Diabetes.
- Others (stress, type A personality, obesity, OCP).

Pathology (the 'response to injury' theory) (Figure 1.3)

- Chronic endothelial injury (hyperlipidaemia, smoking, immune reactions, haemodynamic factors, toxins, viruses).
- Endothelial dysfunction, resulting in increased endothelial permeability, and hence leukocyte and monocyte adhesion.
- Smooth muscle migration from the media to the intima and macrophage activation.
- Macrophages and smooth muscle cells engulf lipids by smooth muscle cell proliferation. Eventually this forms a collagen covering (the atheromatous plaque). The process can then recur leading to atheromatous disease.

a

Adventitia

Media
(smooth muscle)

Intima

Endothelium

b

Leukocyte/monocyte adhesion
damages the endothelium,
resulting in increased
permeability and migration
across endothelium

c

Migration of smooth
muscle cells from
media to intima

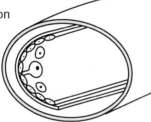

d

Macrophage having
engulfed debris

Plaque

Layer of smooth
muscle cells in intima

Lipid

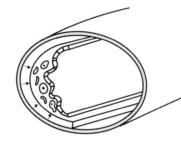

Figure 1.3. Pathology (the 'response to injury
theory'). a) Chronic endothelial injury. b) Endothelial
dysfunction. c) Smooth muscle cell migration. d)
Macrophages and smooth muscle cells engulf lipid
by smooth muscle cell proliferation.

Mechanism of clinical events resulting from atherosclerosis (Figure 1.4)

- Simple occlusion by atheroma.
- Thrombus formation on top of atheroma, causing occlusion.
- Haemorrhage into atheroma, causing occlusion.
- Embolus of atheroma or thrombus, causing occlusion.
- Calcification, particularly of the aorta, results in a 'brittle aorta'.
- Aneurysmal dilatation (pressure atrophy and loss of elastic tissue in the media) with possible rupture.

Transplantation

Types of organ graft

Autograft
Transplant of tissue from self.

Allograft
Transplant of tissue from non-self.

Xenograft
Transplant of tissue from other species.

Cadaveric organ
Examples of sources of cadaveric organs are:

- A young trauma victim.
- A patient on ITU with established brain death.

N.B. Transplant of a cadaveric organ is an example of an allograft.

Types of rejection (hyperacute, acute and chronic)

- Hyperacute. Within a matter of hours, due to pre-formed antibodies in a sensitised patient, e.g. transfusion, pregnancy, previous transplant. The immune response to microvascular endothelium causes thrombosis and hence ischaemic necrosis.
- Acute. Within days to weeks, due to cellular mechanisms (cytotoxic T lymphocytes), causes

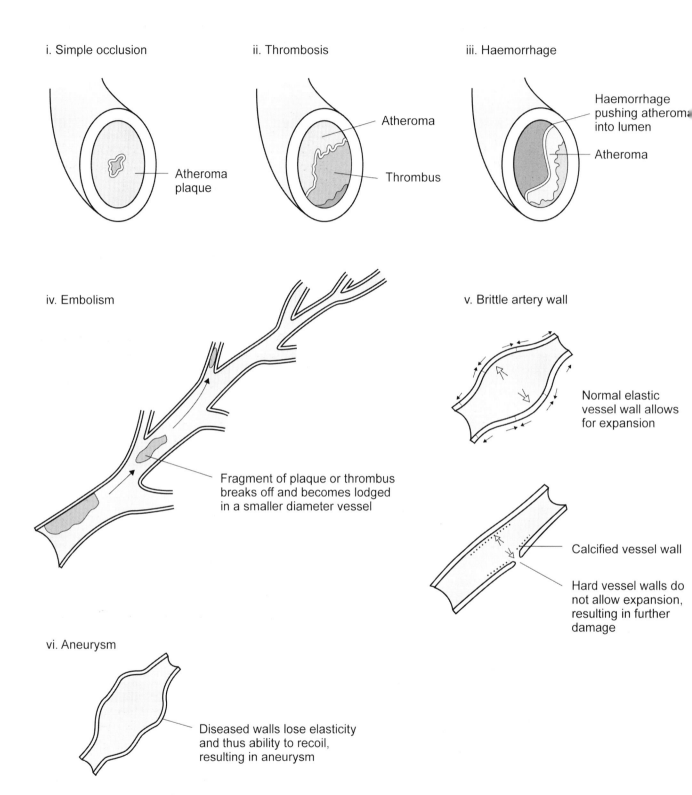

i. Simple occlusion

Atheroma plaque

ii. Thrombosis

Atheroma

Thrombus

iii. Haemorrhage

Haemorrhage pushing atheroma into lumen

Atheroma

iv. Embolism

Fragment of plaque or thrombus breaks off and becomes lodged in a smaller diameter vessel

v. Brittle artery wall

Normal elastic vessel wall allows for expansion

Calcified vessel wall

Hard vessel walls do not allow expansion, resulting in further damage

vi. Aneurysm

Diseased walls lose elasticity and thus ability to recoil, resulting in aneurysm

Figure 1.4. Mechanism of clinical events resulting from atherosclerosis.

prominent vascular damage with fibrinoid necrosis of arterioles.

- Chronic. Within months to years, due to humoral mechansims; however, it is poorly understood.

Note

- The degree of disparity between donor and recipient is related to the severity of the immune response.

Management of rejection

Tissue typing

Major histocompatabilty complex (MHC), located on the short arm of chromosome 6, is responsible for the formation of the human leukocyte antigen (HLA), which is the genetic basis of antibody rejection.

Except for monozygotic twins, no matter how good the tissue match, immunomodulation is still needed (see the 'Immunosuppression' section later).

Types of match in live related donors are:

- Perfect match - 2 haplotype match, 25% chance of this.
- Half match - 1 haplotype mismatch, 50% chance of this happening.
- No match - 25% chance of this happening.

The following tests are also required for prevention of rejection:

- ABO compatibility (a G+S sample tests this).
- Tissue type match (perfect or half match).
- Routine blood tests to be normal.
- HIV, CMV, HepB and HepC negative.
- Mixed lymphocyte culture (MLC) (tests host's lymphocyte response to donor cells; if rejected, the transplant cannot proceed).
- In kidney transplants, an angiography must be performed to ensure the kidney is actually functional (vascularised), and on a technical note, only has one renal artery (occasionally, as an anatomical variant, there are more than one renal arteries, rendering the kidney inappropriate for transplant).
- Intravenous urethrogram (IVU) for abnormalities.

Immunosuppression

Initially, azathioprine and prednisolone were the mainstay of treatment. Now, however, cyclosporin +/- prednisolone are used. Cyclosporin inhibits T cell function and has no effect on B cells or marrow suppression and, therefore, it is safer.

Note

- Cyclosporin has problems with nephrotoxicity.

Azathioprine

Inhibits proliferation of lymphocytes to a stimulus. Side effects are pancytopaenia, lymphoid tumours and infections.

Prednisolone

Prednisolone has a non-specific effect on the immune system; the exact mechanism is not fully understood. It is anti-inflammatory. Side effects of prolonged steroid administration are:

- Cushingoid appearance (moon face, central obesity, peripheral wasting).
- Hypertension.
- Thinning of the skin.
- A propensity to infection.
- Avascular necrosis of bone, e.g. femoral head and humeral head are the two most common.
- Osteoporosis.

Note

- Immunosuppression in the long term results in a 100-fold increase in cancer risk, especially skin tumours (when matched for age and other variables).
- A pre-operative blood transfusion of three units has been shown to have a significant effect on renal graft survival.

Preservation of transplanted organ

There are two concepts: 'warm' and 'cold' ischaemic time. After 20 minutes of warm ischaemia, a degree of necrosis is inevitable, e.g. in a kidney this presents as acute tubular necrosis. When stored at 4°C the kidney can survive for 48 hours safely.

Results of specific organ transplantation

Renal
- 1-year graft survival 85-90%.
- 5-year graft survival 65%.

Liver
- 1-year graft survival 75%.
- 5-year graft survival 55%.

Heart/heart lung
- 1-year graft survival 80%.
- 5-year graft survival 55%.

Suture materials

Absorbable sutures

Catgut
Catgut slides and knots well, and is cheap. There is a marked tissue reaction and an unpredictable loss of strength. However, catgut has now been taken off the market due to the potential to transmit bovine spongiform encephalopathy (BSE).

Note

— Chromic catgut has a longer time maintaining tensile strength. Simple catgut loses 50% of its tensile strength in approximately three days; chromic in 5-7 days.

Vicryl (aka polyglactyl 10)
Vicryl has a predictable strength and less tissue reaction. It slides poorly, but is easy to knot and is short lasting. It loses 50% of tensile strength in 20 days.

PDS/Maxon (aka polydioxone)
A monofilament with predictable strength and longer lasting. It is slippery to knot and can weaken if damaged during knotting. It loses 50% of tensile strength in 28 days. Because it lasts longer than other suture materials it is used for closing the abdomen.

Dexon
Similar to Vicryl with a predictable strength. It slides poorly, is difficult to knot and is short lasting. It loses 50% of tensile strength in 20 days. An important point about absorbable sutures is how long they can be relied upon to maintain their tensile strength *in situ*.

Non-absorbable sutures

Silk
Silk has excellent handling and knotting. It is a braided and biological material; this can result in a fibrotic reaction, which can lead to sinuses.

Nylon
Nylon is strong, slides well and is inert. It is difficult to handle and knot, and can cause wound sinuses near knots.

Prolene
Prolene is excellent for subcuticular and vascular sutures. It is inert, difficult to handle and knot, but is easier than nylon.

Wire
Wire is strong, inert and can be monofilament or braided. It is difficult to handle because of kinking, it can break and sharp ends can cause pain in the future.

Types of needle

- Traumatic/atraumatic (atraumatic is good for vessel repair).
- Straight/curved.
- Cutting (triangular cross-section for cutting tough tissues, e.g. skin).
- Reverse cutting needle (where the apex of the triangle of the needle on a standard cutting needle is on the concave side of the needle, in the reverse cutting needle it is on the convex side. This has the advantage of strengthening the needle and reducing the risk of suture cut-out once placed).

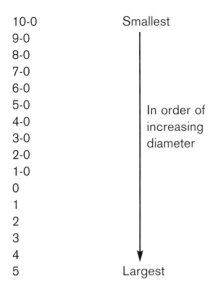

10-0	Smallest
9-0	
8-0	
7-0	
6-0	
5-0	In order of
4-0	increasing
3-0	diameter
2-0	
1-0	
0	
1	
2	
3	
4	
5	Largest

Figure 1.5. Sizes of sutures.

- Roundbodied.
- J needle (can be inserted deep in small holes, e.g. laparoscopy wounds).
- Eyed.

The sizing of sutures is shown in Figure 1.5.

Drains (Figure 1.6)

Drains can be open or closed. A closed drain is attached to a bag or bottle, sealed off from the outside air. They can be positioned superficially or deep and some may also have an underwater seal.

Types of drain:

- Tube drain. Simple, sutured *in situ* and depends on gravity for drainage into a bag or bottle.
- Suction drain. Suction attempts to close a potential space after an operation, for example, after breast surgery or after a thoracotomy.
- Free drainage drain. This, of course, is an example of a tube drain, for example, in urological procedures, negative pressure should not be applied across an anastomosis, e.g. a urinary catheter.
- Corrugated drain. Capillary action, e.g. used in colorectal surgery.

- T-tube drain. This is used in biliary surgery. The two arms of the T-tube are inserted into the biliary duct which has been operated upon, and the stem of the T-tube comes out through the skin to permit drainage. It is made of latex specifically to encourage sinus tract formation, such that when the drain is removed the sinus tract favours flow of any remaining bile away from the abdominal cavity and out to the skin. The sinus then closes with time.
- Sump drain. A sump is a space for storage of fluid. In this case the sump is made from two tubes, one within the other. The outer has perforations to allow inflow of fluid, the sump, and the inner is a simple tube leading from a cavity to the outside world, the drain.
- Rubber drain. Rubber drains cause an intense inflammatory action and granulation tissue forms along the tract. Therefore, when removed, a sinus persists for a while. They are useful for draining pus, e.g. from an empyema.

Drains are positioned into wounds and cavities for varying reasons, e.g. to collect anticipated bleeding, drain seromas, drain bile, etc. The length of time these drains are left in is based on the very reasons the drains were inserted. The following is a guide to how long drains should be left in (the clinical picture should also be taken into account):

- Drains for peri-operative bleeding - remove after 24-48 hours.
- Drains for serous collections - remove after 3-5 days.
- Drains intended to avert later infection - remove after 1-5 days.
- Drains to cover intestinal anastomoses - remove after 5-7 days (many units will perform a gastrograffin study to test for leaks before removal).
- T-tubes - remove after 6-10 days (a T-tube cholangiogram should be performed before removal, again testing for leakage).
- Chest drains for pneumothorax should be taken out after the lung is proven to be re-inflated on X-ray for 24 hours (with no air leak).
- Chest drains for empyemas remain in for variable lengths of time depending on drainage, the clinical picture and radiological appearance.

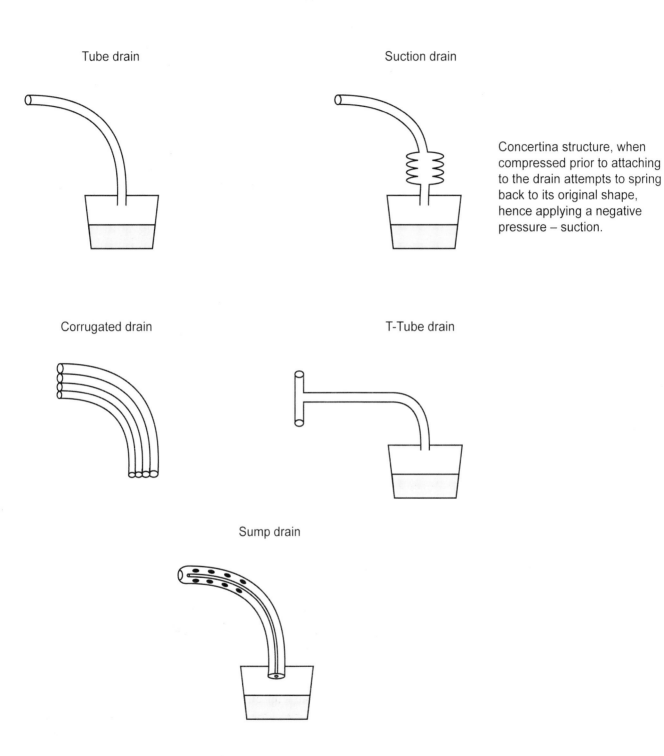

Tube drain

Suction drain

Concertina structure, when compressed prior to attaching to the drain attempts to spring back to its original shape, hence applying a negative pressure – suction.

Corrugated drain

T-Tube drain

Sump drain

Figure 1.6. Types of drain.

LASER

Light amplification by stimulated emission of radiation

The word laser is an acronym; you should be able to recall the definition and answer questions on the basic science behind it.

Energy is pumped into the 'lasing medium' to excite electrons into a higher energy state; when they spontaneously fall back into the ground state a photon is emitted. Photons are bounced between mirrors allowing amplification. A partially reflecting mirror allows some high energy light to escape.

This lasing medium is usually gaseous, e.g. CO_2, argon. But it can be crystalline, e.g. neodynium, NdYAG, aluminium.

Types of LASER

CO_2
Infrared, not visible, low penetration and heals with little scarring quickly.

Neodynium yttrium argon (NdYAG)
Infrared, not visible, slightly more penetration, leaves eschar of scar tissue and is useful for large amounts of coagulation.

Argon
Blue-green colour, therefore it is absorbed by red tissues. It is used in the ophthalmology and dermatology specialties.

DYE (variable wavelength)
Colour and visibility depend on wavelength. DYE laser is used for dermatological removal of tattoos and port-wine stains.

Screening

Screening is the process of examination of a large number of individuals looking for a specific characteristic. In the case of human medicine, one screens for disease or a pre-disease state (e.g. carcinoma *in situ*) that is easier to treat/cure than the established disease state. The following questions need to be asked when implementing a screening program:

- Can the expense be justified?
- Does it provide a better quality of life (QOL) or cure rate, or survival rate for patients? Can the health service afford it even if it is of potential benefit?
- Is the infrastructure available to cope with the numbers involved in it?
- Should economics come into it if society will benefit from and have decided in favour of it?

Breast cancer screening

Mammograms increase the rate of detection of breast cancer. In the UK, it is national policy to perform mammograms in women between the ages of 50 and 65 every three years. Despite the increased pick up rate, as yet, no survival advantage has been shown in the UK after institution of the screening program.

Screening for gastric cancer

Carried out in Japan, with X-rays and oesophago-gastroduodenoscopy (OGD) follow-up. It has reduced mortality by 25% by diagnosing the disease in its early phase, i.e. Stage I.

Screening for colorectal cancer

People considered to be at high risk are screened with colonoscopy or barium enemas. High-risk patients are those with longstanding ulcerative colitis, previous adenoma, familial adenomatous polyposis, and previous colonic cancer.

Since 2006, a programme of screening for colorectal cancer has been in place in the UK. It involves inviting the population aged between 60 and 69 (those over 70 can voluntarily be tested) for faecal occult blood (FOB) testing. If blood is detected by this means in the patient's stools, they are invited for a colonoscopy. Early studies on the UK population have shown an incidence of carcinoma of 1.6 per 1000, 48% of which was Dukes' stage A only. Of this group, only 1% had metastatic cancer.

Euthanasia

Patients have a right to voluntary passive euthanasia, thus a doctor cannot provide life-saving care against a patient's wishes. The exception is if the patient is incompetent to make this decision.

Non-voluntary passive euthanasia (i.e. non-resuscitation) is acceptable providing a representative body of fellow professionals agree it is indicated.

Active euthanasia is illegal as it is viewed as homicide in the eyes of the law. However, proper palliative care which shortens life is permissible. Assisting in voluntary active euthanasia is also illegal under the Suicide Act of 1961.

Note

— Previous to this it was also a crime to take, or attempt to take, your own life.

Withdrawing life-sustaining care is legal, as it is viewed in the eyes of the law to be passive, and not active. It is only illegal if there is thought to be a legal duty for continuing care. If a patient fits the criteria for clinical death, or if there exists an advanced directive made whilst of sound mind, mechanical life support can be switched off.

Note

— There are special issues surrounding the persistent vegetative state which require input from a court of law before being able to withdraw treatment.

Statistics

Sensitivity

The ability of a test to show that which is truly positive. An example is that of a fire alarm. It goes off at a low threshold, but you can be confident that it will always go off when there is truly a fire, even if it sometimes goes off when there isn't. It is, therefore, sensitive.

Specificity

The ability of a test to identify that which is truly negative. An example is that of a speed camera. It may miss some speeders, but if you get caught, then you were definitely speeding. It is, therefore, specific.

P value

Equals the probability, as a proportion of 1, that an event has happened as a result of chance alone. Arbitrarily, $p < 0.05$, i.e. a 20% chance of something happening, has been defined as being statistically significant in medical studies.

Type I error (aka alpha error)

Finding a difference (in your study) where none really exists, i.e. incorrectly rejecting your null hypothesis. To correct a Type I error, you must either increase your sample size (most common), or lower the p value.

Type II error (aka beta error)

Not finding a difference, where really one exists. It is usually due to insufficient numbers in the study. This is the most common type of systematic error in medical studies.

Null hypothesis

A statement that there is no difference between two things (e.g. methods of treatment), and subjecting this null hypothesis to statistical analysis, i.e. obtaining a p value. For example, there is no difference in the outcome of appendicitis, between giving antibiotics alone, or, appendicectomy; then comparing the results.

Parametric data

Represents a sample from a normally distributed population, e.g. height in a large number of people. A normally distributed population is usually represented by a bell-shaped (Gaussian) curve, classically the mode, median and mean. Parametric statistical tests are very powerful.

Non-parametric data

Data which are not normally distributed, e.g. flavour of favourite ice cream in a population. Non-parametric tests are not as powerful as their parametric counterparts.

Examples of parametric and non-parametric tests are shown in the table below.

Examples of parametric and non-parametric tests.

	Parametric	Non-parametric
Unpaired data	Unpaired t-test	Mann-Whitney U test
Paired data	Paired t-test	Wilcoxon Rank test

It is advisable to be aware of these tests for examination purposes.

Mean

The average value, i.e. divide the sum of your results by the total number of results collected.

Median

The central number in a rank of results, i.e. there are an equal number of results above and below the median when the results are presented as an ordered list.

Mode

The number represented by the intersection of a line drawn through the most common result, on a graph, i.e. the peak of the curve.

Variance

The square of the deviance from the mean.

Standard deviation (SD)

Square root of the variance. A standard bell-shaped curve contains 66% of the population within one SD, and 95% within two SDs.

You are not expected to know the maths behind SDs and variance, but simply that they are a measure of the statistical dispersion of the data.

Student's t-test

Compares the means of two samples of a population to show if the two might or might not be from the same population.

ANOVA

Analysis of variance test, which does much the same as the t-test, but with ANOVA (ANalysis Of VAriance) you can perform this analysis on more than two groups, where the t-tests can only be performed on two groups of data (paired or unpaired data).

Regression

Mathematical technique which relates x to y in a 'best fit' style. A good example is Cartesian points on a graph that almost make a straight line. The line of best fit can be defined mathematically and the process of doing this is regression.

Meta-analysis

The process of pooling information from numerous sources to increase numbers of subjects studied to reinforce results.

It requires a ranking of 'power' of trials involved to give greater credence to well performed trials, and less to poorer performed trials.

Clinical audit

Definition

The Department of Health definition of audit is: "The systematic, critical analysis of the quality of medical care, including procedures used for diagnosis and treatment, the use of resources, and the resulting outcome and quality of life of the patient."

The cycle of audit

- Observe current clinical practice.
- Determine a standard of what should be achieved.
- Compare current with standard.
- Implement change to achieve standard.
- Re-audit to see if change has been enough to reach standard ('closing the audit loop').

Medical audit

A doctor auditing their own practice.

Clinical audit

Audit of the entire multidisciplinary team.

Clinical governance

The means by which a company/institution monitors whether the services they provide are of a good quality and comparable to other centres.

It is now a legal requirement and encompasses a system to correct any deficiencies. A poor service is more to do with systems than with individuals. In the UK, there is a centre in Leeds (NHS Executive) to which all the data from hospital admissions, deaths, complications, etc., are sent. They can analyse this by consultant and or department. There exist clinical indicators which flag up variations from the norm. The appropriate team are informed of this and are asked to look into and explain this disparity.

Chapter 2

Physiology and critical care

RESPIRATORY PHYSIOLOGY

Ventilation

Relevant anatomy to respiratory physiology

Air is breathed in through the mouth into the oropharynx. From there it travels through the trachea to the carina, where the trachea splits into two main bronchi. The left and right main bronchi conduct air into each lung. The main bronchi subdivide into lobar bronchi and then further into segmental bronchi, of which there are ten segments for each lung. The final subdivisions of bronchi are termed bronchioles (the difference is the absence of cartilage; this occurs at airway diameters of <1mm). The respiratory bronchioles lead to alveoli. It is at the alveoli that gas exchange takes place, each alveolus having a capillary network surrounding it.

Note

- The pulmonary artery supplies venous blood to the lungs. It is oxygenated and depleted of CO_2 by diffusion at the level of the alveoli, then transported back to the heart (left atrium) by the pulmonary vein, then pumped back into the systemic circulation.

Mechanics of ventilation

The thorax is considered as being made up of three separate structural units: the ribcage, pleura and lungs.

Ribcage

The tendency of the ribcage is to expand. A useful visual exercise that demonstrates this well is to split the sternum vertically; when this is done the ribs are seen to 'spring open'. This tendency to expand results in a small negative intrathoracic pressure.

Pleura

There are two layers of pleura in the thorax: the parietal pleura lines the inside of the ribcage and the visceral pleura lines the outside surface of the lungs. Between the pleura is a small amount of liquid, the surface tension of which attracts the two layers together and also acts as lubrication for the movements of respiration. As mentioned previously, there is a negative pressure between the two pleural layers, i.e. between the ribcage and the lungs.

Lungs

These can be thought of as pyramids, attached to the midline at the level of the pulmonary hilae (containing main bronchi, pulmonary artery, pulmonary vein and lymphatics surrounded by a cuff of pleura). The lungs, due to the effects of gravity, are more dense inferiorly, and are less so at their apex. This is because the vascular pressures in the lung are low, and hence they are relatively more susceptible to the effects of gravity than the higher pressure systemic circulation. As a result, in the upright patient, the blood flow to the apex is at low pressure (less flow) and to the base is at high pressure (high flow) but also more congested. The net result is that the mid zone of the lung has the optimal ratio of ventilation and blood flow for oxygen exchange. These are the pulmonary zones of 'West' (I at the apex, II in the midzone, III at the base).

Note

— In postoperative basal atelectasis, what appears on X-ray as a small proportion of the lung volume actually represents a large proportion of the functional part of the lung, and results in a greater desaturation as a result.

— The ribcage contains interthoracic muscles responsible for resting inspiration and expiration movements. The accessory muscles of respiration are pectoralis major, latissimus dorsi and rectus abdominis. These are used in forced expiration and inspiration, as well as sneezing and coughing.

Control of ventilation

There are a range of systems present by which respiration is controlled. It should be remembered that, for the most part, respiration is under subconscious control, but that it is possible to overide this by voluntary means.

Chemoreceptors

Central

These detect changes in pCO_2 and H^+ ion concentration behind the blood-brain barrier and respond by increasing or decreasing respiratory rate, e.g. increased pCO_2 or H^+ ion concentration results in increased respiratory stimulation.

Peripheral

There are chemoreceptors found within the aortic body that respond to pCO_2 and H^+ ion concentrations in a similar fashion as the central chemoreceptors.

Note

— A cycle exists, mediated centrally, as a result of detection of stretch in thoracic stretch receptors which reduces the stimulus to inspire as stretch increases and vice versa. Thus, a sinusoidal inspiratory/expiratory pattern is generated at rest. This is termed the Hering-Breuer reflex.

Respiratory neurons in the medulla

The medulla contains two different types of neurons: inspiratory and expiratory neurons. These in turn stimulate inspiration and expiration in a cyclical fashion.

Ventilation - the functional residual capacity (FRC)

FRC and the resting state

It is a poorly emphasised point that the most important spirometric measure, with respect to normal ventilation, is the functional residual capacity (FRC).

The FRC is the amount of air left in the lungs at the end of tidal volume expiration (2-2.4 litres; approximately 40% of the maximum lung volume).

The FRC represents the gas present in the lungs in which gas exchange takes place during normal resting ventilation. Its constituents vary with each inspired tidal volume (TV). However, the TV is smaller than the FRC, thus only a proportion of the FRC is renewed with each breath. At rest, therefore, only a small proportion of the O_2 is renewed and only a small proportion of the CO_2 is expired. This is the normal resting state that you should be aware of, on a background of which changes can occur, be they physiological (e.g. exercise), or pathological (e.g. pulmonary oedema).

Factors involved in O_2 uptake

- Alveolar minute-volume.
- Diffusion capacity.
- Blood flow in the lung.

Factors involved in CO_2 excretion

◆ Alveolar minute-volume.
◆ Diffusion capacity (although to a much lesser extent than for O_2, as CO_2 is 20 times more easily diffused than O_2).
◆ Blood flow in the lung.
◆ Carbonic anhydrase function.

Lung volume measurements (spirometry)

Volumes

Anatomical dead space

This is the volume contained within the airways from the nose and mouth to the terminal bronchioles (approximately 0.15 litres) and is called 'dead space' because no gas exchange takes place.

Tidal volume

The amount of air expelled during resting quiet breathing (approximately 0.5 litres).

Functional residual capacity

The amount of air left in the lungs at the end of tidal volume expiration (2-2.4 litres, approximately 40% of maximum lung volume).

Residual volume

The amount of air left in the lungs after forced expiration (1-1.2 litres).

Total lung capacity

Total amount of air that can be inspired (5-6 litres).

Vital capacity

Total lung capacity minus residual capacity (TLC-RC), i.e. from maximal inspiration to maximal expiration (4-5 litres).

FEV1

Forced expiratory volume in one second.

FEV1 to FVC (forced vital capacity) ratio

This is used for identifying restrictive or obstructive defects. Restrictive gives a high value (>70%); obstructive gives a low value (<70%).

Hysteresis curves

These are dynamic representations of the respiratory flow loop depicted in Cartesian graph format. They give more information than the above volume measures about the origin of any pathological process occurring with respiration.

Oxygen transport

As a basic principle, O_2 is mainly transported in the arterial circulation (from the heart and lungs to the body) and CO_2 is mainly transported in the venous system (from the body to the heart and lungs).

Haemoglobin has four 'haem' groups capable of binding O_2. The speed at which each haem group binds an O_2 molecule determines the sigmoid shape of the O_2 curve, i.e. the first part is slow, the next two are increasingly fast, and the last one is slightly slower than the third.

O_2 is bound reversibly to haemoglobin. The reaction time of O_2 binding is milliseconds, and it needs to be for adequate binding and off-loading of O_2 in the pulmonary and peripheral circulation, respectively.

Note

— Hb concentraton, if low, has a bearing on O_2 transport (it is regulated by renally secreted erythropoietin in response to chronic renal hypoxia).

Factors affecting the O_2 dissociation curve (the Bohr effect)

The 'P50' is the pO_2 at which 50% saturation of haemoglobin occurs.

When comparing the pulmonary circulation with the systemic circulation, there are key differences that stimulate different behaviour of the haemoglobin molecules with respect to binding and off-loading O_2.

It is important that conditions in the pulmonary circulation facilitate O_2 uptake by haemoglobin and, conversely, that conditions in the peripheral circulation facilitate off-loading of O_2.

In the peripheral circulation the factors that stimulate a greater tendency for O_2 off-loading are:

- Increased acidity.
- Increased pCO_2.
- Increased temperature.
- Increased 2,3 diphosphoglycerine (2,3 DPG), which is a by-product of anaerobic metabolism found especially in RBCs, which have no mitochondria.

The above factors shift the O_2 dissociation curve to the right, thus the term right shift.

Conversely, in the pulmonary circulation, the factors that stimulate a greater tendency for O_2 uptake, are:

- Decreased pCO_2.
- Decreased acidity.
- Decreased temperature.
- Decreased 2,3 DPG.

The above factors shift the O_2 dissociation curve to the left, thus the term left shift. You can see, therefore, that O_2 is released to peripheral tissues and taken up in the lung because of this mechanism.

Oxygen reserves of the body

O_2 has poor solubility in solution (unlike CO_2), therefore, little O_2 is found as dissolved stores.

O_2 is stored by the following mechanisms:

- Physical solution (plasma).
- In RBCs.
- Left in the alveoli of the lung.
- In myoglobin (found in skeletal and cardiac muscle cells).

Factors affecting respiratory gas diffusion

- Need a large surface area (many alveoli).
- Short distance to travel across (one cell thickness of the alveolar membrane).
- Membrane/concentration gradient to flow down.
- Partial pressure difference to flow down (alveolar pO_2/pulmonary arterial pO_2).
- High diffusivity of molecule (both O_2 and CO_2 are highly diffusible molecules).

Note

- Although O_2 is a smaller molecule than CO_2, CO_2 is more water-soluble and hence has a greater diffusibility (20 times greater than O_2).

CO_2 transport

CO_2 is transported by three mechanisms:

- Dissolved in physical solution.
- In blood, CO_2 is found bound to Hb (as carbaminohaemoglobin). It is also present in sodium bicarbonate by virtue of the Henderson-Hasselbach equation which states $NaHCO_3$ is equivalent to $CO_2 + H_2O$ (a reaction catalysed by carbonic anhydrase, which is present in RBCs).
- Bound to circulating proteins (as 'carbamino' compounds).

Note

- Carbon monoxide has a 200-fold greater affinity for haemoglobin than does O_2; therefore, it competitively inhibits O_2 transport, i.e. it is toxic, causing anaemic-type symptoms.

Lung compliance

Compliance is the ease with which the lungs can be distended. Thus, increased compliance equates to easily distended lungs and vice versa. Chronic obstructive pulmonary disease (COPD) causes raised lung compliance. Restrictive airway diseases cause reduced lung compliance.

Note

- There are three different anatomical structures which are relevant to the overall compliance: lung, chest wall, and a combination of the two.

Surfactant

Its chemical composition is dipalmitoyl-phosphatidyl-choline. It is a detergent molecule (i.e. hydrophobic, thus repels water) that, by its effects on surface tension, keep the alveoli from collapsing during expiration.

Effect of breathing on airway dimensions

Airways are both distensible and collapsible. Inspiration causes distension. Expiration causes collapse if the intrathoracic pressure rises above the critical collapsing point of the airways.

Note

–   COPD causes increased compliance and, hence, an increased ease of collapsibility during high expiratory airway pressures.

Dyspnoea

This is the sensation of difficulty in breathing (usually shortness of breath) that is inappropriate to the level of exercise by the patient (usually at rest).

Tests of airflow

Peak flow
This is the highest airflow sustained for ten milliseconds; the maximal forced expiration from the maximal inspiratory point.

Forced expiratory volume in one second (FEV1)
From TLC, expiration to RV.

Forced expiratory ratio
FEV1/FVC, should be >0.7 in normal airway calibre (<0.7 in COPD, >>0.7 in restrictive airways disease).

Note

–   In patients with Type II respiratory failure (i.e. low pO_2, high pCO_2), it is the hypoxia causing their respiratory drive. As a result, if too much FiO_2 (forced inspiratory oxygen) is given, this then raises their pO_2, removing their drive to respire, and hence causing them to hypoventilate. They become progressively more hypercarbic and, hence, acidotic.

Artificial ventilation

Advantages
◆   Eliminates CO_2.

◆   Reduces respiratory work and, hence, O_2 consumption of respiratory muscles.
◆   Allows high inspiratory O_2 concentrations.
◆   Recruitment of collapsed alveoli, using positive end expiratory pressure (PEEP), i.e. a 'blast' of pressure at the end of each respiratory cycle by the ventilator, which would otherwise have been dead space.

Disadvantages
◆   Usually requires some degree of sedation (propofol, midazolam, opiates).
◆   Barotrauma, i.e. can cause pneumothorax, surgical emphysema.
◆   Misplaced endotracheal (ET) tube.
◆   Tracheal stricture (occurring as a late complication).
◆   Circulatory embarrassment (a high intrathoracic pressure can impede venous return).
◆   Favours the survival of micro-organisms, resulting in ventilator-associated pneumonia.
◆   Accidental disconnection of ventilator.
◆   Haemodynamic repercussions.

Mechanical ventilation

This is taken to mean assisting or replacing spontaneous respiration mechanically, i.e. with the aid of a machine.

Indications include:

◆   Neurological causes (15%).
◆   Type I (hypoxic) acute respiratory failure (66%).
◆   Type II (hypoxic and hypercarbic) acute respiratory failure (13%).

This obviously does not take into account elective ventilation in surgical cases, merely the medical causes likely to necessitate mechanical ventilation.

Standard ventilator modes in current use are:

◆   Continuous mandatory ventilation (CMV). Provides complete ventilatory support, requiring deep sedation (or the patient 'resists' the ventilator). It is used during the acute phase of respiratory failure.
◆   Assist control ventilation (ACV). Lighter than CMV.

- Synchronised intermittent mandatory ventilation (SIMV). Gives the opportunity for spontaneous respiratory cycles by the patient, as well as mandatory cycles when required. It does not require such a deep level of sedation and is particularly useful in weaning the patient from the ventilator.
- Continuous positive airway pressure (CPAP). Used in the non-invasive treatment of respiratory failure (i.e. not requiring intubation), or in weaning from the ventilator. Avoids the need for intubation by use of a face mask strapped to the patient's head, making a seal around the nose and mouth. The continuous pressure of oxygen provides additional support to the airway pressures in the patient's lungs, opening up more airways and allowing the patient's respiratory muscles to work less hard.

Pulse oximetry

Pulse oximetry is a non-invasive means of monitoring the percentage saturation of arterial blood. A probe is placed over a fingertip, a toe tip, or an ear lobe. The one thing these body parts have in common is the ability for a beam of infrared light to shine through them fairly easily.

Pulse oximetry relies on the different capacity of haemoglobin, when oxygenated, compared with deoxygenated, to be able to absorb specific wavelengths of infrared light.

The probe shines infrared light of two separate wavelengths (650nm and 805nm) from one of its sides. The other side is a receiver, and quantifies the amount of these two wavelengths through the tissue, i.e. how much has been absorbed.

Pulsatile bloodflow is necessary for this to work for arterial oxygen saturation. This is because the oxygen saturation of muscle (and other soft tissues) is to all intents and purposes the same as that for venous blood. Pulsatile flow is arterial, and is detected by the oximeter. It is the infrared absorption of the pulsatile blood that is measured, hence the oxygen saturation of arterial blood.

The factors that can interfere with this mechanism are as follows: overly bright ambient light; nail varnish; haemoblobin to which carbon monoxide is bound (carboxyhaemoglobin which inactivates the oxygen-carrying capacity of the molecule, but not its infrared absorption ability); venous congestion; and sluggish blood flow.

Remember that oxygen saturation is only one factor in assessment of the patient. Pulse oximeters give no information on CO_2 levels in the blood, which can be just as important in a respiratory-compromised patient.

Adult respiratory distress syndrome

This is a frequently examined topic in physiology as well as critical care areas of viva examinations. You should have the following lists ready at the front of your mind.

Definition

- CXR shows diffuse opacifications in over two of four quadrants.
- PaO_2 to FiO_2 ratio is <200.
- Pulmonary wedge pressure is <18cm H_2O (low).

Causes

Direct (lung trauma)
- Physical trauma.
- Pneumonia.
- Gastric aspiration.
- Inhalation of toxins.
- Thermal respiratory tract injury.
- Viral.
- Radiation.

Indirect
- Sepsis.
- Pancreatitis.
- Major multiple trauma.
- Haemorrhage.
- DIC.
- Massive blood transfusion.
- Burns.
- CABG.
- Pre-eclampsia.

Clinical phases

There are four clinical phases:

- I. Tachypnoea and tachycardia.
- II. Dyspnoea and cyanosis (may hear early/mild lung creps).
- III. Worsening dyspnoea and cyanosis, marked chest crepitations and visible CXR bilateral irregular opacifications.
- IV. Other organ system involvement (reduced urine output, hypotension, acidosis, hypoxia), restlessness, lethargy, coma.

Type IV imparts a bad prognosis, worsening with each extra organ system to fail, e.g. three organ failure results in over 90% mortality.

Pathology

A stimulus results in complement activation, with an influx of macrophages and neutrophils to the alveoli and endothelium. Release of toxic mediators causes alveolar oedema, and necrosis of endothelial and epithelial cells (may set off DIC). Later in the natural history, hyaline membranes lining the alveolar ducts are formed (affects surfactant). This is followed by proliferation of fibroblasts and Type II pneumocytes, which results in diffuse interstitial fibrosis. However, if the patient survives the primary insult, this fibrosis is usually reversible within four to six months (if steroid therapy is instituted from an early stage).

Note

— Mortality ≥50%.

Pulsus paradoxus

Defined as a greater than 10mmHg reduction of arterial pressure brought on by inspiration. It is usually seen in the hyperinflated lungs of patients with severe COPD. The high intrathoracic pressure at the end of inspiration causes a reduced end-diastolic volume and therefore a reduced stroke volume.

CARDIAC PHYSIOLOGY

Physiology

The cardiac cycle

This is the sequence of events during the normal beating of the heart. For simplicity the left heart structures have been considered here, but the cycle is analagous for the right heart.

The cardiac cycle occurs in the following order:

- Atrial systole. The left atrium contracts, ejecting blood into the ventricle. The mitral valve closes as the pressure of the ejected blood in the left ventricle equals that in the left atrium.
- Isovolumetric contraction of the left ventricle. The left ventricular myocardium contracts. It must first overcome the pressure of the blood still in the aorta before the aortic valve opens, thus the contraction until this point is said to be isovolumetric. The closing stage of isovolumetric contraction is the opening of the aortic valve.
- Rapid ejection of blood from the left ventricle.
- Reduced ejection. As the left ventricle empties into the aorta, the pressure across the aortic valve equalises and the aortic valve closes to end this phase.
- Isovolumetric relaxation. The mitral valve opens at the end of the relaxation phase.
- Rapid ventricular filling, i.e. atrial systole, see step 1.

Cardiac action potentials

Action potential
This is a rapid change in membrane potential (depolarisation) that occurs following stimulation of an excitable cell. It is followed by a rapid return to resting membrane potential (repolarisation).

Action potentials (AP) in myocardial cells are distinct from those in other cell types. They need to be for obvious reasons. The heart must continue to beat, and beat regularly, throughout one's lifespan. The following are the steps that determine the shape of the myocardial AP curve.

Cardiac action potentials are composed of phases
0 - 4 (Figure 2.1).

1. SLOW RESPONSE FIBRE (i.e. has pacemaker activity)

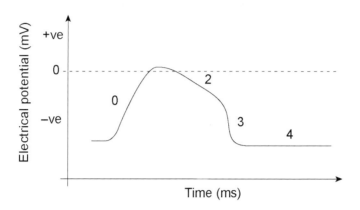

Note the absence of
a phase one, i.e. no
'brief repolarisation
phase' before a plateau

2. FAST RESPONSE FIBRE (i.e. conduct the electrical signal, a series of depolarisations rapidly through the myocardium, resulting in a heart beat)

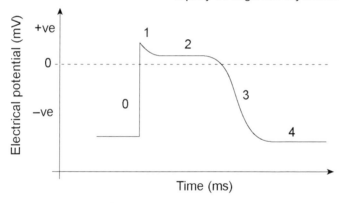

3. AN EXAMPLE OF NERVE ACTION POTENTIAL (non-cardiac)

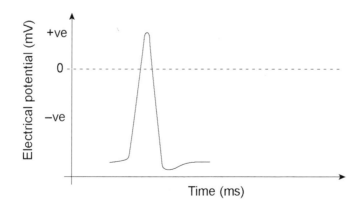

Note the much shorter time it
takes for the AP, no plateau
phase and a brief refractory phase.
This all takes about 2ms, compared
to 200ms for cardiac APs.

Figure 2.1. Cardiac action potentials.

0 is the upstroke of the AP, the depolarisation (stimulated by the conduction of the electrical impulse, originally from the sino-atrial [SA] node, by cell-to-cell conduction. This activates the fast sodium [Na^+] channels, Na^+ flows rapidly into the myocyte, making it more positively charged).

1 is a brief period of repolarisation (inactivation of fast Na^+ channels). Also, there is a transient efflux of potassium (K^+) from inside the cell.

2 is a plateau that persists for approximately 0.2s (balance of charged ions flowing in and out of cell).

3 is repolarisation which is more slow than the depolarisation phase 0 (repolarisation takes the form of efflux of K^+ and Na^+ is greater than their respective influx).

4 is the resting membrane potential (dependent on the ratio of K^+ concentration between intracellular and extracellular compartments).

Note

- Cell-to-cell conduction is faster in the Purkinje fibres than in normal myocyte-to-myocyte conduction, i.e. the wave of signal flows down the Bundle of His, made up of Purkinje fibres, spreading outwards into the ventricular myocardium using the bundle as a starting point.
- The above is the description of APs in fast reponse fibres, but slow response fibres exist. They are in the SA and AV nodes and are of a different shape, effectively depolarising at a greater rate than the rest of the heart, i.e. they have pacemaker behaviour (whichever group of cells has the greatest baseline rate of action potential stimulation, by conductance, will necessarily dictate the rate at which other myocardial cells contract, by 'jump-starting' the phase 0 depolarisation, hence acting as a pacemaker).
- Normal myocytes have pacemaker behaviour of their own, but a ventricular myocyte will only beat at 30/minute.

Heart sounds

Whilst having a grasp of cardiac anatomy and the cardiac cycle, it is not immediately apparent from these first principles what the origins of the heart sounds are. Thus, the following is important to learn.

The first heart sound begins during systole, and is the result of closure of the atrioventricular (AV) valves, i.e. mitral and tricuspid.

The second heart sound results from closure of the semilunar valves at the end of systole, i.e. aortic and pulmonary valves.

The third and fourth heart sounds are not usually heard, and their origins are complex and poorly understood (they are heard only during heart failure, or as a result of some high-flow states).

Cardiac output

Cardiac output is defined as the volume of blood pumped by the heart in a unit of time (ml/min).

The equation that defines cardiac output (CO) is the heart rate (HR) times the stroke volume (SV), thus:

$$CO = HR \times SV$$

Regulatory factors of cardiac output are:

- Preload. Stretching force on the ventricle during diastole, i.e. central venous pressure (CVP).
- Afterload. Resistance against which the ventricle contracts, i.e. systemic vascular resistance (SVR).
- Myocardial contractility.
- Heart rate.

Control of rate
The heart rate is controlled by the following factors:

- Sympathetic innervation (this is responsible for increasing the HR).
- Parasympathetic innervation (this is responsible for decreasing the HR).

♦ To a lesser extent, the level of circulating catecholamines (adrenaline and noradrenaline, both of which are responsible for increasing the HR).

Stroke volume

The stroke volume is the volume of blood ejected from either the left or right ventricle at the end of a beat. The SV does not differ between left and right heart; they are necessarily the same.

Determinants of stroke volume are:

♦ Preload. The stretching force on the ventricle during ventricular filling. It is equivalent to the CVP.
♦ Afterload. The resistance against which the ventricle contracts, i.e. SVR.
♦ Myocardial contractility. The ability of the heart to pump with the necessary force as stimulated by the preload. It is also defined as the work of the ventricle (dP/dT). This becomes particularly relevant to the heart damaged by myocardial infarction, or the heart that is being supplied with insufficient oxygen (shock). If it is incapable of beating with sufficient force to expel the normal venous return, then a vicious cycle ensues resulting in cardiac failure due to insufficient contractility.
♦ Myocardial kinetics. Starling's law of the heart states that strength of contraction of the myocyte is directly proportional to the myocyte fibre length at rest on the previous beat.

Pressures in cardiac chambers

The values of cardiac chamber pressures are occasionally asked in physiology and critical care sections of viva examinations. These are as follows:

♦ Right atrium: 0-4mmHg (this is the filling pressure of the heart, and is related to the CVP).
♦ Right ventricle: 20/0mmHg.
♦ Left atrium: 5-10mmHg (the left atrium pressure is related to pulmonary artery

pressure, which can be measured by use of a pulmonary artery balloon-tipped catheter, e.g. Swan-Ganz).
♦ Left ventricle: 120/0-10mmHg.

Monitoring cardiac output in the clinical setting

There exist many different methods to calculate the cardiac output (CO). High speed MRI, or aortic root Doppler are useful, but in the ITU setting the following catheter-based technique is more easily used. The CO is the product of the heart rate (beats/min) and the stroke volume (amount of blood ejected by the heart in one beat, mls), i.e. CO = HR x SV.

A pulmonary artery catheter (PAC) (commonly known as a Swan-Ganz catheter) is a cannula placed in the venous system by the usual central line route, i.e. usually the internal jugular vein, and advanced through the inferior vena cava into the right heart, and into the pulmonary artery. It has more than one channel, one of which opens before the end of the cannula, i.e. 'upstream'. If you inject cold water into this, then a thermoreceptor at the tip of the cannula, i.e. 'downstream', picks up the change in temperature. The time it takes from release to detection over a known distance allows you to calculate the rate of flow of blood, i.e. the cardiac output. More modern cannulae have a small heating element upstream which changes the temperature allowing a similar calculation to be made. It also enables pretty continuous CO monitoring, if needed.

Frank-Starling relationship

Force developed by the heart ventricle can be related to the initial fibre length (of its myocytes), i.e. increased preload results in an increased force of contraction. However, the graph plateaus and then decompensates beyond a threshold preload (heart failure begins).

Cardiac muscle behaves as a syncytium: a single multinucleated cell formed from many fused cells.

Intracellular calcium is responsible for increasing the contractility of the myocardium, and the ease with which it can be activated (inotropes have their effect by increasing the intracellular Ca^{2+}).

Contractility can be regulated by the autonomic nervous system, mechanical factors (pre-load and afterload), and humoral factors (adrenaline [Adr]).

Factors that influence coronary blood flow

♦ Aortic pressure.
♦ Metabolic rate of the heart results in release of vasodilatory mediators to the coronary vessels, thus increasing their diameter and hence flow.

Note

— There is no coronary blood flow during the high pressure component of systole (extra-coronary resistance). An important consequence of this is that coronary blood flow takes place during diastole.

— An intra-aortic balloon pump takes advantage of this by the effect of counterpulsation. It sits in the aorta and inflates during diastole (increasing coronary blood flow) and deflates during systole (reducing afterload).

— During tachycardia more time is spent in systole, less in diastole, hence, one would assume there is less coronary blood flow. However, the metabolic rate of the heart is increased in tachycardia and coronary vasodilation takes place as a result increasing coronary blood flow. These two effects cancel each other out such that the heart receives as much coronary blood as it needs.

Equations and basic principles

Arteries conduct blood, and act as a reservoir as well, so that flow can continue in capillaries during diastole.

Arterial compliance diminishes during life. The less the compliance the greater the work the heart must do to pump a given cardiac output, resulting in a greater pulse pressure, i.e. the difference between systolic and diastolic pressure.

The mean arterial pressure varies directly with cardiac output and total peripheral resistance. Pulse pressure varies directly with stroke volume (SV), but inversely with arterial compliance.

$CO = HR \times SV$
$BP = CO \times SVR$ (systemic vascular resistance)

HR is influenced by the innervation of the cardiac plexus, made up of sympathetic (C8-T5, noradrenaline, beta receptors) and parasympathetic (vagal, acetylcholine [muscarinic]) fibres that have opposite effects (sympathetic = increased HR; parasympathetic = decreased HR).

Note

— The resting HR in an average human is 60-80 bpm, but if the vagal input is completely abolished, a resting HR rises to 100. Therefore, parasympathetic innervation predominates *in vivo*.

— It is on SA and AV nodes that all the above mechanisms act to regulate HR (and contractility).

Baroreceptor reflex

The carotid sinus and aortic bodies contain baroreceptors which are responsive to changes in pressure. A raised blood pressure (BP) detected by baroreceptors causes reduced sympathetic and increased parasympathetic (vagal) tone, resulting in a reduced HR and contractility. The converse is also true.

Bainbridge reflex

Atrial stretch receptors (present at veno-atrial junctions in both the left and right heart) sense increased stretch (e.g. after infusion of IV fluid, therefore increasing intravascular volume), and, via the vagus, reflexly increase the HR. This reflex acts independently of the baroreceptor reflex, although *in vivo* both are present.

Note

— Increased atrial stretch stimulates increased urine flow. The mediators of this are atrial natriuretic peptide and antidiuretic hormone (ANP and ADH).

Respiratory arrhythmia

Inspiration increases HR, and expiration reduces HR. This is mostly achieved via increasing and reducing vagal tone. The effects of the sympathetic system are negligible.

Note

— Inspiration causes reduced intrathoracic pressure, hence an increased venous return, an increased atrial stretch, and then the Bainbridge reflex causes reduced vagal tone, which leads to an increased HR.
— There is also a central component cycling the vagal tone with inspiration and expiration, independent of the above factors.

Contractility of the myocardium

This is regulated by neural, intrinsic (e.g. Frank-Starling) and humoral factors. N.B. An inotrope is a substance which increases the force of contraction. A chronotrope is a substance which increases the rate of contraction.

The humoral factors are:

♦ Adrenaline (+ve inotrope and +ve chronotrope).
♦ Insulin (+ve inotrope).
♦ Thyroid hormone (+ve chronotrope).
♦ Blood gases (via chemoreceptors in the carotid body affect the HR, e.g. hypoxia stimulates +ve

chronotropy and +ve inotropy. Also, a rise in pCO_2 has exactly the same effect).

Note

— Acidotic intracellular pH also has a direct effect on myocardial contractility. It diminishes influx of Ca^{2+}, and is thus a -ve inotrope.

'Coupling' of the heart and the blood vessels

The four factors that control cardiac output (HR, contractility, preload and afterload) all combine *in vivo*. An important point to remember is that preload and afterload depend on both cardiac and vascular factors. They are therefore called coupling factors.

There are two function curves involved in regulation of CO:

♦ The cardiac function curve, the Frank-Starling curve, relating the preload (vascular filling or CVP) and cardiac output, i.e. the cardiac output is directly proportional to the preload.
♦ The vascular function curve shows that the CVP varies inversely with cardiac output, as a result of vascular factors such as arterial and venous compliance, peripheral resistance and blood volume.

Note

— There is a maximum CO, no matter how strong the pump, at which the venous return can no longer fall, i.e. the veins collapse, limiting the CO.

This is the point at which the straight line relating CVP to CO crosses the zero axis.

Note

— Incidentally, the compliance of arteries is 19 times less than in veins. Superimposing the vascular and cardiac function curves one on the other gives an overview of how the heart responds to changes in venous return or cardiac output.

'Coupling' can be summarised by the following apparently contradictory statements:

- As the CVP rises (increased preload), CO increases in proportion.
- As CO rises, the CVP falls in proportion.

Other factors affecting cardiac output

- Gravity (venous pooling).
- Muscle pumps (increase venous return).
- Respiratory effects (inspiration results in decreased intrathoracic pressure and hence increased venous return, termed the 'thoracic pump').

Shock

The definition of shock is important to remember: inadequate tissue perfusion secondary to a drop in blood pressure.

Types of shock

- Hypovolaemic.
- Cardiogenic.
- Septic.
- Neurogenic.
- Anaphylactic.

Note

– Treat the cause of shock, as well as providing supportive fluid management.

Compensatory mechanisms in shock

This is important to remember for physiology and critical care sections of viva examinations. It is vital to learn the following in detail.

Baroreceptors

These are found in the aorta. They cause decreased vagal tone and increased sympathetic tone, resulting in vasoconstriction and venoconstriction.

Chemoreceptors

These are found in the aortic and carotid bodies, augmenting vasoconstriction, in response to hypoxia or hypercarbia.

Renal conservation of Na^+ and H_2O

Decreased renal blood flow, therefore leading to a reduced urine output. Also, aldosterone leads to Na^+ reabsorption.

Reabsorption of tissue fluids

Reduced plasma hydrostatic pressure, flow of fluid from tissues to plasma at capillary level, leading to a consequent increase in plasma volume associated with a reduction in plasma oncotic pressure (dilution).

Vasoconstrictor release

Adrenaline, noradrenaline, vasopressin and renin lead to angiotensin being released.

Cerebral ischaemia responses

Systolic pressure <40mmHg results in cerebral stimulation of adrenaline and noradrenaline release, and more intense vasoconstriction. However, this eventually results in increased vagal tone, producing a counterproductive bradycardia.

Note

– There are also decompensatory mechanisms in shock. These include:
  • cardiac failure (reduced BP causes reduced coronary flow which in turn causes reduced CO);
  • acidosis (decreased tissue perfusion causes increased build up of H^+ which is poorly excreted by the hypoperfused kidney. Acidosis causes cardiac depression);
  • disordered coagulation (first, a hypercoagulable state is followed by a hypocoagulable state);
  • an impaired reticulo-endothelial system (decreased function of immune defence allows passage of micro-organisms through the GIT and past the liver into the circulation; endotoxins cause further hypotension).

Clinical signs of shock

- Cool peripheries.
- Poor filling of peripheral veins.
- Capillary refill time >2 seconds.
- Increased respiratory rate.
- Increased core peripheral temperature gradient (peripheral shutdown).
- Poor signal on pulse oximetry.
- Poor urine output.
- Restlessness or decreased level of consciousness.
- Metabolic acidosis (increased lactate).

Haemorrhagic shock

Defined as the acute loss of circulating blood volume.

Class I
Blood loss up to 15%.

Class II
Blood loss between 15-30%. Uncomplicated shock, where fluid resuscitation is required.

Class III
Blood loss between 30-40%. Complicated shock, where at least crystalloid, and sometimes blood, is required.

Class IV
Blood loss greater than 40%. Considered a pre-terminal event unless aggressive measures are undertaken involving blood replacement plus or minus the use of inotropes, as well as arresting the source of haemorrhage. Otherwise, this is a rapidly terminal event.

Sepsis

SIRS

The systemic inflammatory response syndrome (SIRS) comprises two or more of the following:

- Pyrexia >38°C (or <36°C).
- Tachycardia >90 beats per minute.
- Tachypnoea >20 beats per minute.
- White cell count (WCC) >12 giga per litre.

Sepsis

Sepsis is specifically the presence of SIRS (as defined above) with a documented source of infection.

Severe sepsis

Severe sepsis is defined as the presence of sepsis (as defined above) with evidence of associated organ failure, e.g. renal failure.

- Cardiovascular system (CVS): lactate >1.2mmol/l.
- SVR <800 dyne/s/cm^3.
- Respiratory: PaO$_2$ <9.3 kPa.
- Renal: urine output <120ml in four hours.
- Central nervous system (CNS): Glasgow Coma Scale (GCS) <15 in the absence of sedation/lesion.

Note

– One of the most useful things to remember about severe sepsis is that the physiological abnormalities mentioned in the list above can generally be corrected by simple fluid resuscitation (filling).

Sepsis syndrome

As for severe sepsis but with no confirmed source of infection.

Note

– In the case of septic shock (as opposed to severe sepsis), simple refilling does not correct the tissue perfusion problem, and vasopressor therapy is required.

Septic shock

Refractory hypotension causing inadequate tissue perfusion.

Body fluids and compartments

Total body water

Body water is the solvent in which numerous biological processes can occur. Total body water is two thirds intracellular and one third extracellular, and of the proportion that is extracellular, two thirds are interstitial and one third is vascular.

There is a category of body fluid that, under non-pathological conditions, occupies a negligible volume of water compared with total body water. This is the transcellular water, e.g. intrapleural, cerebrospinal fluid (CSF), abdominal cavity fluid, etc.

Solute

Solute represents the chemicals that exist within the solvent that is the body water in its various compartments. An important concept to grasp is that different body fluid compartments contain different proportions of specific solutes. The different proportions are responsible for gradients and forces across barriers between the fluid compartments, and hence provide energy for a huge variety of biological reactions within the body. The maintenance and use of this source of energy is a very fundamental principle of biological life.

Intracellular
◆ High in potassium (K^+) and protein.

Extracellular
◆ Interstitial fluid is high in electrolytes and low in protein.
◆ Vascular fluid is high in electrolytes and high in protein.

Measurement of solute
Solute is measured by its osmolality. Osmolality is the 'total solute content': the number, not the charge, of molecules within the fluid compartment.

Forces that move water and electrolytes

◆ Diffusion. Molecules have a tendency to flow down their concentration gradients.

◆ Osmolality. Water will flow from a compartment of low osmolarity to one of high osmolarity, across a semipermeable membrane.
◆ Gibbs-Donnan equilibrium. The higher presence of negatively-charged extracellular protein in plasma than interstitial fluid results in water being attracted towards the protein, i.e. from the interstitial to the vascular compartment. This is an important concept, i.e. that the presence of protein, which is too large a molecule to diffuse across a cell wall, enables a degree of control on the amount of ionic diffusion out of the vascular compartment.
◆ Ion pumps. The classic example of an ion pump is the sodium-potassium-adenosine triphosphatase pump. It uses energy (adenosine triphosphate [ATP]) to pump Na^+ out of cells in exchange for K^+ into the cells.
◆ Endocrine. For example, antidiuretic hormone or aldosterone have specific actions on renal water and ionic re-uptake and diffusion.

Starling's hypothesis (Figure 2.2)

Starling's hypothesis states that 90% of all fluid filtered from arteriole and capillary into interstitial fluid is returned back into the capillary and venule. This is

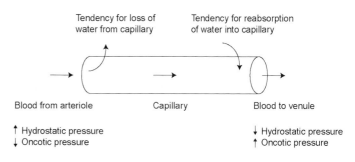

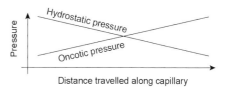

The mechanism by which 90% of water is reabsorbed in the capillary.

Figure 2.2. Starling's hypothesis.

because of the gradually increasing oncotic and reducing hydrostatic pressure from the arteriole (relatively high intravascular pressure and relatively low oncotic pressure), to the venule (relatively low intravascular pressure, but because of the loss of water [but not protein] to the interstitial compartment, a relatively high oncotic pressure), i.e. the conditions favour water loss from the vascular to the interstitial compartment at the level of the arteriole, but, by the time the blood has flowed through the capillary to the venule, the conditions have reversed to favour water gain from the interstitial to the vascular compartment.

Clinical applications of body fluid compartment dynamics

Tonicity of intravenous fluid regimes

The tonicity of a fluid refers to its ionic concentration compared with that maintained as normal by the human body. You will often see normal saline represented as 0.9% sodium chloride (NaCl). Thus, an isotonic solution is one in which the sodium concentration is a match for that of the intravascular compartment.

Remembering that water will flow from a low to a high osmolality, one can deduce the following useful heuristics:

- Administration of an IV of a hypotonic solution results in cell swelling.
- Administration of an IV of a hypertonic solution results in cell shrinkage.
- Administration of an IV of an isotonic solution results in no change in cell volume.

Important characteristics of common fluid regimens

Normal saline

Contains 150mmol of Na^+ in one litre. The daily requirement of Na^+ is only 70mmol, therefore, only 500ml of normal saline is needed for Na^+ replacement.

5% glucose

Glucose is absorbed immediately in the first-pass hepatic metabolism, leaving only water, thus 5% glucose is a hypotonic fluid.

Dextrose saline

Dextrose saline is one-fifth strength saline (and glucose, which as explained is absorbed in first-pass hepatic metabolism), therefore, 2.5 litres are needed over one day for Na^+ replacement.

Hartmann's solution

Hartmann's solution is isotonic with extracellular fluid (ECF) (as is normal saline), but Hartmann's contains other electrolytes found in the ECF, whereas normal saline only contains Na^+ and Cl^-).

Note

- If plasma (not blood) is lost, then the concentration of haemoglobin (represented by the haematocrit [Hct]) will rise, but if ECF is lost then the Hct will rise in addition to protein (albumin) concentration. This is because in plasma loss, there is also loss of protein, which therefore remains at the same concentration.
- Rule of 70s: a 70kg man needs 70mmol of K^+ and 70mmol of Na^+ every 24 hours.

Physiology of the arterial system

Compliance (Figure 2.3)

Compliance is a property of the elasticity of arteries, responsible for damping of the pulsatile nature of blood flow through capillaries. With age, arteries harden (arteriosclerosis), and lose this damping property. It is the compliance of arteries that is responsible for the biphasic pressure wave trace seen when an arterial line is *in situ*. The author finds it easiest to visualise the aorta to understand this concept, although the principle is the same for all major arteries in the body. The heart beats (completes ventricular systole) and pumps blood into the aorta (this is the first peak of the biphasic wave trace). The compliance of the stretched artery causes it to recoil inwards after the heart stops its pump action, which results in a rise again (slight) in the intraluminal pressure (this is the second peak of the biphasic wave trace).

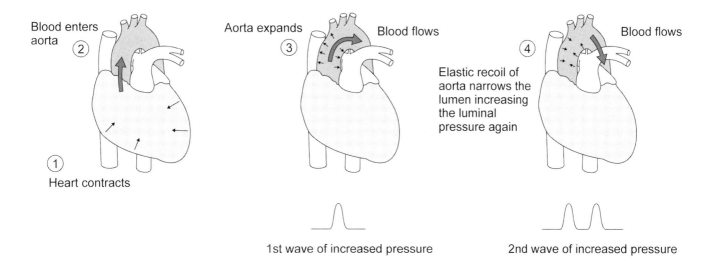

Blood enters aorta ② Aorta expands ③ Blood flows Blood flows ④

Elastic recoil of aorta narrows the lumen increasing the luminal pressure again

① Heart contracts

1st wave of increased pressure   2nd wave of increased pressure

Figure 2.3. Compliance.

Strangely, this is a common question in viva examinations. This may be because the two waves are a useful phenomenon when performing portable duplex in the clinical setting; arterial blood signals will have a biphasic sharp staccato signal, which is different from a venous signal which is monophasic and slow.

Blood pressure

The hydrostatic pressure exerted by blood on the wall of the blood vessel.

Mean arterial pressure (MAP)

The equation for MAP is 1/3(SP-DP) + DP. The reason for this is that blood pressure is a product of both systolic (SP) and diastolic (DP) phases, and spends more time during diastole, e.g. MAP in a patient with a BP of 120/80 will be approximately 93mmHg.

Determinants of arterial pressure

If right atrial pressure does not vary, then the MAP is determined by the rate at which blood enters the system, i.e. cardiac output (CO), and the rate at which blood leaves the system, i.e. systemic vascular resistance (SVR). These are important definitions to know for the physiology section of viva examinations, i.e. MAP-P(ra) = CO × SVR (where P(ra) is the pressure in the right atrium).

Relationship of pressure and flow

An analogy exists with Ohm's law (V = IR), in that flow is proportional to the pressure difference times the resistance, i.e. Q = Delta P × RC.

Note

— The above two equations show that resistance is a strong modulator of flow, therefore, in the body the resistance of the arterioles is used to influence the flow (and hence cardiac output) by their ability to contract the smooth musculature of their media layer, and the fact that there are a great number of arterioles covering a large surface area.

Pulmonary circulation

This parallels the systemic circulation, in that cardiac output is necessarily the same. The pressure gradient accross the pulmonary vasculature can be represented by the difference in pressure between the pulmonary artery (pa) and the left atrium (la). The determinants of this pressure gradient are CO and pulmonary vascular resistance, i.e. P(la) - P(pa) = CO × PVR (peripheral vascular resistance).

Note
- The greatest cross-sectional area blood is exposed to and where there is the lowest blood flow is in the capillaries. This is vital for gas, nutrient and metabolic byproduct exchange.
- Capillary vascular beds are arranged in parallel, therefore, individual beds can have their blood flow regulated independently (useful in homeostasis).

Other determinants of vascular resistance

Blood viscocity (increased viscocity is proportional to increased resistance) and vessel radius (vascular resistance is proportional to one over the radius to the power of four) are both represented in Poiseuille's equation (you are not expected to know the full equation, which is highly detailed, however, you are expected to remember it is proportional to $1/r^4$). The best example of an application of this equation is in the use of a short and wide-bore cannula, which enables a greater flow rate.

Velocity and flow

Velocity is the speed in metres per second (m/s) of travel of blood. Flow is the volume of fluid travelling per unit of time. To relate the two, you need to know the cross-sectional area through which the blood is flowing (units: litres or ml per second, i.e. flow rate = velocity x cross-sectional area).

Arterial stenosis

Normally there is effectively no pressure drop across a major artery. However, in the presence of a stenosis, a pressure drop exists.

If flow rate in that vessel remains constant then the velocity must rise in proportion to the cross-sectional area reduction, i.e. stenosis.

Critical stenosis

If stenosis increases to more than 70%, then the flow rate cannot remain constant. From this point on Poiseuille's equation determines the rate of fall in flow. Where flow decreases, the stenosis is then called a critical stenosis.

Collateral circulation

Collaterals develop as a result of stenoses. They are NOT new vessel formation; they are in fact dilatation of existing vessels from the stem artery in response to increased blood flow forced through them. Collaterals take several weeks to form, and thus, they are not very useful in acute stenosis.

Disadvantages of collaterals with respect to stem arteries

- Increased vascular resistance.
- Run-off arteries are already at maximal dilatation, therefore, there is no reserve for exercise.
- Do not compensate well for multiple stenotic lesions.

Measurement of blood flow

- Duplex (Figure 2.4).
- Using a pulmonary artery catheter as a receiver and a central line as an injection source, inject a detectable chemical (or cold fluid), and then

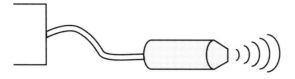

Ultrasound wave. Major property in this context is its ability to rebound off layers between changes in density of tissue (e.g. vessel walls/bones/bowel gas, etc.). The reflected wave is then detected.

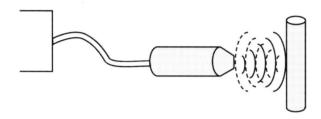

The Doppler effect: a change in pitch of sound proportional to the velocity of the moving (or in the case of vascular ultrasound, reflecting) object is used to measure blood flow.

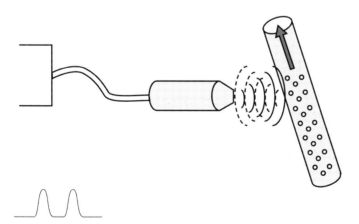

The flow of blood in a vessel reflects the ultrasound waves back at a different frequency than they started. The change of frequency can be used to calculate flow.

Biphasic flow wave
of arterial blood

Figure 2.4. Measurement of blood flow: duplex.

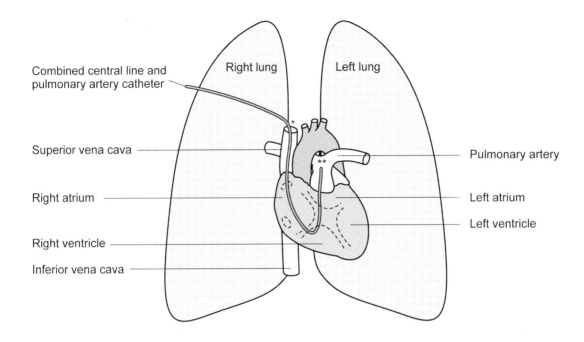

Combined central line and
pulmonary artery catheter

Right lung

Left lung

Superior vena cava

Right atrium

Right ventricle

Inferior vena cava

Pulmonary artery

Left atrium

Left ventricle

*   Chemical (or cold fluid) injected here. (SVC or jugular vein).
     Time of injection recorded by machine (T_1).

** Chemical (or cold fluid) is detected as it arrives here (pulmonary artery).
     Time of detection recorded by machine (T_2).

$T_2 - T_1$ = time it took blood to flow from one known
location to another. Thus, blood flow can be calculated.

Figure 2.5. Measurement of blood flow: using a pulmonary artery catheter.

measure its change in concentration (or
temperature) when it reaches the pulmonary
artery (Figure 2.5).
- Plethysmography (measuring limb diameters
  after applying a cuff at venous pressure,
  therefore, this relates to arterial filling of the
  limb).
- PET scans.

Cutaneous circulation

- Skin requires little in the way of nutrients.
- The major determinant of cutaneous blood flow
  is thermoregulation.
- Skin contains mainly arterioles and
  arteriovenous anastomoses under sympathetic
  control.

Skeletal muscle circulation

Determined by neural, hormonal, and metabolic
byproducts.

Inotropes

An inotrope is a drug that is capable of affecting the
contraction of the heart. Where you see reference to
alpha and beta, this is based on the knowledge that
there are two major types of adrenoreceptors. A
simplification of where the different types of
adrenoreceptors can be found is as follows:

- Cardiac - alpha receptors. Increase
  contractility of the myocardium when
  stimulated.

◆ Vascular smooth muscle - some vessels contain alpha receptors, which cause contraction (increasing SVR) when stimulated. Others contain beta receptors, which cause relaxation (decreasing SVR) when stimulated.

Dobutamine

◆ Beta-1 agonist (+ve inotrope).
◆ Some beta-2 effect (reduces BP).
◆ Slight alpha effect increases BP by increasing SVR.
◆ Used in myocardial failure.
◆ 5-10μg/kg/min (can be given via a peripheral line, but preferably via a central route given the choice).

Dopamine

◆ Beta-1 agonist.
◆ Dopamine agonist.
◆ Dose-dependent stimulation of alpha receptors.
◆ Used in shock/hypotension.
◆ 1-5μg/kg/min (must be via a central line).

Norepinephrine (aka noradrenaline)

◆ Not technically an inotrope, more of a vasoactive substance.
◆ Alpha agonist (increases SVR and therefore increases BP).
◆ Used in hypotension in septic shock.
◆ Not to be used in hypovolaemic states.

Epinephrine (aka adrenaline)

◆ Alpha agonist.
◆ Beta-1 agonist.
◆ Positive inotrope.
◆ Positive chronotrope.
◆ Potent vasoconstrictor.
◆ Used in low cardiac output states.

Central line insertion

Internal jugular vein (IJV)

Central lines can be inserted as the IJV runs deep to the two heads of sternocleidomastoid, at a needle to skin angle of approximately 30°, aiming towards the ipsilateral nipple.

Subclavian vein

Central lines can be inserted infraclavicularly, approximately 2cm below the midclavicular point, aiming towards the jugular notch.

Both techniques require ECG monitoring throughout and a CXR post-procedure, to look for the line's position before using it, as well as to exclude some of the pulmonary complications (see below).

Femoral vein

A quick and easy route, especially useful in emergency central access. The landmark is the palpation of the femoral arterial pulse and move one centimetre medially, which leads you to the femoral vein (as in the mnemonic 'NAVY'; from lateral to medial in the groin the order of structures is Nerve, Artery, Vein, Y-front).

Complications

Early
◆ Pneumothorax (in IJV and subclavian lines, not femoral).
◆ Air embolism (in IJV and subclavian lines, not femoral).
◆ Thrombus.
◆ Haematoma.
◆ Exsanguinations.
◆ Arterial damage.
◆ Arrhythmias.
◆ Chylothorax (leak of lymph from the thoracic duct). (In IJV and subclavian lines, not femoral).

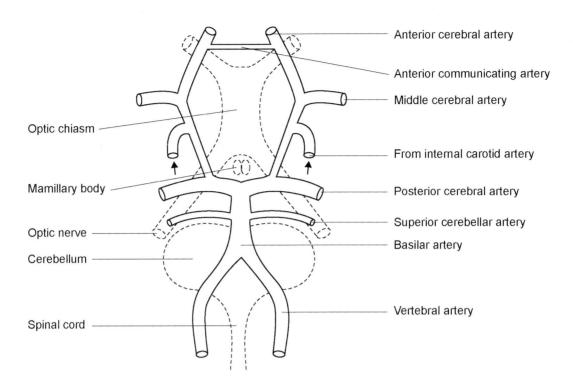

Figure 2.6. The dual artery supply of the cerebrum (referring to left and right internal carotid arteries).

Late

- Line infection.
- Line migration.
- Sepsis.
- Endocarditis.

Cerebral blood flow (Figure 2.6)

The brain has a very high blood flow compared with its size. The importance of blood flow to the brain is emphasised by the fact that there is autoregulation of its circulation.

Mechanisms of brain autoregulation

- Dual arterial supply, i.e. both internal carotids.
- Resistance to vasoconstriction caused by sympathetic outflow.
- PCO_2 acts as a vasodilator.
- Broad range of BP over which autoregulation occurs.

- Arterial baroreceptors located in the carotid sinus, i.e. in the artery responsible for cerebral perfusion.

Fick principle

This can be used to measure blood flow to the brain, which relies on conservation of mass. If a chemical is administered into the blood, its concentration can be measured. You also know the quantity administered.

Note

- Concentration = Quantity/Volume, therefore Quantity = Concentration x Volume. If time is introduced into the equation then Quantity per unit time = Concentration x Volume per unit time (we know that volume per unit time is the same as flow).
- For the purpose of the calculation here, quantity is represented as 'Q.' and concentration as 'C.'

This allows us to calculate the flow of blood into the brain by measuring Q.in and Q.out, and C.in and C.out, giving us:

Flow = (Q.in-Q.out) / (C.in-C.out).

In vivo N_2O gas is used as the substance for measuring cerebral blood flow with the Fick principle.

RENAL PHYSIOLOGY

Kidneys

Functions of the kidneys

- Regulation of body fluid osmolality and volume. Osmolality is a measure of the number of solute particles in a specific volume of water.
- Regulation of electrolyte balance.
- Regulation of acid-base balance.
- Excretion of metabolic products and foreign substances.
- Production and secretion of hormones (renin, PGs, kinins, 1,25 dihydroxy D3, erythropoietin).

It is important to know the above list, as it commonly arises during examinations. It forms the stem of a large proportion of questions in physiology, and is the basis of the explanations you will be asked for in the critical care section of viva examinations.

Some renal trivia

Blood flow to the two kidneys is 20% of the cardiac output, despite constituting only 0.5% of the body weight (blood flow is eight times greater than coronary blood flow). Each kidney contains 1.2 million nephrons, the functional unit of the kidney, which are one cell thick. The right kidney is lower than the left due to the displacing presence of the liver.

Constituents of the nephron (functional unit of the kidney) (Figure 2.7)

- Renal corpuscle (the glomerulus, a specialised capillary) and Bowman's capsule which surrounds it.
- Proximal tubule.
- Loop of Henle.
- Distal tubule.
- Collecting duct system.

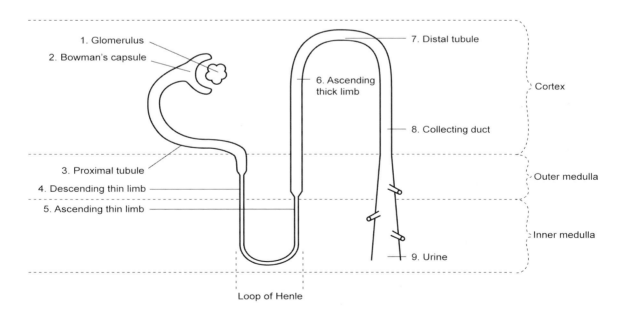

Blood is filtered from the glomerulus into Bowman's capsule. The filtrate then travels via 2–9. See following sections for changes that occur at each level.

Figure 2.7. Constituents of the nephron (functional unit of the kidney).

Ultrafiltration

This is the process of passage of a protein-free fluid from the glomerular capillary to Bowman's space.

Renal function

Renal clearance

Renal clearance is a quantitative measure of the rate at which waste products are removed from the blood by the kidneys. The units are litres of blood per minute, i.e. the volume of blood that could be completely cleared of the substance in question in one minute.

Clearance = $(U \times V)/P$.

Where U is the concentration in urine, V is flow, and P is the concentration in the plasma.

Renal clearance is dependent on three processes:

♦   Glomerular filtration rate (GFR=160 litres/24 hours; this value is often asked for in viva examinations). The definition of GFR is the volume of blood that is filtered by the kidney per unit of time. Unlike clearance it refers not to a chemical but only to the volume of blood passing through the filtration system of the kidneys.

Note

—   Not all blood that is pumped into the kidney is filtered.

♦   Reabsorption (from the tubular fluid into the blood).
♦   Secretion (from the blood into the tubular fluid).

One substance that can be used to measure GFR is inulin, as it is not made by the body and is not secreted or reabsorbed by the kidneys. It is simply filtered, i.e. amount filtered = amount excreted.

However, the reason creatinine is used in practice to measure GFR is that it is produced at a relatively constant rate from muscle, and is very minimally secreted in the proximal tubule, introducing an error of approximately 10%, but for practical purposes it is a useful index of GFR.

Filtration fraction

Not all blood that enters the kidney is filtered; in fact, only 15-20% is filtered.

Autoregulation

The renal blood flow within the kidney is regulated by changes in the arterioles such that it remains constant, despite changes in systolic pressure between 90 and 180mmHg.

Haemorrhage results in increased sympathetic outflow. This stimulates renal arteriolar constriction, and increases angiotensin II and renin secretion, which also act to increase the renal arteriolar constriction hence further reducing renal blood flow, thus counteracting the fall in BP due to the haemorrhage.

Glomerular filtration rate

In the normal adult male this is 120-125ml/min.

Juxtaglomerular apparatus (Figure 2.8)

The juxtaglomerular apparatus is a collection of cells located next to the glomerulus that is responsible for autoregulation of renal blood flow.

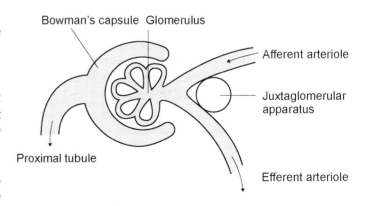

Figure 2.8. Juxtaglomerular apparatus.

The apparatus is made up of:

◆   Macula densa.
◆   Renin-producing juxtaglomerular cells.
◆   Extraglomerular mesangial cells.

Regulation of urine composition

◆   Ultrafiltration.
◆   Secretion.
◆   Reabsorption (approximately 65-70% of the GFR is reabsorbed).

Renal tubular function

The renal tubules are responsible for transport of H_2O and Na^+ along the nephron in the kidney.

Transport of chemicals against their concentration gradient requires energy. This can be in the form of primary active transport (direct coupling of the process with a Na^+-K^+-ATPase pump), or secondary active transport (indirect coupling to an energy source, e.g. energy stored in an ion gradient).

Water is always transported as a passive process down its concentration gradient, from low to high osmolality.

The Na^+-K^+-ATPase pump forces Na^+ out of the cell, and K^+ into the cell.

A symporter carries molecules in the same direction across a cell membrane. An antiporter carries molecules in the opposite direction across a cell membrane. The Loop of Henle reabsorbs approximately 25% of filtered $NaCl^-$ and K^+, and also, approximately 15% of filtered water (but only in the descending thin limb, because the ascending limb is impermeable to water).

Furosemide inhibits the Na^+-Cl^--K^+ symporter, thus more $NaCl^-$ is lost in the urine, also resulting in a reduction in the lumen's positive voltage, which is the mechanism by which K^+ is normally reabsorbed, therefore more K^+ is lost in the urine.

The distal tubule is under the influence of antidiuretic hormone (ADH) which controls the amount of water excreted.

Thiazide diuretics inhibit $NaCl^-$ reabsorption in the distal tubule and are therefore diuretic.

Amiloride and spironolactone inhibit $NaCl^-$ reabsorption in the distal tubule and collecting duct by inhibiting aldosterone.

Angiotensin II

A potent stimulator of reabsorption of $NaCl^-$ and hence water in the proximal tubule. (N.B. angiotensin II is stimulated by the drop in extracellular fluid volume).

Aldosterone

Synthesised in the adrenal gland (zona glomerulosa of adrenal cortex), aldosterone stimulates $NaCl^-$ reabsorption in the thick ascending limb of the loop of Henle, and the distal tubule and collecting duct. It also stimulates the secretion of K^+ by the distal tubule (aldosterone is stimulated by a rise in angiotensin II and by a rise in serum K^+).

Antidiuretic hormone (ADH)

Secreted by the posterior pituitary gland, ADH is responsible for most of the control of body water. It is secreted in response to increased plasma osmolality or decreased ECF volume, acting on the wall of the collecting duct making it more permeable to water, therefore, water flows along the osmotic gradient into the blood.

Potassium regulation

Two overall systems relating to K^+ exist for regulation:

- $[K^+]$ ECF ('[ ]' represents 'concentration' of the bracketed chemical).
- Total amount of K^+ in the body, i.e. ingestion vs excretion (renal).

K^+ in the body is 98% intracellular, 2% extracellular ($[K] = 4$ mEq/l).

The Na^+-K^+-ATPase pump is responsible for maintaining this potential difference across cell membranes (critical for nerve excitability, muscle contractility, etc.).

A meal contains K^+ in abundance, resulting in rapid absorption of K^+ from the GIT to the blood stream. This rise has to be buffered and then matched by excretion. Adrenaline, aldosterone and insulin cause an increased cellular uptake of blood K^+ by direct or indirect stimulation of Na^+-K^+-ATPase, therefore, buffering the post-prandial increase.

Note

- A decrease in $[K^+]$ results in inhibition of release of these hormones. Aldosterone also causes increased renal excretion of K^+ in the distal tubule and collecting duct. This, however, is slow, taking approximately six hours.
- Metabolic acidosis results in increased serum $[K^+]$, as K^+ and H^+ are swapped across the cell membrane to buffer the acidosis.
- Plasma osmolality, when increased, increases plasma $[K^+]$.
- Cell lysis increases $[K^+]$, as does exercise.

The kidneys are responsible for excretion of 90-95% of ingested K^+; small amounts are lost in the stool and sweat (unregulated); it is in the distal tubule and the collecting duct that K^+ is secreted into urine (N.B. aldosterone control).

Calcium homeostasis

Ca^{2+} is important for bone formation, cell division and growth, and coagulation.

- 99% of Ca^{2+} is stored in bone, 1% is in intracellular fluid, and 0.1% is in extracellular fluid.
- Low Ca^{2+} results in increased excitability of cells and tetany.
- High Ca^{2+} can cause decreased cellular excitability, hence the potential for cardiac arrhythmias.

Arrhythmias

Regulation of Ca^{2+} is balanced between GIT ingestion and renal excretion. 1,25-dihydroxyvitamin D3 is responsible for stimulating increased GIT uptake of Ca^{2+} and increased bone resorption of Ca^{2+}.

Parathyroid hormone

- Stimulates bone resorption of Ca^{2+}.
- Stimulates renal resorption of Ca^{2+}.
- Stimulates increased 1,25-dihydroxyvitamin D3 secretion.
- Overall effect, therefore, is to increase $[Ca^{2+}]$.

Calcitonin

- Secreted from the medullary cells of the thyroid.
- Inhibits osteoclast activity, thus causing a fall in circulating Ca^{2+}.

Acid-base balance

The hydrogen ion

The single most important fact to convey in explaining acid-base balance is that it all relates simply to following the course of the hydrogen (H^+) ion. This may seem an obvious statement, but as the subject increases in complexity, it is easy to become confused. At this time it is worth remembering this simple premise: it is all about following the H^+ ion.

The H^+ ion can be represented when present in the body in one of two ways:

- As a concentration, i.e. in nM/l. The average concentration of H^+ in blood is 40nM/l.
- As a pH. Although pH is universally taught, and used, in clinical practice, it is a difficult concept to understand. pH comes from the German 'potenz hydrat ion', or the 'potential of the hydrogen ion'. It is a calculated value based on a logarithmic scale.

Specifically, $pH = 6.1 \times \log ([HCO_3^-]/pCO_2)$.

Thus, relatively small changes in the pH represent relatively large changes in the concentration of H^+. The normal range for the pH in human blood is 7.35-7.45 (there are no units).

The Henderson-Hasselbach equation:

This equation explains how the body deals with ingested hydrogen ions by buffering with bicarbonate, allowing the formation of CO_2 in the lungs that can be 'blown off', preventing acidosis.

$$\overset{(1)}{} \qquad \overset{(2)}{}$$
$$H^+ + HCO_3^- = H_2CO_3 = CO_2 + H_2O.$$

The important implications of this equation that should be understood are:

- $H^+ + HCO_3^- = H_2CO_3$ is a reaction that favours formation of H_2CO_3 by 20:1, i.e. it does not require a catalyst. An example of the usefulness of this point *in vivo* is: after the ingestion of a large H^+ load, contact between circulating HCO_3^- and H^+ results in rapid removal of H^+ from the circulation and formation of H_2CO_3, i.e. H^+ is buffered (remember from early chemistry lessons that a buffer is a 'proton acceptor', also that an acid is a 'proton donor').
- $H_2CO_3 = CO_2 + H_2O$ is a reaction that requires a catalyst. The catalyst, in this case, is carbonic anhydrase (CA). In the presence of CA, circulating H_2CO_3 is converted to water and CO_2. Where better in the body than in the lungs to form CO_2 (so it can be 'blown off', i.e. expired), thus CA is present in high levels in the lungs.

The anion gap

Caused by the presence of protein in the circulation, calculated by:

$Na^+ - (Cl^- + HCO_3^-)$, i.e. the difference between sodium (the major source of +ve ions) and chloride + bicarbonate (the major source of -ve ions).

The implication of a high anion gap is the presence of a metabolic acidosis (also implies the presence of an acid other than H^+, e.g. keto-acid or lactic acid).

The normal range for the anion gap is 12-20.

The base deficit

This is the amount of acid/alkali required to restore one litre of blood to a normal pH when pCO_2 is 5.3 and the temperature is 37°C.

The normal range is from -2 to +2mmol/l.

Sources of hydrogen ions

- Diet. H^+ is present on side chains of all organic molecules, as these are broken down in the process of digestion, and large quantities of H^+ are released into the circulation, e.g. after a meal.
- Respiratory. Under normal circumstances the lungs 'blow off' CO_2, but during times of hypoventilation, CO_2 builds up. From the Henderson-Hasselbach equation, it can be seen that an excess of CO_2 will react with H_2O to form H_2CO_3, thus a relative increase in H^+ will result. This, as will be explored in greater detail, is a respiratory acidosis.
- Renal. Under normal circumstances the kidneys excrete H^+ in exchange for Na^+ and/or K^+. But during times of renal insufficiency (failure), the kidneys are unable to excrete as much H^+ as before, thus it builds up in the circulation. This is an example of a metabolic acidosis.
- Ketoacids and hydroxybutyrate. This is the classic case of formation of acidic compounds for use as cellular nutrients when glucose is in short supply (diabetics), and thus reduces pH. This is much less common than the above as a cause of acidosis in clinical practice.

◆ Bicarbonate loss in stool. HCO_3^- loss equals a H^+ gain, overall. This, it should be remembered, is so rare as to be virtually ignored by all but the specialists.

Buffering of hydrogen ions

Definition of a buffer

As previously mentioned, a buffer is a 'proton acceptor', i.e. a molecule that when exposed to H^+ reacts favourably with it to form a stable compound, thus effectively removing H^+ from the circulation in its ionic form.

Molecules that are buffers

◆ The most important buffer of all is the bicarbonate ion (HCO_3^-). Bicarbonate is produced in significant quantities by the kidney, secondary to excretion of H^+ in exchange for Na^+ or K^+, using the Henderson-Hasselbach equation; losing H^+ from the '$H^+ + HCO_3^-$' section leaves only HCO_3^- to circulate in the blood as a buffer. A less important source of HCO_3^- is as a result of H^+ secretion into the stomach by the proton pump; again HCO_3^- is a byproduct of this reaction.
◆ Haemoglobin molecules are capable of buffering H^+ ions.
◆ Circulating proteins are capable of buffering H^+ ions.
◆ Phosphate (PO_4^{3-}) ions are capable of buffering H^+ ions.
◆ Sulphate (SO_4^{2-}) ions are capable of buffering H^+ ions.

Excretion of hydrogen ions

From the Henderson-Hasselbach equation it can be surmised that H^+ and CO_2 are equivalent, i.e. loss of one from the circulation can be regarded as loss of the other from the circulation. From this statement, it follows that when the lungs 'blow off' a CO_2 molecule, this is equivalent to excreting a H^+ molecule. Because the H^+ has effectively become one of the two Hs in H_2O this will then be excreted in the urine. Thus, a major form of H^+ excretion is respiratory excretion.

Remember that carbonic anhydrase is present in high levels in the lungs. It catalyses H_3CO_3 (which can be considered H^+ buffered by HCO_3^-) to H_2O and CO_2, thus the CO_2 can be 'blown off' (or expired).

Also, as previously mentioned, H^+ can be excreted by the kidneys, hence renal excretion. In the collecting duct portion of the nephron, H^+ ions are exchanged for Na^+ and/or K^+ ions, i.e. H^+ is excreted in the urine, and Na^+ and/or K^+ are reabsorbed from the filtrate back into the circulation.

Abnormalities of hydrogen ion levels

Acidosis

Two different types of acidosis occur in the clinical setting:

◆ Volatile (respiratory) acidosis. This is insufficient excretion of CO_2 by the lungs due to hypoventilation:
  • breathing too slowly (low minute-volume, e.g. opiate overdose, or exhaustion);
  • ventilation-perfusion mismatch, e.g. PE results in a localised area of hypoperfusion of the lung even though it is still being ventilated, or pulmonary oedema in which case the lung is still being well perfused but the presence of fluid in the airways increases the distance across which [O] and [CO_2] must diffuse, thus causing a relative decrease in ventilation;
  • insufficient excretion of CO_2 means CO_2 builds up in the circulation, and as per the Henderson-Hasselbach equation, CO_2 is equivalent to H^+, thus an acidosis ensues.
◆ Non-volatile (metabolic) acidosis. Due to renal failure the kidneys are unable to excrete H^+ ions from the circulation, thus they build up, and an acidosis ensues.

Alkalosis

As for acidosis, there are two types of alkalosis in the clinical setting:

◆ Volatile (respiratory) alkalosis. Hyperventilation (breathing too fast, high minute-volume) effectively 'blows off' more CO_2 than is the norm. This results in low circulating concentrations of CO_2, and, as per the Henderson-Hasselbach equation, CO_2 is equivalent to H^+, thus low circulating levels of H^+ ensue. This is an alkalosis.

- Non-volatile (metabolic) alkalosis. This is rare in the clinical setting. Causes include the following specific instances:
  - H^+ loss, e.g. GI (vomiting) or from urine acidosis (diuretics, Conn's);
  - HCO_3^- gain, e.g. dietary or iatrogenic (over-treating acidosis).

Management of acute renal failure

Oliguric patient

- Check if the catheter is blocked; if so, change it.
- Check for signs of hypovolaemia; if so, rehydrate.

Note

- Hypovolaemia signs are tachycardia, cold peripheries, hypotension, low CVP. Measure urine osmolality - if it is double plasma osmolality this is not renal failure. However, if it is iso-osmolar with plasma this could be renal failure (the ability to concentrate urine means the kidneys are working).

Management
- Dopamine may improve renal perfusion without fluid overloading.
- Restrict fluid intake.
- Monitor K^+ level carefully.
- If K^+ is >6, the patient needs insulin and dextrose, and may require dialysis. This is not a decision you are qualified to make, so call a nephrologist.

Dialysis

This replaces the excretory function of kidneys in patients with acute or chronic renal failure.

Note

- Dialysis only achieves approximately 10% of normal renal function.
- Dialysis has no endocrine function (unlike the normal kidney).

Dialysis is based on two principles:

- Diffusion. Urea and creatinine are in a high concentration in blood, and low in dialysate, therefore, they are excreted. Bicarbonate and calcium are low in concentration in blood but high in dialysate, therefore they are absorbed.
- Ultrafiltration. Relies on hydrostatic or osmotic gradients to force fluid from blood into the ultrafiltrate.

Haemodialysis machines can vary the pressure using a blood pump, but in peritoneal dialysis the heart is the pump responsible for the difference in pressure between vascular and peritoneal compartments.

Note

- High glucose concentration in the dialysate results in a high osmotic pressure and hence increases ultrafiltration.

Vascular access

AV shunt
A prosthetic which is susceptible to infection, and restricts bathing and swimming for the patient.

AV fistula
This is a side-to-side anastomosis between the artery and vein in the forearm. There is a less infective risk, and the patient can bathe and swim. However, it can result in steal syndrome in the hand, cause an aneurysm and, rarely, can cause heart failure.

The principle of an arteriovenous fistula is to expose vein to arterial BP to distend the vein, which then arterialises. It is therefore easier to cannulate with large-bore needles (faster dialysis) and is less susceptible to thrombosis.

Peritoneal dialysis

A catheter (Tenkhoff) is placed between the symphysis pubis and the umbilicus (through skin into the abdominal cavity). The dialysate must be changed every four hours. It is advantageous because the patient can be more independent and it provides continuous dialysis for improved fluid balance.

Complications include catheter blockage, tract infection, peritonitis and retroperitoneal fibrosis. It is also an expensive treatment.

Haemofiltration

Useful in the ITU setting, it passes blood through an ultrafilter, and can also put a dialysis solution around the ultrafiltrate. This is usually performed with a central line.

Note

–   Haemofiltration is veno-venous haemofiltration.
–   As there is no endocrine function in the dialysis machine for patients in chronic renal failure, erythropoietin is needed to prevent chronic anaemia, and also phosphate binders, vitamin D, and 1,25 dihydroxy-cholecalciferol are needed to prevent renal osteodystrophy (osteoporosis, osteomalacia, and hyper-parathyroidism).
–   Because beta-2-microglobulin is poorly excreted in dialysis, there is the eventual risk of amyloidosis.
–   There is an eventual risk of acquired multicystic kidney disease on dialysis, which may lead to haemorrhage and occasionally malignancy.

GASTROINTESTINAL PHYSIOLOGY

GI tract histology

Development

The GI tract originates from a simple tube of endoderm initially closed by an oropharyngeal membrane and cloacal membrane. Both disintegrate in early development.

Wall structure (from luminal surface to deep)

◆   Epithelium.
◆   Lamina propria.
◆   Muscularis mucosa.
◆   Submucosa.
◆   Muscularis externa (circular smooth muscle and longitudinal smooth muscle).
◆   Serosa (in abdominal cavity), adventitia (outside abdominal cavity).

Mucosa

The epithelium is non-keratinised, stratified and squamous in the mouth, oesophagus and anal canal (for protection and transport, not for absorption).

Simple cuboidal mucosa exists in the stomach and small intestine (for absorption and secretion).

Lamina propria

This is connective tissue containing many blood and lymphatic vessels. It also contains scattered lymphatic nodules and mucosa-associated lymphoid tissue (MALT). These may be arranged in patches (Peyer's patches).

Muscularis mucosa

This is connective tissue, highly vascularised containing some lymphatics and glands. It also contains Meissner's plexus (a submucosal plexus of the autonomic nervous system) innervating the muscularis mucosa and blood vessels and secretory cells of the mucosal glands.

Muscularis externa

This is mainly skeletal muscle found in the mouth, pharynx, upper third of the oesophagus and the external anal sphincter. The rest is smooth muscle (inner circular and outer longitudinal), containing the Auerbach's plexus (also known as the myenteric plexus), which provides motor and secretomotor innervation to the muscle and lining glands.

Serosa

A superficial layer of connective tissue and simple squamous epithelium.

Gastric function

Acid secretion is an active process using the hydrogen-potassium ATPase pump (proton-pump) (Figure 2.9).

The varying stomach cell types and their functions as well as hormonal action are tabulated below.

Stomach cell types.

Chief cells (zymogenic)	Secrete pepsinogen	Pepsin (activated form) breaks certain peptide bonds in proteins
	Secrete gastric lipase	Splits short-chain triglycerides into fatty acids and monoglycerides
Parietal cells (oxyntic)	Secrete HCl	Kills microbes in food Denatures protein Converts pepsinogen to pepsin Inhibits gastrin secretion Stimulates CCK and secretin secretion
	Secrete intrinsic factor	Needed for absorption of Vit B12 (required for erythropoiesis)
Mucous cells	Secrete mucus	Forms protective barrier that prevents autodigestion of stomach wall
Entero-endocrine cells	Secrete gastrin	Stimulates parietal cells to secrete HCl
G-cells		Stimulates chief cells to secrete pepsinogen Contracts oesophageal sphincter Increases motility of stomach Relaxes pyloric sphincter

Hormonal control of digestion.

Hormone	Site of secretion and stimulus	Action
Gastrin	Entero-endocrine cells Distension of stomach Partially digested protein Alkaline pH	Increase H$^+$ Increase pepsin Constricts lower oesophageal sphincter Relaxes pyloric and ileocaecal sphincter
Gastro-inhibitory peptide	Entero-endocrine cells in small intestine Fatty acids in small intestine	Release of insulin by pancreatic B cells Inhibits H$^+$ and pepsin Slows gastric emptying
Secretin	Entero-endocrine cells in small intestine Acidic pH in small intestine	Stimulates secretion of pancreatic juice Stimulates secretion of bile
CCK	Entero-endocrine cells in small intestine Amino acids in small intestine Fatty acids in small intestine	Stimulates secretion of pancreatic juice Ejection of bile from liver Opens sphincter of Oddi Induces satiety

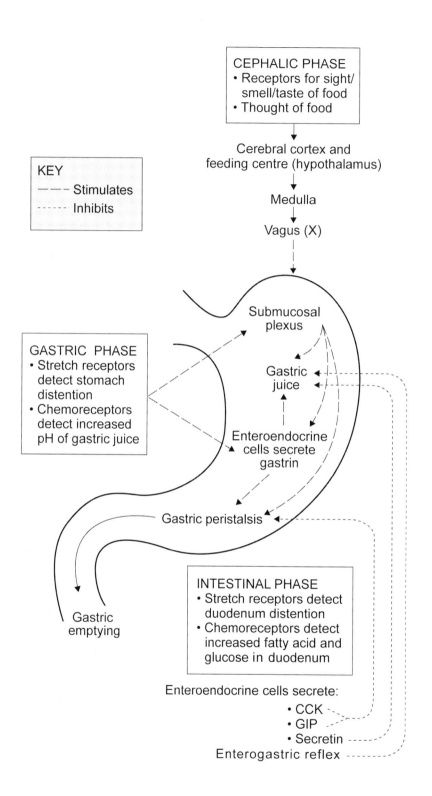

Figure 2.9. Phases of gastric acid secretion. CCK = cholecystokinin; GIP = gastro-inhibitory peptide.

Pancreas

Exocrine function

The pancreas is 99% composed of cells in clusters (acini), which excrete pancreatic juice.

Endocrine function

◆ 1% is organised into Islets of Langerhans.
◆ Secretes glucagon, from the alpha cells, stimulating the liver to release glucose from glycogen stores by glycogenolysis and gluconeogenesis. It is therefore catabolic.
◆ Secretes insulin from beta cells, stimulating glycogen synthesis in the liver (reducing blood glucose levels). Stimulates fatty acid stimulation and inhibits proteolysis and lipolysis. Inhibits gluconeogenesis in the liver and is therefore anabolic.
◆ Secretes somatostatin from delta cells, which is an inhibitory hormone that inhibits growth hormone, thyroid stimulating hormone (TSH) and gastric hormones (gastrin, CCK, secretin, motilin, GIP). It also inhibits gastric emptying, insulin and glucagon synthesis, as well as the exocrine functions of the pancreas.
◆ Secretes pancreatic polypeptide from P cells, which inhibits CCK and stimulates gastric secretions.

Pancreatic juice

Pancreatic juice is made up of various different constituents that have the following functions:

◆ Water.
◆ Salts.
◆ Sodium bicarbonate (alkaline buffer).
◆ Several enzymes:
  ● pancreatic amylase (breaks down starch);
  ● procarboxypeptidase → (trypsin) → carboxypeptidase (a proteolytic enzyme);
  ● chymotrypsinogen → (trypsin) → chymotrypsin (a proteolytic enzyme);
  ● proelastase → (trypsin) → elastase;
  ● pancreatic lipase (a proteolytic enzyme);
  ● ribonucleases and deoxyribonuclease (break down RNA and DNA, respectively).

Liver

Functions

◆ Carbohydrate metabolism - maintains blood glucose level by glycogenolysis, gluconeogenesis and lipogenesis.
◆ Lipid metabolism - stores some triglycerides:
  ● beta oxidation (fatty acids → acetyl CoA);
  ● ketogenesis (excess acetyl CoA → ketone bodies);
  ● synthesis of lipoproteins;
  ● cholesterol synthesis by hepatocytes (used to make bile salts).
◆ Protein metabolism - synthesis of plasma proteins including globulins, albumin, clotting factors:
  ● transamination (transfer of amino groups);
  ● deamination (removal of NH_2 from amino acids for use in ATP production);
  ● conversion of toxic NH_3 to urea.
◆ Removal of drugs and hormones.
◆ Excretion of bilirubin.
◆ Synthesis of bile salts.
◆ Storage:
  ● glycogen;
  ● vitamins (A, B12, D, E, K);
  ● minerals (iron, copper);
  ● iron (as ferritin = iron and apoferrin).
◆ Phagocytosis - Kupffer's cells phagocytose worn out red and white blood cells, and some bacteria.
◆ Activation of vitamin D - skin, liver and kidneys all participate in this.

Enterohepatic circulation of bile

The reticulo-endothelial system breaks down red blood cells into haem groups which are then reduced to bilirubin and carried in the blood stream bound to albumin as unconjugated bilirubin. It is then carried to the liver where it is conjugated with glucuronic acid into the water-soluble molecule, diglucuronide. This is excreted in bile and is subsequently reduced by intestinal bacteria in the colon to urobilinogen and stercobilin (gives stool its characteristic brown pigment). A small amount of both is reabsorbed by the colon and is either recycled by the liver or enters the systemic circulation as urobilinogen (a colourless compound which can then be excreted into the urine).

Haemolysis

Haemolysis results in:

- Increased unconjugated bilirubin.
- Jaundice without bilirubin in the urine as the unconjugated bilirubin bound to albumin in the blood is too large to be filtered by the kidney.
- Increased urobilinogen.
- Increased stercobilin.

Obstructive jaundice

Obstructive jaundice is caused by a blockage of the drainage of bile in the biliary system (for example, by gallstones). It results in:

- Increased conjugated bilirubin which is obstructed from being excreted into the intestine.
- Increased bilirubin in the urine.
- Decreased stercobilin in the stool.

Jaundice

Jaundice can be defined as yellow pigmentation of the skin, sclerae and mucosae due to a plasma bilirubin >35mmol/L.

Haemoglobin breakdown pathway

Haemoglobin is broken down to bilirubin. The addition of glucuronic acid to bilirubin (called conjugation, occurring in the liver) produces conjugated bilirubin. Some of the conjugated bilirubin is excreted (in bile) into the gut; the rest circulates in blood and is excreted renally. Bacteria in the gut reduce conjugated bilirubin to urobilinogen, and then to stercobilinogen, which is then lost in the stool.

Hyperbilirubinaemia (jaundice) can be classified as:

- Conjugated/unconjugated hyperbilirubinaemia.
- Pre-hepatic/hepatic (hepatocellular)/post-hepatic (cholestatic/obstructive).

Pre-hepatic jaundice (or unconjugated hyperbilirubinaemia)

This is unconjugated bilirubin which is not water-soluble and is therefore not excreted in the urine. In Gilbert's syndrome, there are high levels of unconjugated bilirubin normally found on blood testing, but it is usually asymptomatic. The levels rise during fasting or during mild illness. Dubin-Johnson syndrome and Rotor's syndrome also involve high levels of unconjugated bilirubin.

With this disorder, the patient is jaundiced, but has no pale stools as the biliary circulation is unaffected (allowing some conjugated bilirubin, as the liver is still capable of conjugating a proportion of the excess bilirubin, to enter the bowel lumen) and no dark urine, as the lion's share of the bilirubin in the circulation is unconjugated (hence non-water-soluble) and thus unable to be filtered by the kidney into the urine. Remember, urobilinogen is one of the pigments responsible for darkening urine.

Post-hepatic (or obstructive/cholestatic) jaundice

Cholestatic jaundice causes jaundice with pale stools and dark urine as the serum bilirubin is conjugated (water-soluble and hence can be filtered by the kidney into the urine), but cannot enter the bowel lumen as the biliary circulation is by definition obstructed in the following ways:

- Intrahepatic: swelling/oedema of hepatocytes in parenchymal liver damage (hepatocellular).
- Extrahepatic: large duct obstruction at any point in the biliary tract distal to the bile canaliculi.

Causes

Pre-hepatic (haemolysis)
Ineffective erythropoiesis, Gilbert's syndrome, sickle cell anaemia, Dubin Johnson syndrome and Rotor's syndrome.

Hepatic (hepatocellular)
Virus (hepatitis A, B, C, E and Epstein-Barr Virus), leptospirosis (Weil's disease), and chronic liver disease.

Post-hepatic (cholestatic)
Can be intrahepatic (e.g. primary biliary cirrhosis, cholangitis, cholangiocarcinoma) or extrahepatic (e.g. gallstones, carcinoma compressing the bile duct, carcinoma of the head of the pancreas, or a peri-ampullary tumour).

Note

- Look out for the slightly strange concept of intra- and extrahepatic causes of post-hepatic causes of jaundice. The post-hepatic refers to the fact the liver has finished its actions upon the bilirubin (in this context, conjugation). The intrahepatic refers to the fact that the cause of cholestasis (blockage to bile flow) is located within the liver itself.

Tests

- Urine for bilirubin and urobilinogen.
- Blood for liver function tests (LFTs), gamma glutamyl transpeptidase (GammaGT), bilirubin, prothrombin time, serum albumin, FBC, urea and electrolytes (U&Es), creatinine, glucose, EBV and CMV serology, and hep A, B and C.
- Liver ultrasound scanning (USS) (shows whether the bile ducts are dilated, hence cholestasis).
- Endoscopic retrograde cholangiopancreatography (ERCP) or percutaneous transhepatic cholangiography (PTC).
- CT (a CT cholangiogram is a less common investigation).

If the bile ducts are not dilated then a liver biopsy should be performed.

Volumes of GI secretions

This is a useful series of values to have at your disposal, as it occasionally comes up as a question, which is often followed with further questions relating to GI physiology.

- Gastric - 2000ml/day.
- Saliva - 1500ml/day.
- Pancreatic - 1500ml/day.
- Small intestine -1500ml/day.
- Bile - 500ml/day.
- Small bowel reabsorbs - 8500ml/day.
- Large bowel reabsorbs - 400ml/day.

ENDOCRINE PHYSIOLOGY

Regulation of hormone secretion

As a general rule hormone secretion from glands can be stimulated or inhibited by:

- Nerve impulses.
- Chemical changes in blood.
- Other hormones (levels in blood).

Hypothalamus

This is a small region of the brain which is the main link between the nervous and endocrine system. It receives input from the higher centres of the brain and sensory signals from the organs. It controls the autonomic nervous system (ANS) and is an important endocrine gland. The anterior lobe of the pituitary gland's secretions are controlled by hypothalamic hormones released by neurosecretory cells. There are five releasing hormones and two inhibitory hormones.

- Growth hormone releasing hormone (GHRH) - stimulates release of human growth hormone (hGH).
- Growth hormone inhibitory hormone (GHIH) - inhibits release of hGH.
- Thyrotrophin releasing hormone (TRH) - stimulates secretion of thyroid stimulating hormone (TSH), also known as thyrotropin, and hGH.
- Gonadotrophin releasing hormone (GnRH) - stimulates release of gonadotrophins, luteinising hormone (LH) and follicular stimulating hormone (FSH).
- Prolactin releasing hormone (PRH) - stimulates secretion of prolactin.
- Prolactin inhibiting hormone (PIH) - inhibits secretion of prolactin.
- Corticotrophin releasing hormone (CRH) - stimulates secretion of adrenocorticotrophic hormone (ACTH), also known as corticotrophin, and melanocyte stimulating hormone (MSH).

Pituitary

A pea-sized gland beneath the hypothalamus which is divided into the anterior pituitary (adenohypophysis) and posterior pituitary (neurohypophysis).

Anterior pituitary

The anterior pituitary is derived from an infolding of the ectoderm from the mouth (Rathke's pouch). Release of anterior pituitary hormones is stimulated by hypothalamic-releasing factors and suppressed by inhibitory factors.

The pituitary gland is made up of five different cell types that are responsible for the synthesis of seven different hormones in all:

♦ Somatotrophs - somatotropin (human growth hormone [hGH]).
♦ Thyrotrophs - thyrotropin (TSH).
♦ Gonadotrophs - FSH and LH.
♦ Lactotrophs - prolactin.
♦ Corticotrophs - corticotropin (ACTH) and melanocyte stimulating hormone (MSH).

hGH

This is the most abundant anterior pituitary hormone, which causes body cells to grow and regulates metabolism by:

♦ Increased protein synthesis.
♦ Decreased protein breakdown.
♦ Increased lypolysis.
♦ Slowing down the use of glucose for ATP production.

TSH

Stimulates secretion of T3 (tri-iodothyronine) and T4 (thyroxine).

FSH

Female

Initiates development of follicles in the ovaries and stimulates the follicles to produce oestrogens.

Male

Initiates spermatogenesis.

LH

Female

Stimulates ovulation, corpus luteum formation, and progesterone (together with FSH).

Male

Stimulates interstitial cells to produce testosterone.

Prolactin

Female

Initiates and maintains milk secretion by the mammaries (together with other hormones).

Male

Function unknown but hypersecretion leads to impotence.

ACTH

Controls synthesis and secretion of glucocorticoids from the adrenal cortex.

MSH

Melanocyte stimulating hormone (function not fully understood).

Posterior pituitary

The posterior pituitary does not synthesise hormones but it does store and release two hormones. They are stored in the cells of neurosecretory cells and travel to axon terminals by fast axonal transport.

Oxytocin

Pregnant female

Uterine contraction and milk ejection. Function in non-pregnant females and males is unknown.

Antidiuretic hormone (ADH)

Retains body water by decreased sweating and increased water reabsorption by the kidneys. At high concentrations it causes vasoconstriction (hence the old name - vasopressin).

Thyroid physiology

Under the action of TSH the follicular cells of the thyroid gland produce T4 and T3. The parafollicular cells produce calcitonin.

The thyroid gland is the only gland that stores its secretory product in a large quantity (approximately 100 days supply).

Thyroid hormones are produced by attaching iodine atoms to tyrosine.

Iodide trapping

Iodine is transported to the follicular cells, which is an active process as the concentration of iodine inside the cells is 20-40 times that of blood.

Thyroglobulin synthesis
- Oxidation of iodide. Iodide ions combine to form iodine (I2).
- Iodination of tyrosine. I2 binds to tyrosine producing either T1 or T2.
- Coupling of T1/T2, producing either T3 or T4.
- Secretion of thyroid hormones. T3 and T4 are lipid-soluble, therefore they can diffuse through the plasma membrane into the blood.
- Transport in the blood. Thyroid hormones are usually carried in blood bound to thyroid-binding globulins.

T4 is secreted in a greater quantity than T3 (but T3 is more potent). T4 circulates in the blood and enters cells as T4 but is converted into T3 within the cell.

The main functions of thyroid hormones are the regulation of:

- Oxygen use and basal metabolic rate.
- Cellular metabolism.
- Growth and development.

Calcitonin
Calcitonin acts in conjunction with parathyroid hormone and calcitriol to maintain calcium homeostasis. It exerts its effect by decreasing the concentration of calcium ions in the blood, as well as decreasing the concentration of phosphate ions.

Parathyroid physiology

Parathormone is secreted by the principal (chief) cells of the parathyroid gland. It acts to increase both the number and activity of osteoclasts. It also increases the rate at which the kidneys reabsorb calcium and magnesium ions, and inhibits the reabsorption of phosphate ions by the kidneys. It also promotes the formation of calcitriol (synthesised from vitamin D), which increases the absorption of calcium, phosphate and magnesium ions from the gut.

Adrenal physiology

The adrenal gland (suprarenal) is composed of an innermost medulla and an outer cortex which comprises three layers: the outermost zona glomerulosa, the zona fasciculata, and the zona reticularis.

Cortex

Zona glomerulosa
The main secretions are the mineralocorticoids which control water and electrolyte balance. Although there are several types of mineralocorticoid, over 95% of their action is due to aldosterone.

Aldosterone
- Increases the concentration of Na^+ in the blood (leading to an increased reabsorption of water).
- Decreases the concentration of K^+ in the blood.
- Forms part of the renin-angiotensin-aldosterone pathway.

Zona fasciculata
The main secretions are glucocorticoids which regulate metabolism and resistance to stress. Again there are several types, but over 95% of their activity is due to cortisol (hydrocortisone).

Cortisol
- Increases protein breakdown (except in the liver).
- Stimulates gluconeogenesis and lipolysis.
- Has an anti-inflammatory effect.
- Can depress the immune system in high doses.

Zona reticularis
The main secretions are androgens, male sex hormones that exert masculinising effects. The major androgen secreted by the adrenal gland is dihydroepiandrosterone (DHEA).

Adrenal medulla

The medulla consists of chromaffin cells which surround blood vessels. These cells receive direct innervation from preganglionic neurones of the sympathetic nervous system. Chromaffin cells are therefore neuroendocrine post-ganglionic cells that secrete noradrenaline (norepinephrine) and adrenaline (epinephrine). Therefore, hormone release in this way is very rapid. The main types of hormone released are the catecholamines, adrenaline and noradrenaline.

Both these hormones are sympathomimetic and are responsible for the fight/flight response:

- Increase heart rate and contractility.
- Cause vasoconstriction.
- Increase blood pressure (as a result of the previous two effects).
- Dilate the airways.
- Decrease digestion.
- Increase blood glucose.
- Stimulate cellular metabolism.

Calcium metabolism

99% of body calcium (Ca^{2+}) is in the form of hydroxyapatite in bone.

Calcium is vitally important for:

- Cell membrane stability.
- Nerve conduction.
- Muscle contraction.
- Enzyme and hormone activation.
- Blood coagulation.
- Bone mineral deposition.
- Milk synthesis.

Note

- The above is an important list to remember as it often comes up as an exam question.

Fifty percent of circulating Ca^{2+} is bound to protein (80-90% to albumin, 10% to globulins). Osteo**c**lasts (**c**hew bone to) increase Ca^{2+} in plasma. Osteo**b**lasts (**b**uild bone to) decrease Ca^{2+} in plasma.

Parathyroid hormone (PTH) is secreted by the parathyroid gland, which stimulates osteoclast activity to raise plasma Ca^{2+}, and also acts on the kidney to increase Ca^{2+} reabsorption (and PO_4 secretion), thus increasing plasma Ca^{2+}. PTH is subject to negative feedback control, i.e. a high Ca^{2+} in plasma causes decreased PTH secretion and vice versa.

Vitamin D is ingested in the diet and synthesised by the skin in response to sunlight. It is subject to numerous hydroxylation reactions in the liver which activate it to vitamin D3. D3 is cholecalciferol. The first hydroxylation reaction takes place in the liver (25,OH D3); the second in the kidney (1,25, OH D3). In bone this acts to increase osteoclast activity, causing bone resorption, hence increased [Ca]. In the gut it promotes increased absorption of Ca, hence increased [Ca]. Its actions are parallel to those of PTH which also increase dietary absorption of Ca^{2+}.

Calcitonin is secreted by the C cells of the thyroid gland in response to a high plasma Ca^{2+}. It acts to reduce plasma Ca^{2+} by its action on osteoclasts (which it inhibits). However, the effect of calcitonin is by far weaker than that of PTH in calcium homeostasis.

Therefore, Ca^{2+} levels depend on dietary intake, PTH, vitamin D, calcitonin, bone reabsorption and formation, renal excretion and reabsorption, GIT absorption, sunlight, liver function and renal function.

GENERAL PHYSIOLOGY TOPICS

Nociception

Nociception is detection of a noxious stimulus.

Pathophysiology

The following definitions apply to already damaged tissue.

Allodynia
Pressure causing pain at a lower threshold than it otherwise would.

Primary hyperalgesia

Pain as a result of pressure is more intense than it otherwise would have been.

Hyperpathia

Pain lasts longer than the stimulus would normally have caused.

Secondary hyperalgesia

Pain at an adjacent site in response to pressure where there would otherwise have been none.

Normal nociception and the main components

Nociception occurs in the following series of steps:

- Transduction. Translates damage into a signal in nociceptive fibres.
- Transmission. Carries impulse along A-delta (fast) and C-fibres (slow) to the spinal cord dorsal column, and thence on to the pain centre in the thalamus.
- Modulation. Gate theory of pain modulation. A-delta and C-fibres bring nociceptive information to the spinal cord at this level. This signal can be inhibited by A-beta fibres which are activated peripherally (e.g. by rubbing the affected part of the limb), thus, inhibiting some of the nociceptive information before it reaches (is perceived by) the brain.
- Perception. Signal reaches brain and is 'felt'.

Note

- NSAIDs block cyclo-oxygenase which normally catalyses the formation of prostacyclins, prostaglandins and thromboxane A2 (these chemicals sensitise inflamed tissue to pain, thus their inhibition reduces this effect).

Pain

Pain is defined as an unpleasant sensory or emotional experience associated with actual or potential tissue damage.

Classification

Classification can be done by 'timing': acute or chronic (defined as pain which persists after all possible healing of any injury has occurred and long after pain could serve any useful or protective functions), or by 'origin':

- Nociceptive - representing tissue damage.
- Neuropathic - representing nerve damage.
- Psychogenic - which is predominantly psychological.

Principles of pain management

- Placebo response (can account for as much as 30% of response).
- Remove cause.
- Prevent initial excitation of nociceptors (ice packs, anti-inflammatories).
- Interrupt peripheral nociceptive transmission (local anaesthetic [LA] nerve block).
- Alter spinal modulation of nociceptive transmission (TENS, acupuncture, opiates).
- Interrupt spinal cord nociceptive transmission (cut spinothalamic tract).
- Alter central processing of nociceptive information (opiates and nitrous oxide).
- Alter emotional response to pain (psychiatric strategies and antidepressants).
- Alter behavioural response to pain.

Analgesic ladder

A graduated system of administration of analgesics of increasing clinical efficacy is known as the analgesic ladder:

- Step one - non-opioid, e.g. paracetamol or aspirin.
- Step two - weak opioid, e.g. cocodamol, codydramol, codeine.
- Step three - strong opioid, e.g. morphine, diamorphine.

Non-steroidal anti-inflammatory drugs (NSAIDs) can be added at any step as can adjuvant analgesics. Adjuvant analgesics are drugs which contribute to pain relief in certain situations without being classic analgesics.

Opioids are less effective at controlling neuropathic pain so the following drugs can help, e.g. amitriptyline, gabapentin and carbamazepine.

Local anaesthetics

'Ana' means no and 'aesthesia' means sensation; thus, no sensation in a local area.

Local anaesthetics work by the membrane-stabilising effect of blocking sodium (Na^+) channels in all nerves, which prevents action potential (AP) progression. It is important to realise that the smaller the nerve the faster the effect, e.g. 'A' fibres for pain, i.e. pain is rapidly blocked, leaving the larger fibres relatively unaffected such that pressure and touch can still be felt.

The pKa concept

It is important to understand that the pKa is the pH at which a local anaesthetic (LA) is exactly 50% dissociated.

Dissociated means present in its ionic form, i.e.
(H^+) + (Base-) = (H)(Base)
Dissociated   Undissociated

The relevance of this concept is that only an undissociated base can penetrate the nerve to have its clinical effect.

The nerve fibre cell wall is a phospholipid bi-layer, thus repelling ions, i.e. a dissociated base. The Na^+ channel is located inside this layer. It is at this point that the LA blocks the channel.

However, it is only as a dissociated base that the LA is able to block the channel, i.e. it crosses the nerve cell wall undissociated, then it dissociates and blocks the Na^+ channel.

Relevance of sodium channels in action potentials

Remember that cells capable of action potentials have a negative resting potential. It is the influx of positively charged Na^+ ions into the nerve cell that raises the potential from negative to positive. This is the action potential. It is by this mechanism that information (e.g. pain information) is transmitted along nerves.

Block the Na^+ channel and you block the action potential; thus, you block the transmission of information along that nerve. In the case of small diameter 'A' pain fibres, you thus block pain.

Duration of action of LA agents

Two factors are of major importance in determining the duration of action of LAs:

♦   Re-association of the LA molecule.
♦   Clearance of the LA molecule from the nerve fibre.

Another important concept at this point is that bases become highly dissociated at acid pHs. Lignocaine, for example, is stored at a pH of 6.8, i.e. an acidic pH. Thus, lignocaine is highly dissociated.

When lignocaine is injected into human tissue (pH ~7.4), it becomes more undissociated, i.e. more readily travels across the nerve membrane. Then, as some of it dissociates (in the relatively more acidic environment of the nerve) it blocks the Na^+ channels, resulting in its anaesthetic effect.

Note

–   An important exception to know about LA function is that of infected tissue; infected tissue is highly acidic. Thus, it prevents dissociation, and hence the ability of the LA molecule to travel across the nerve membrane (this is especially true of abscess cavities).

Addition of adrenaline to local anaesthetic agents

The use of adrenaline and LA mixtures is common in practice. This helps to reduce bleeding, e.g. suturing of scalp wounds which have a tendency to bleed. Adrenaline has this effect by causing contraction of vascular smooth muscle. This is particularly relevant to end arteries, e.g. in the digits, and therefore should not be used here due to the risk of resulting ischaemia (and hence gangrene).

But this is not the only function of adrenaline. The duration of action of LAs is dependent upon the speed of clearance of the LA molecule from its active position in the nerve fibre. By reducing the clearance (which takes place in the blood), adrenaline thus prolongs the duration of action of LAs.

It also effectively doubles the safe amount of LA that can be administered to a patient due to its reduction of vascular clearance time, and hence concentration of LA absorbed into a given volume of blood. It is this concentration, which, if it rises above a certain threshold, is responsible for the side effects of LAs.

Side effects of local anaesthetics

These side effects only occur if LA is accidentally given as an IV, or an overdose given. In both circumstances it is evident that LA is present in the vascular compartment in high concentration.

The vascularity of the site of injection determines the amount of LA possible to inject without rising to intravascular toxic doses, i.e. the greater the vascularity of the tissue, the greater the absorption of LA from the injection site into the vascular compartment, thus the greater the intravascular concentration, and the greater the chance of side effects. Obviously the converse is also true, e.g. the buttock is not particularly vascular, whereas the scalp is.

Side effects occur in a very specific order, as follows:

- Metallic taste in mouth.
- Tinnitis.
- Circum-oral paraesthesiae.
- Slurred speech.
- Agitation.
- Convulsions.
- Cardiac arrhythmias.
- Cardiovascular collapse.

Note

— Hypoxia and hypercarbia increase the likelihood of serious side effects, and, therefore, they must be prevented, i.e. give O_2 via a mask, maintain BP with IV fluids, and apply a cardiac monitor to look for dysrhythmias.

Clearly the cardiac side effects are the most serious, and potentially life-threatening. These occur as a result of the same membrane-stabilising effect (i.e. AP prevention) that LAs have on sensory nerves, but this time it is in cardiac myocytes.

Methaemoglobinaemia

Prilocaine is a special case amongst local anaesthetics in that it has no cardiac side effects in overdose. Thus, it is useful in Bier's blocks, i.e. when the tourniquet is released and, potentially LA is released into the circulating volume. Prilocaine does not affect the myocardium, whereas other LA agents do to varying extents.

However, in overdose (OD), prilocaine causes methaemoglobinaemia. This means that the Hb molecule undergoes a conformational change that detrimentally affects its ability to bind its usual four molecules of O_2. Thus, O_2 transport is reduced, and cyanosis characteristically ensues.

Fortunately methaemoglobinaemia is reversible, using methylene blue administered intravenously. A simple way of remembering this is that in methaemoglobinaemia the patient becomes cyanotic, i.e. goes blue. Administration of another blue dye, methylene blue, renders the patient pink again.

EMLA

A eutectic mixture of local anaesthetics (EMLA) is a mixture of 80% LA (lignocaine and prilocaine) in a lipid medium. EMLA is used as a topical local anaesthetic. It is placed on the region of skin you wish to anaesthetise under an impermeable dressing, and is left in place for approximately 20 minutes. Minor operative procedures can be carried out by this means, e.g. excision of a skin lesion. The most popular use of EMLA is as a 'magic cream' in paediatrics at sites of intended venepuncture or cannula insertion.

Maximum doses of local anaesthetic

As has already been alluded to in the section on side effects of LAs, the maximum dose before which toxic intravascular levels are reached is dependent upon the vascularity of the tissue into which it has been injected. The greater the vascularity, the greater the rate the LA is cleared into the vascular compartment, and hence the greater its intravascular concentration.

It is expected that clinicians should have a general idea of the maximum volumes of LA that can be administered. Thus, it is important to remember the following:

- 1% lignocaine maximum dose = 20ml or 200mg (with adrenaline 50ml or 500mg).
- 2% lignocaine maximum dose = 10ml or 200mg (with adrenaline 25ml or 250mg).
- Prilocaine maximum dose = 400mg (with adrenaline 600mg).
- Bupivacaine (also known as marcaine) maximum dose = 150mg (with adrenaline 200mg).

The unit that is seen on the LA bottles in the UK is a percentage. This is intended to represent grams (gm) per millilitre (ml), i.e. gm/ml. Thus, it does not represent a true percentage. This can actually cause some confusion, but so long as it is remembered that it is gm/ml this can be converted to a percentage and the correct amount of LA given.

Examples of specific uses of LAs

Ring block (Figure 2.10)
This is the injection of local anaesthetic agent into the lateral bases of digits (fingers, thumbs or toes) as a form of nerve block (digital nerves are located laterally and slightly volar/palmar/plantar). The result is anaesthesia in the length of the digit. One can choose, or not, to use a small tourniquet for a bloodless field. Adrenaline should be avoided in digits

as there are end arteries, and digital gangrene can occur if blood supply is compromised.

Haematoma block (Figure 2.10)
This is injection of local anaesthetic agent into a haematoma for analgesic purposes. The most common use of this procedure in clinical practice is for the manipulation of distal radial fractures. Using the X-ray as a guide, one feels the ridge formed by the fracture on the dorsum of the wrist, passes the needle across the skin obliquely into the fracture site waiting for a flush-back of haematoma-blood before injecting lignocaine alone (or mixed 50:50 with marcaine, for prolonged analgesia post-manipulation).

Bier's block
This is achieved by placing a cannula in a vein in the distal portion of a limb, applying a tourniquet proximally in a limb and inflating it. A calculated dose of LA agent (calculation based on weight) is injected intravenously. The preferred agent is prilocaine due to its lack of cardiotoxic effects. (N.B. There is a potential for methaemoglobinaemia). Wait for adequate analgesia before performing any intended manoeuvre. The cuff should be deflated only after 30 minutes post-injection (and no earlier) to prevent a high dose of anaesthetic agent flooding into the systemic circulation.

General anaesthesia

General anaesthesia (GA), as the name implies, does not act locally (as for LAs), but its effect is intended to encompass the entire body. Remember 'ana' means no and 'aesthesia' means sensation.

In fact, the aims of GA are slightly more complex than this, but they can be summarised with simplicity as follows:

- Unconsciousness.
- Analgesia ('ana' = no, and 'algesia' = pain, a slightly different concept to anaesthesia).
- Muscle relaxation.

For the surgeon, the following concepts are the most important relating to GA. To go too deeply into the pharmacology here is beyond the remit of this book.

Ring block

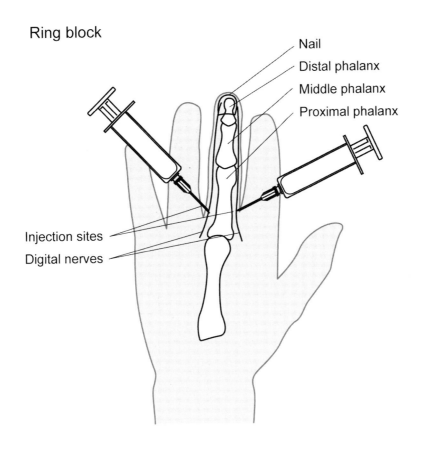

Nail
Distal phalanx
Middle phalanx
Proximal phalanx

Injection sites
Digital nerves

Haematoma block (lateral view of wrist)

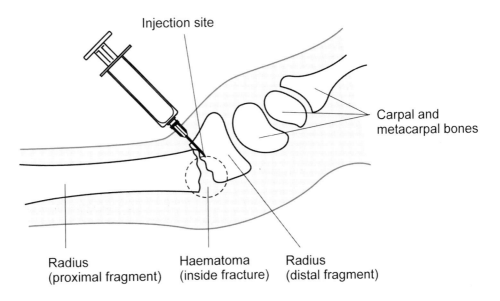

Injection site

Carpal and
metacarpal bones

Radius
(proximal fragment)

Haematoma
(inside fracture)

Radius
(distal fragment)

Figure 2.10. Local anaesthetics: ring and haematoma blocks.

Pre-assessment

This is the identification of anaesthetic risks before the patient is due for theatre.

In general, pre-assessment takes two basic forms:

◆ That performed by a member of the surgical team as an outpatient-type procedure.
◆ That performed by the anaesthetist, generally the day before, or on the morning of, surgery.

Patient factors to identify relevant to operative risks are:

◆ Diabetes is a multi-system disorder increasing both anaesthetic and post-surgical risks.
◆ Cardiac disease is a significant anaesthetic risk, especially in the case of previous myocardial infarction, hypertension (or hypotension), unstable angina, aortic stenosis, and valvular diease.
◆ Respiratory disease is a significant risk for postoperative complications, e.g. pneumonia and cough that may cause increased pain and dehiscence rates in abdominal wounds.
◆ Previous thrombotic events, e.g. DVT or PE.
◆ Immune deficiency states and postoperative wound infection risk.

Pre-medication

The two main concepts to emphasize with modern-day pre-medication are as follows:

◆ Anxiolysis ('anxio' = anxiety, and 'lysis' = to split [in this context though, it means to reduce anxiety]). Generally, benzodiazepines are used for this purpose, a common agent being lorazepam.
◆ Pain relief is commonly in the form of morphine or other opiate derivatives.

Maintenance of anaesthesia

General anaesthetic agents have complex mechanisms of action. They are thought to have the bulk of their effect centrally on GABA (gamma-aminobutyric acid) receptors, resulting in analgesia at the level of the spinal cord, and a reduced level of consciousness at the level of the brain.

Anaesthesia is maintained by mixing volatile anaesthetic agents with the inspired O_2 via the patient's endotracheal (ET) tube. The same effect (maintenance of anaesthesia) can be achieved by infusion of hypnotic agents, e.g. midazolam or propofol.

Analgesia is often given in the form of intravenous opiates during the procedure.

Muscle relaxation

Muscle relaxants come in two different forms: depolarising and non-depolarising.

Depolarising (e.g. suxamethonium)

Used only for crash induction (see later section on this subject), not for maintaining muscle relaxation during a procedure. This is because its effect only lasts 5-10 minutes. It is made up of two linked acetylcholine (ACh) molecules. It has its mechanism of action by occupying the ACh receptors on the post-synaptic membrane of the neuromuscular junction, initially activating them, i.e. causing depolarisation, hence the name. But then, remaining bound to these receptors, does not allow any further motor stimulation, hence, muscle relaxtion. This initial depolarisation results in contraction of all affected musculature, transiently, i.e. a violent shake or series of shakes, which then resolves.

Non-depolarising

Almost purely the group of muscle relaxants of choice, with the exception of crash induction mentioned above. These competitively inhibit ACh at the neuromuscular junction, thus achieving muscle relaxation.

Reversal of muscle relaxation

This is achieved by neostygmine. This is a chemical that blocks cholinesterase. Under normal circumstances, cholinesterase breaks up the ACh molecules present at the neuromuscular junction, thus reducing their number, and hence effect. One can see then, that blocking cholinesterase will result in less breakdown of ACh, more ACh present at the neuromuscular junction and thus a gradual reversal of its effects.

Pre-operative fasting

This is obviously relevant to the on-call doctor in all surgical specialties. Current advised periods of time for fasting before safe induction of general anaesthesia are:

- Food - 6 hours.
- Milk - 4 hours.
- Water - 2 hours.

It must be borne in mind that fatty acids delay gastric emptying, and hence food and milk stay in the stomach longer than water, but perhaps more important to remember is that trauma (in its many guises) also delays gastric emptying, thus increasing the above numbers.

The anaesthetist must then take a part in the decision making as to when normal intubation is safe, but this may be a source of unacceptable delay with respect to the clinical condition, e.g. an open fracture or emergency laparotomy. When anaesthesia needs to be given before the stomach can reliably be considered empty, the anaesthetist then proceeds to crash induction.

Crash induction is a manoeuvre designed to minimise the risk of aspiration of gastric products into the respiratory airways. This is a risk when there are gastric contents present and the anaesthetic agent (which has some emetic properties) is given. As consciousness level decreases, the gag reflex is lost. The combination of these three reasons results in an increased aspiration risk. The manoeuvre is cricoid pressure after induction of anaesthesia with a fast-acting, low half-life, relaxing agent (e.g. suxamethonium) and fast-acting anaesthetic agent (e.g. thiopentone) given. The cricoid pressure is maintained until successful intubation and inflation of the cuff is performed. Only at this point are the airways considered protected. The cricoid pressure is intended to push the trachea against the oesophagus, compressing it, and hence preventing passage of gastric contents.

The intention is to produce unconsciousness, analgesia and muscle relaxation.

Anaesthetic agents

- Thiopentone (barbiturate, short half-life, used in crash induction).
- Propofol (very short half-life, used in day-case surgery).
- Fentanyl (opiate).

Diathermy

Basic science

Composed of alternating current (AC) electricity. Increasing current results in increased tissue damage and neuromuscular stimulation. However, increasing the frequency combined with high currents only damages tissue (which is the intention for diathermy coagulation), and does not result in neuromuscular stimulation, i.e. activating nerves (which is not the intention).

High current and high resistance results in high current density, i.e. high heat, and hence, the cautery effect.

Different types of diathermy (Figure 2.11)

Unipolar diathermy (also known as monopolar diathermy)
One electrode and one 'earth' (patient-electrode-pad).

Bipolar diathermy
One pair of forceps with each 'prong' as one electrode. Bipolar diathermy cannot be used for 'cutting', and the bipolar forcep tips cannot be applied to a metallic instrument (e.g. another pair of forceps in the wound) to cauterise tissue (which can be done with unipolar diathermy).

UNIPOLAR DIATHERMY (also known as monopolar diathermy)

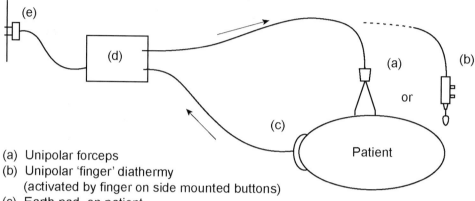

(a) Unipolar forceps
(b) Unipolar 'finger' diathermy
     (activated by finger on side mounted buttons)
(c) Earth pad, on patient
(d) Diathermy machine
(e) Mains electricity

BIPOLAR DIATHERMY

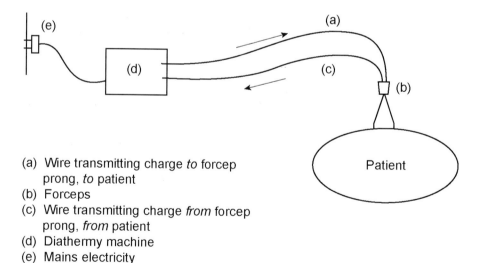

(a) Wire transmitting charge *to* forcep
     prong, *to* patient
(b) Forceps
(c) Wire transmitting charge *from* forcep
     prong, *from* patient
(d) Diathermy machine
(e) Mains electricity

Figure 2.11. Different types of diathermy.

— Can have a pair of forceps as one electrode in unipolar.

Cutting diathermy
The cutting mode involves the use of AC unipolar electricity.

Coagulating diathermy
The coagulation mode is achieved by the use of AC unipolar 'pulsed' electricity.

Blend diathermy
'Blend' diathermy is a combination of the above types, i.e. it cuts and coagulates.

Risks of diathermy

- Burns where earthed metal comes into contact with skin.
- Pacemaker can stop functioning.
- Pacemaker lead can send current to myocardium, burn heart, or cause MI, or VF.
- In laparoscopic use, diathermy touching metal instruments in contact with bowel can cause bowel perforation.

Direct coupling
Current passed onto a laparoscopic port results in a burn.

Capacitance coupling
The field produced by diathermy charges the laparoscopic port, which can result in a burn.

Nutrition

The usual energy requirements of a 70kg adult male is 1800kcal/day. The brain uses carbohydrates as its sole fuel in the fed state (approximately 100g of glucose a day). Unused glucose replenishes glycogen stores in the liver and the rest is converted into fat.

Amino acids in the diet are used to replace those lost in the normal daily turnover. The rest are metabolised by the liver, which converts the carbohydrate portion into fuel and the nitrogenous component into urea for excretion.

Metabolic phases

After feeding
High levels of insulin and low levels of glucagons.

12 hours fasting
Low levels of insulin and high levels of glucagons. The liver begins to convert stored glycogen (approximately 200g stored) to glucose for use by the brain. Glycogen stored in muscle is converted to lactate then exported to the liver for conversion to glucose (Cori cycle). Muscle protein breakdown begins to contribute amino acids for formation of glucose in the liver.

48 hours fasting
Approximately 75g of muscle protein is broken down each day. Fatty acids from lipolysis provide the main metabolic fuel for many tissues.

The brain adapts to using ketone bodies as fuel (from the breakdown of fatty acids) thereby sparing approximately 55g of muscle protein breakdown per day.

Summary of effects of prolonged fasting
- Low levels of insulin and high levels of glucagons.
- Hepatoglycogenolysis.
- Muscle and visceral protein catabolism.
- Hepatic gluconeogenesis.
- Lipolysis.
- Ketogenesis.
- Fall in metabolic rate (to approximately 1500kcal/day).

Indications for parenteral (i.e. intravenous) nutritional support

- Inadequate oral intake for >3 days.
- Severe dysphagia.
- Massive enterectomy.

- Distal enterocutaneous fistula.
- Major injury, e.g. head injury.
- Prolonged recovery.
- Severe inflammatory bowel disease.
- Any indication for nutritional support where the enteral route is contraindicated.
- Small bowel obstruction which needs pre-operative feeding.
- Short bowel syndrome.

Disadvantages of parenteral nutrition
- Expensive.

Catheter-related complications
- Mechanical:
  - blockage;
  - central vein thrombosis;
  - migration/dislodgement.
- Infection:
  - skin entry site infection;
  - line sepsis;
  - infective endocarditis.

Physiological disadvantages
- Barrier function (of the bowel) is lost.
- Decrease in villous height (leading to diarrhoea).
- Deranged LFTs (biliary stasis, excessive calories).
- Hyperglycaemia.
- Hypertriglyceridaemia.
- Hyperchloric acidosis.
- Septic complications (including pulmonary).

Burns

Definition

Injury to skin resulting in erythema or formation of eschar. The severity of burn injury depends on:

- Aetiology of the injury.
- Percentage body surface area of skin damage.
- Depth of the burn.

Incidence

0.5-1% of the UK population sustains burns each year; 10% require admission and of these, 10% are life-threatening. The kitchen and bathroom are the commonest locations for injury at home. Acid burns tend to occur mostly in people working in the plating or fertilising industry; for alkali burns, oven cleaners and soap manufacturers.

Anatomy and classification

Erythema
Epidermis only, no blisters, sunburn, not included in area of burn assessment.

Superficial partial thickness
Epidermis and part dermis, blisters.

Deep partial thickness (also known as deep dermal)
Dermis and some adnexal structures (hair follicles and sweat glands).

Full thickness
Destruction of epidermis, dermis and adnexal structures.

Assessment

Mainly by history, examination and pin-prick test (shows anaesthetised or non-haemorrhagic areas, both indicative of a deep burn).

Depth

See table overleaf.

Size (% of total body surface area)

It is important to be able to quantify the area of skin involved with the burn, both for communication, and to aid treatment:

- Lund and Browder chart.
- Wallace 'Rule of Nines'. A useful system that represents easily remembered values for each part of the body based on the number 9: each arm is 9%; each leg is 18%; the front of the

Depth of burns.

	Superficial	Superficial dermal	Deep dermal	Full thickness
Cause	Steam/hot liquids	Steam/hot liquids	Flame/boiling liquids	Flame/boiling liquids/electric/chemical
Symptoms	Very painful	Painful	Some pain	Often painless
Blisters	None	Present	+/-	Absent
Colour	Red	Pale pink	Blotchy red	White
Sensation	Present	Present	Reduced	Absent
Pressure	Blanches	Blanches	No blanching	Fixed staining

trunk is 18%; the back of the trunk is 18%; the head is 9%; and the perineum plus genitals is 1%. N.B. Children have larger heads and smaller limbs in terms of body surface area compared with adults.

♦ The patient's palm approximates to 1% of their body surface area - useful for children and smaller burns.

Treatment

Initial management
♦ Resuscitation ABC.
♦ Address other life/limb-threatening injuries.

First aid
♦ Cool the burn to reduce oedema and protein extravasation.
♦ Irrigation for chemical burns is essential.

Burn blister
If large, over joints and produces functional impairment, then de-roof.

Escharotomies
This is required if there are circumferential full-thickness burns of the chest, limbs or digits. These are relaxing incisions along the long axis of the burned limb through the circumferential burn tissue.

Subsequent management
Dependent upon:
♦ Patient's age, general status.

♦ Burn depth and size:
  • erythema - usually resolves in a few days with complete healing;
  • superficial partial thickness - heal spontaneously from epithelial remnants within two weeks and leave little/no residual scarring;
  • deep partial thickness - if treated conservatively heal by a combination of epithelialisation from epithelial remnants and granulation tissue formation and wound contraction. Often need skin grafting;
  • full thickness - requires excision and split-skin grafting.
♦ Anatomical site. Burns on the face, ears, anterior chest, genitalia, and buttocks are treated conservatively if possible.
♦ Resuscitation formulae are guides - it is essential to titrate input with haemodynamic and cardiovascular status. Intravenous fluids are given to children with >10% total body surface area (TBSA) involvement and to adults with >15% TBSA. The Parkland formula is the most commonly used in the UK, i.e.:

First 24 hours:
Hartmann's given at:
3-4ml × weight (kg) × %TBSA

Half is administered in the first eight hours, back to the time of the injury, and the remainder in the next 16 hours, plus a maintenance fluid regime is also given in children (dextrose saline).

Next 24 hours:
Albumin given using the Brooke formula:
0.5ml 5% albumin/kg/%TBSA.

Specific clinical situations

- Erythema - topical soothing lotions, analgesia and protection from sunlight.
- Superficial partial thickness - debride blisters under sedation if large areas are involved or under a general anaesthetic in children. Use non-adherent dressings. If a late presentation then apply topical Silvadene (1% silver sulphadiazine).
- Deep partial thickness - conservative management can be prolonged with overly frequent dressing changes, infective complications and hypertrophic scarring. Small areas in children and the elderly can be treated conservatively. An early surgical approach of excision and split-skin grafting is recommended for larger areas.
- Full thickness - requires excision and split-skin grafting. Early surgery minimises the risk of infection and results in better healing

Difficult areas

- Face, ears and eyelids.
- Trunk and breast.
- Buttocks and genitalia.
- Hands and feet.

Inhalational injury

- Potentially fatal.
- Must be excluded in all cases of burn injuries.
- Signs include facial burns, singed nasal hairs and respiratory distress.
- Confusion and carboxyhaemoglobin are present.
- Treatment is via a secure airway, humidified oxygen and ventilatory support.

Electrical burns

- Low voltage (<1000v):
  - local tissue necrosis, tetany and dysrhythmia/cardiac arrest.
- High voltage (>1000v):
  - deep muscle injury, compartment syndrome and haemoglobinuria.

Chemical burns

- From acids, alkalis and organic hydrocarbons.
- Treatment is with analgesia, copious irrigation and wound debridement.

Complications

Early

- Airway. N.B. Inhalation injury.
- Concomitant injuries.
- Dehydration and renal failure.

Intermediate

- Infection (toxic shock syndrome).
- Electrolyte imbalance.
- GI haemorrhage.
- Hypercatabolism.

Late

- Scarring and contracture.
- Disfigurement.
- Psychological.

Myocardial infarction

Myocardial infarction (MI) is irreversible damage to myocardial tissue as a result of a prolonged period of ischaemia.

Note

- MI can be subendocardial (limited to the tissue on the inside of the muscular layer of the heart) or transmural (damage across the entire thickness of the heart muscle).

Natural history of MI

- Coagulation necrosis and inflammation (30 minutes).
- Granulation tissue (4 hours to 10 days).
- Resorption of necrotic myocardial tissue (as above).
- Organisation into fibrous scar tissue (7-8 weeks).

Note

- The resorption phase after granulation takes place due to a large infiltrate of macrophages and neutrophils.

The position of the MI is determined by the coronary artery affected: if it is the left anterior descending (LAD) artery, then the damaged part of the myocardium is the anterior wall or apical part (meaning at the apex of the heart); if it is the right coronary artery, it is the posterior wall of the left ventricle; and if the left circumflex artery, it is the lateral wall of the left ventricle.

Complications of MI (especially when transmural)

◆ Sudden death (frequently as a result of VF).
◆ Papillary muscle dysfunction (therefore mitral valve dysfunction).
◆ External rupture of MI (causes haemopericardium or a left to right shunt when the interventricular septum is involved).
◆ Mural thrombus (risk of CVA, embolic).
◆ Acute pericarditis.
◆ Ventricular aneurysm (increased risk of mural thrombus, can also lead to left ventricular failure [LVF]).
◆ Post-infarct dysrhythmias.

Note

— Cardiac enzymes rise post-MI as a result of tissue damage: specifically, CK MB fraction within six hours of MI; lactate dehydrogenase (LDH) within 24 hours of MI; and troponin within 12 hours of MI. This is highly cardio-specific.

Risk of postoperative MI

Time since infarct:

◆ 0-6 months - 55%.
◆ 1-2 years - 22%.
◆ 2-3 years - 6%.
◆ Greater than 3 years - 1%.

It is important to remember these figures, as they are relevant when considering patients for surgery as this increases their GA risk.

APACHE II score

(Acute Physiology And Chronic Health Evaluation), Knaus *et al*, 1985.

This is a predictor of risk of surgery and was initially designed to predict the outcome of patients on the ITU. APACHE II and ASA scores (see next section) are scoring systems used to quantify risk of patients undergoing GA for surgery (in this context, obviously they have other uses, not least of which is for audit purposes). Every single point in the list need not necessarily be remembered, but the meaning of the acronyms, their general use, and the interpretation of the scores should be understood.

Acute physiology score (APS)

◆ Rectal temperature.
◆ Mean arterial pressure.
◆ Heart rate.
◆ Respiratory rate (RR).
◆ Alveolar - arterial O_2 gradient if $FiO_2 >0.5$, or PaO_2 if $FiO_2<0.5$.
◆ Arterial pH.
◆ Na^+.
◆ K^+.
◆ Cl^-.
◆ Haematocrit.
◆ WCC.
◆ GCS.

Age points

Are graded from <44 to >75.

Chronic health points

◆ 2 points for elective operation.
◆ 5 points for emergency operation.
◆ Non-operative admission.
◆ Immunocompromised patient.
◆ Chronic liver, cardiovascular, respiratory and renal disease.

ASA score

(American Society of Anaesthesiologists).

This is a predictor of risk of surgery and statistical mortality for ITU patients. It was initially intended to predict outcome of patients on the ITU.

- I. Healthy patient.
- II. Mild systemic disease, no functional limitations.
- III. Severe systemic disease, definite functional limitation.
- IV. Severe systemic disease, constant threat to life.
- V. Moribund, life expectancy is 24 hours with/without surgery.

Brainstem death criteria

Pre-requisites for considering testing brainstem death criteria in a patient

- Patient must have no sedative drugs in his system.
- A known (non-malignant) diagnosis.
- Temperature >35°C.
- No metabolic disturbance.

The reason to test for brainstem death criteria is for potential organ salvage for transplantation purposes.

Tests of brainstem death criteria

Cranial nerves (because their nuclei lie in the brainstem)
- I - cannot test.
- II - cannot test.
- III - pupillary and consensual reflex.
- IV - doll's eyes.
- V - corneal reflex.
- VI - doll's eyes.
- VII - cannot test.
- VIII - cold water in the auditory canal results in nystagmus.
- IX - gag reflex.
- X - catheter to carina to stimulate cough.

- XI - cannot test.
- XII - cannot test (although positive gag involves XII).

Note

- The doll's eyes reflex, also known as the oculocephalic reflex, is a persistent forward gaze when the head is turned to the left or the right. This reflex is lost in brain dead patients. As you cannot ask the patient to look left or right to test for the ocular muscle and, hence, relevant cranial nerve function, the movement of the head left and right, with the presence of the doll's eyes reflex confirms the function of the cranial nerves mentioned in the above list. The absence of the reflex, conversely, implies brainstem death (in the context of the other tests mentioned).

Respiratory effort
Brainstem death is implied if no respiratory effort is made after withdrawal of artificial ventilation and pCO_2 is >10 (some books quote >6.7).

Pain stimulation
If there is no response or withdrawal response to a painful stimulus, e.g. crushing nailbed, brainstem death is implied.

Paediatric general principles

Paediatric surgery is an extensive subject, for the most part outside the remit of this book. But there are some general principles to be aware of which may be asked in exams.

Definitions of the stages of childhood

- Premature - before 38/52s gestation.
- Neonate from birth to 1 month old.
- Infant - <1 year.
- Pre-school child - <4 years.
- Child - 5-12 (or 14) years.
- Adolescent - 12-18 years.

Main priorities of general care of the newborn

♦ Temperature control.
♦ Respiration.
♦ Nutrition.

Hypothermia intra-operatively delays onset of spontaneous respiration postoperatively.

Ileus or intestinal obstruction in infants is an aspiration risk, therefore a nasogastric (NG) tube should be inserted with regular suction, to prevent this.

With fluid replacement care should be taken to avoid overhydration as the neonatal kidney cannot compensate. It causes oedema and prolonged wound healing and increases dehiscence.

Neonates require vitamin K pre-operatively due to immature liver physiology.

The infant abdomen is broader than it is long, therefore better access is achieved by a horizontal incision, which gives a more acceptable cosmetic scar.

Note

— Total body water in infants is 75% (compared with 60% in adults).
— For nutrition, infants require 100 calories/kg/day; therefore, a normal full-term infant (3kg) requires 300 calories/day.
— The minimum weight of a term infant is 2.5kg; beneath this is by definition underweight.

Respiratory function

Infants have half the number of alveoli as adults, therefore less reserve. Infants do not increase their tidal volume, they increase their respiratory rate (RR). Infants have a higher RR than adults due to their increased metabolic rate.

Circulation

Changes at birth:

♦ Cessation of placental blood flow results in decreased right atrial pressure.
♦ Beginning to breathe, therefore decreased pulmonary artery pressure and increased left atrial pressure.
♦ The above changes result in a reversal of the pressure balance in the infant heart such that the foramen ovale closes.
♦ The ductus arteriosus gradually closes over the first eight weeks of life.

A newly born infant has 300ml of blood in total, a normal heart rate of >140 bpm, and only 10% of circulating blood loss results in circulatory failure, i.e. 30ml.

Fluid resuscitation in children

Firstly decide on the degree of dehydration, (mild, moderate, severe):

♦ Mild (5%) - thirst, dry mucous membranes, oliguria. Requires oral rehydration or maintenance IV (crystalloid).
♦ Moderate (5-10%) - lethargy, sunken fontanelle, reduced skin turgor, reduced capillary return, tachycardia. Requires 10ml/kg colloid over one hour, then maintenance crystalloid.
♦ Severe (10-20%) - drowsiness, hypotension. Requires 20ml/kg colloid, half as an initial 'push', then maintenance crystalloid.

Note

— Bile-stained vomiting in a neonate demands admission and investigation(s). Look for Hirshprung's disease, a fistula, duodenal atresia, meconium ileus (90% association with cystic fibrosis).

IV fluid regimes for children

Dextrose saline (maintenance)
This is determined by the child's weight:

- 1st   10kg   100ml/kg).
- 2nd   10kg   50ml/kg) Over 24 hours.
- 3rd   10kg   25ml/kg).

Always add 10mmol of KCl to every 500ml bag of dextrose saline.

Chapter 3

Anatomy

ABDOMINAL ANATOMY

Anterior abdominal wall

The anatomy of the arcuate line (Figure 3.1)

The rectus abdominis is surrounded in its superior half by the rectus sheaths (anterior and posterior). The anterior rectus sheath is formed from the aponeurosis of external oblique and part of internal oblique (split). The posterior rectus sheath is made up from the aponeurosis of transversalis abdominis and part of internal oblique (split). However, in its inferior half, the rectus abdominis only has rectus sheath anteriorly. The line, posteriorly, of transition from the posterior rectus sheath to no posterior rectus sheath is called the arcuate line. Therefore, incisions through the muscle bellies of rectus abdominis above the arcuate line will include anterior and posterior rectus sheath layers (e.g. Kocher's). Incisions beneath the arcuate line will include only an anterior rectus sheath layer (e.g. paramedian laparotomy scar).

Abdominal wall incisions

Common types of abdominal incisions (Figure 3.2)

- Midline laparotomy scar.
- Paramedian scar.

- Right iliac fossa (McBurney's) appendicectomy scar.
- Kocher's scar (open cholecystectomy or other hepatobiliary surgery).
- Rooftop scar (hepatic surgery).
- Groin crease scar (inguinal hernia repair).
- Thoraco-abdominal (used in gastrectomy surgery for greater access).
- Femoral hernia repair scars:
  - inguinal ('high'; above and parallel to the inguinal ligament);
  - crural ('low'; in the groin crease, below and parallel to the inguinal ligament);
  - preperitoneal (McEvedy's, essentially a vertical incision parallel to the rectus abdominis fibres).
- Stoma scars:
  - either containing the stoma, or simply a post-reversal-of-stoma scar;
  - right iliac fossa (usually an ileostomy);
  - left iliac fossa (usually a colostomy).
- Laparoscopic scars (umbilical, or numerous other port sites, usually only 1-2cm in length).

Midline incisions

Midline incisions go through the following layers: skin, subcutaneous fat, Scarpa's fascia, linea alba, transversalis fascia, pre-peritoneal fat, and the peritoneum.

(a)

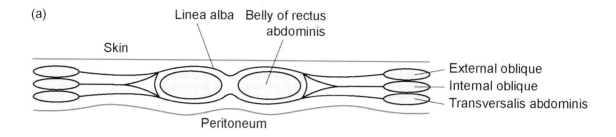

(b)

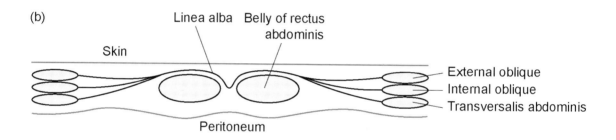

(c)

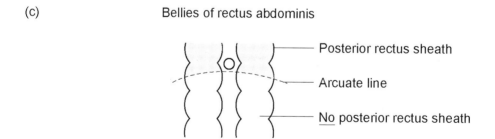

Figure 3.1. Anatomy of the arcuate line: (a) above the arcuate line; (b) below the arcuate line; (c) view from the abdominal wall from behind, with the peritoneum removed.

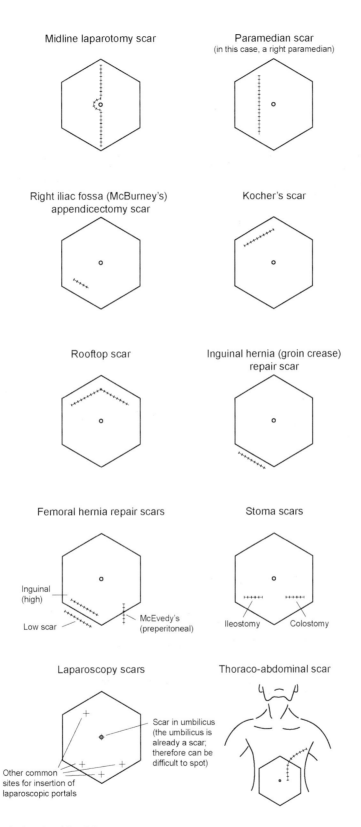

Figure 3.2. Types of abdominal incisions.

Note

— Questions relating to the layers crossed in midline abdominal incisions represent a common exam topic, so it is important to get every part of it right. Follow-on questions will probably relate to different types of incision.

Gridiron (McBurney's)

A gridiron incision (McBurney's) goes through the following layers: skin, subcutaneous fascia, external oblique in line with fibres including its aponeurosis, internal oblique and transversus in line with their fibres, transversalis fascia, and the peritoneum.

Posterior abdominal wall structures

The posterior abdominal wall structures are:

♦ Liver.
♦ Kidneys.
♦ Suprarenal glands.
♦ Spleen.
♦ Pancreas.
♦ Duodenum, ascending and descending colon, rectum (see relevant sections).

Anatomy of the liver

The liver is the largest organ in the body lying across the right hypochondrium, epigastrium and left hypochondrium. It is covered in peritoneum apart from the following:

♦ Gallbladder fossa.
♦ Bare area (between the coronary ligaments).
♦ Fissure for the ligamentum venosum (which gives attachment for the lesser omentum).

It may be divided anatomically into left and right lobes by the falciform ligament. The area between the bare area and the falciform ligament is called the caudate lobe. The area between the fissure for the ligamentum venosum and the ligamentum teres is called the quadrate lobe. The posterior surface is connected to the diaphragm over the right lobe by the coronary ligament. The ligamentum venosum is the fibrous remnant of the ductus venosus which lies in its eponymous fissure. It joins the left branch of the portal vein to the IVC. The ligamentum teres is the remnant of the left umbilical vein.

The porta hepatis is the gateway to and from the liver. It contains the common hepatic ducts, hepatic artery and portal vein. It also contains lymph nodes (which may lead to obstructive jaundice if they become enlarged).

The liver may be divided functionally into left and right lobes by a plane that passes through the gallbladder fossa and IVC fossa. It can then be further subdivided into segments based on blood supply and biliary drainage.

The liver is drained by three hepatic veins: right, middle and left, which lead to the IVC.

The blood supply to the liver is mainly via the portal vein and a relatively small proportion via the right and left hepatic arteries from the coeliac trunk.

The liver is a major lymph-producing organ which drains to the coeliac nodes, cysterna chylae and thoracic duct.

Nerve supply is from the hepatic nerve plexus which accompanies the hepatic artery and portal vein. The sympathetic nervous system is from the coeliac plexus; the parasympathetic nervous system is from the vagus.

The anatomic relations of the liver are as follows:

♦ Superior: pleura, lungs, pericardium, heart (via diaphragm).
♦ Inferior: oesophagus, stomach, duodenum, colon (hepatic flexure), right kidney and the suprarenal gland.

Anatomy of the kidneys

The kidneys are retroperitoneal organs (approximately 11cm x 6cm) which are mostly under cover of the costal margins (N.B. there is a risk of pneumothorax when doing a renal biopsy, so it is advisable to aim for the lower pole). The renal hilae lie between L1 and L2. The kidney is surrounded by a renal capsule, which is surrounded by perinephric fat. The fat is surrounded by renal fascia, known as Gerota's fascia. At the upper pole of the kidneys, above the renal fascia, lie the adrenal (suprarenal) glands.

The anatomic relations of the left kidney are the spleen, splenic flexure of the colon, and the tail of the pancreas. The relations of the right kidney are the right lobe of the liver, the hepatic flexure of the colon, and the duodenum.

The order from anterior to posterior of the hilar vessels emerging from the kidney is vein, artery, ureter (VAU). Because the IVC is on the right of the aorta ('I'VCR'), the left renal vein is longer than the right.

Each kidney has a renal pelvis, which contains two or three major calyces. The renal pelvis is lined with the same transitional epithelium as the bladder and ureters. Each kidney is divided into five arterial segments. The renal artery and its branches are all end arteries.

The lymph drainage of each kidney is to the para-aortic lymph nodes at the level of the renal arteries (L2).

Structure of the kidneys (Figure 3.3)

- Cortex.
- Medulla.
- Minor calyx.
- Major calyx.
- Nephron (1.2 million per kidney).
- Glomerulus.
- Juxtaglomerular apparatus.

The ureters

Each ureter is 25cm (ten inches) long. The points of narrowest calibre are: the pelvi-ureteric junction and the vesico-ureteric junction, half way down as it crosses the pelvic brim (crosses the iliac arteries at this point).

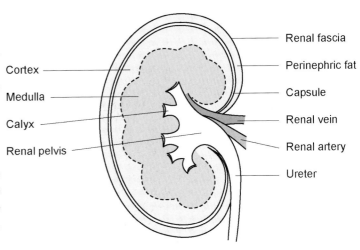

Figure 3.3. Structure of the kidney as seen from its posterior aspect.

Ureters are identified at surgery by virtue of being white, non-pulsatile, and show peristaltic activity when grasped with forceps.

The line of the ureter in a KUB (kidneys, urethra, bladder) X-ray is along the transverse processes of the lumbar vertebrae (slightly medial), entering the pelvis at the sacro-iliac joint, then heading towards the pubic tubercle and turning medially towards the bladder.

The blood supply of the ureters is as follows:

- Upper one third from a branch of the renal artery.
- Middle one third from the gonadal artery.
- Lower one third from the branches of the vesical (inferior and superior), and medial rectal artery (and the uterine artery in women).

Suprarenal glands (adrenal glands) (Figure 3.4)

The suprarenal glands lie on the upper pole of each kidney. The right adrenal is pyramidal; the left adrenal is crescentic.

Blood supply is from the following three sources:

- Branch of the renal artery.
- Phrenic artery.
- Direct branch from the aorta (right adrenal artery; the left adrenal artery is in fact a branch of the left renal artery).

The adrenal gland is made up of two distinct macroscopic layers: the outer cortex making up 90% of the gland's mass and the medulla making up 10% of its mass.

The cortex contains three regions:

- Zona glomerulosa - secretes aldosterone.
- Zona fasciculata - secretes cortisol.
- Zona reticularis - secretes sex steroids.

The medulla's sympathetic neuro-ectodermal (chromaffin) cells secrete the catecholamine hormones, adrenaline and noradrenaline.

Anatomy of the spleen

The spleen is a small organ lying in the left side of the lower thorax. It is found at the level of the 9-11th

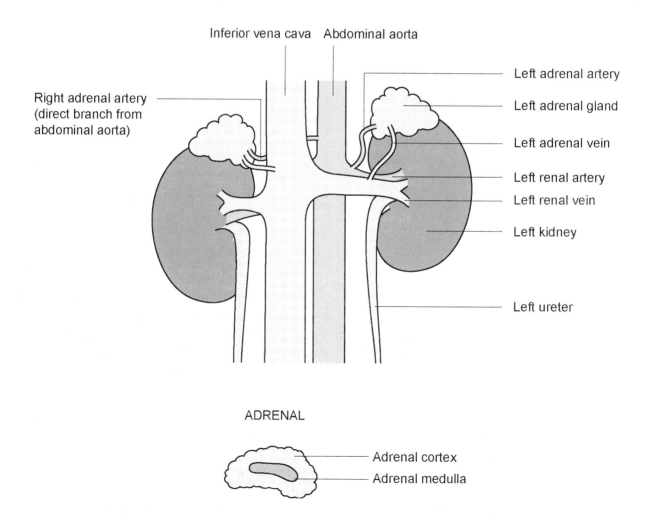

Figure 3.4. The adrenal glands.

ribs. It is attached to the posterior abdominal wall by the lienorenal ligament ('lieno' denotes spleen, 'renal' obviously denotes kidney). Thus, that portion of the posterior abdominal wall that this ligament joins is directly anterior to the left kidney.

It is also attached to the stomach (which lies directly anterior to it) by the gastrosplenic ligament. Both these ligaments contain blood vessels, which are particularly relevant to splenectomy surgery. The lienorenal ligament contains the splenic artery and vein which enter the spleen at the splenic hilum. The gastrosplenic ligament contains the short gastric arteries (these run from the splenic artery to the stomach).

The anatomic relations of the spleen are:

- Thorax laterally.
- Stomach anteriorly.
- Diaphragm superiorly.
- Left kidney posteriorly.
- Splenic flexure of descending colon inferiorly.

The spleen has a fibrous capsule and is adherent to the surrounding peritoneum. The spleen is a reticulo-endothelial organ (the largest in the body).

Anatomy of the pancreas

The pancreas is an abdominal organ lying in the transpyloric plane, in the bed of the 'C' shape of the duodenum. It has a head, neck, body and tail (also an uncinate process; uncinate means hook-shaped). The tail lies entirely within the lienorenal ligament (this places it at risk during splenectomy).

The pancreas contains a duct which runs the length of the gland. The pancreatic duct and the bile duct together enter the second part of the duodenum at the sphincter of Oddi.

It is supplied arterial blood by both superior and inferior pancreaticoduodenal arteries. Lymph from the pancreas follows the splenic artery. The vagus nerve (Xth cranial nerve) innervates the pancreas.

It is a combined endocrine and exocrine organ, i.e. it secretes hormones into the blood system (insulin from alpha cells and glucagons from beta cells), and

secretes pancreatic enzymes into the bowel (cholecystokinin), respectively.

The anatomic relations of the pancreas are:

- Bile duct, portal vein, inferior vena cava, aorta, superior mesenteric artery, left adrenal gland; all lie posterior to the pancreas.
- Stomach and the gastroduodenal artery lie anterior to the pancreas.

GI tract anatomy

Blood supply to the foregut (stomach) (Figure 3.5)

The aorta gives off the coeliac trunk, which divides into three branches:

- The left gastric artery. Supplies the lesser curve of the stomach, and anastomoses with the right gastric artery.
- The splenic artery. Gives off the short gastric artery and the left gastroepiploic artery which anastomoses with the right gastroepiploic artery and supplies the greater curvature of the stomach.
- The common hepatic artery. Gives off the gastroduodenal artery and right gastric artery which anastomoses with the left gastric artery, supplying the lesser curvature of the stomach. It continues as the right and left hepatic arteries.

The gastroduodenal artery branches into the superior pancreaticoduodenal artery and the right gastroepiploic artery which anastomoses with the left gastroepiploic artery and supplies the greater curvature of the stomach.

Nerve supply of the stomach (relevant to vagotomies)

Vagotomies used to be a widely discussed subject before the advent of proton pump inhibitors, which have reduced the incidence of peptic ulcer disease to such a great extent that the operation is now uncommon.

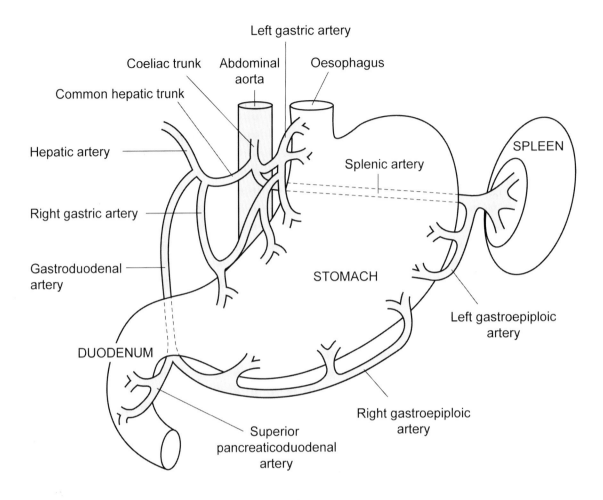

Figure 3.5. Blood supply to the foregut (stomach).

Nerve supply to the stomach is via the anterior and posterior vagal nerve trunks. (If the trunks, only, are cut, this is a truncal vagotomy).

There are further coeliac and hepatic divisions which, if spared, are called a selective vagotomy (the hepatic division innervates the first part of the duodenum).

Highly selective vagotomy cuts only those branches of the vagus that supply the body of the stomach from the anterior and posterior vagal trunks (sparing the 'crows feet' that innervate the pylorus), thus there is no need for a pyloromyotomy.

Note

— Pyloromyotomies were needed before the advent of highly selective vagotomies, as the innervation of the pylorus was interrupted affecting its function. A longitudinal incision is closed transversely, permanently opening the pylorus allowing it to drain freely.

Complications of vagotomy

The 'dumping syndrome' is divided into early or late types.

Early dumping

A rapid influx of hyperosmotic gastric contents into the small bowel, resulting in a net third space loss, flushing, pain and faintness approximately half an hour after consuming food.

Late dumping

This occurs three to four hours after consuming food, due to hypoglycaemia and causes similar symptoms. There may also be post-vagotomy diarrhoea, alkaline gastritis and chronic gastroparesis (inactivity of the stomach musculature leading to distension, and incomplete emptying).

Blood supply to the midgut (Figure 3.6)

The aorta gives off the superior mesenteric artery (SMA) 1cm below the coeliac trunk (at the level of the L1 vertebra). The SMA has five branches:

♦ Inferior pancreaticoduodenal artery. Supplies the duodenum beyond the entrance of the bile duct, and the pancreas, anastomosing with the superior pancreaticoduodenal artery.
♦ Jejunal and ileal arteries. Supply the ileum and jejunum in an arcade pattern.

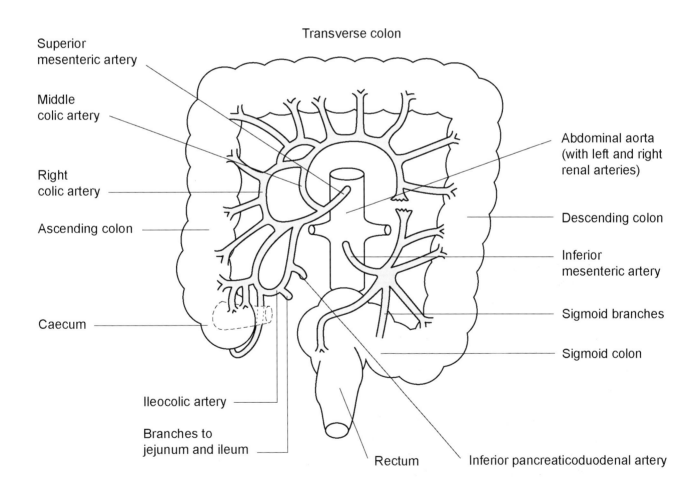

Figure 3.6. Blood supply to the midgut and hindgut.

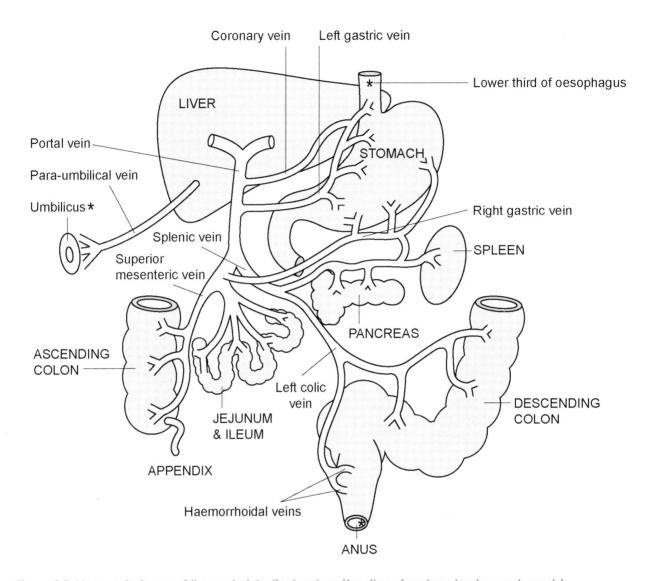

Figure 3.7. Venous drainage of the gastrointestinal system (* = sites of portosystemic anastomosis).

- Ileocolic artery. Supplies the ileum, caecum and some of the ascending colon in an arcade pattern.
- Right colic artery. Supplies the rest of the ascending colon.
- Middle colic artery. Located in the transverse mesocolon and supplies the transverse colon.

Each branch of the mesenteric artery anastomoses with its neighbour above and below establishing a continuous chain of anastomoses known as the marginal artery. Blood supplies of the inferior mesenteric artery (IMA) and SMA meet at a point just proximal to the splenic flexure making this location the most common place for ischaemic colitis to occur.

Blood supply to the hindgut (Figure 3.6)

The aorta gives off the IMA at the level of the L3 vertebra; it has two branches and continues itself to supply the upper third of the rectum:

- Left colic artery. Supplies the descending colon.

- Sigmoid arteries. Three or four branches supply the sigmoid colon.

Note

- The remainder of the hindgut is supplied by the IMA (upper third of the rectum); the lower two thirds of the rectum are supplied by the middle and inferior rectal arteries (branches from the internal iliac arteries).

Venous drainage (Figure 3.7)

The portal vein is formed from two tributaries: the superior mesentric vein and splenic vein. It also receives blood from the right and left gastric veins (thus blood from the lower end of the oesophagus as well as from the stomach), and the superior pancreaticoduodenal vein.

The portal vein carries venous blood from the intestinal circulation into the liver (at the porta hepatis). At this level it divides into two in a 'T-shape' (left and right branches).

Note

- The five sites of porto-systemic anastomosis are:

  - lower end of the oesophagus;
  - upper end of the anal canal;
  - bare area of the liver;
  - peri-umbilical region;
  - retroperitoneal areas.

  This is occasionally asked as a question in the clinical or viva setting.

Lymph drainage

This follows the arteries back to the para-aortic lymph nodes.

Gastroepiploic foramen (of Winslow)

The gastroepiploic foramen joins the greater and lesser sacs of the abdominal cavity.

The anatomic relations are as follows:

- Posterior - IVC.
- Superior - caudate process of the liver.
- Inferior - first part of the duodenum.
- Anterior - both leaves of the lesser omentum.
- Palpable within the foramen of Winslow are the portal vein, hepatic artery and biliary tract.

Note

- The lesser omentum runs from the liver to the stomach, the anterior boundary of the lesser sac.
- The lesser sac contains the portal vein, hepatic artery and biliary tract as they travel to the liver hilum.
- Knowledge of this is necessary for Pringle's manoeuvre (digital compression of the portal vein and hepatic artery in repairing lacerations of the liver).

Referred pain follows sympathetic supply. The concept of referred pain is an important one to grasp. The following list describes where pain will be felt according to the fore/mid/hind gut origins of the organs that are at the source of the pain.

The sympathetic nerves are key to the area in which pain is felt:

- Foregut - T8-T9. Great splanchnic nerve.
- Midgut - T10-T11. Lesser splanchnic nerve.
- Hindgut - T12-L2. Least splanchnic nerve.

This is particularly relevant to the inflamed appendix (pain felt in the T10-11 distribution, lesser splanchnic nerve, i.e. pain felt centrally in the abdomen, peri-umbilical). But when the peritoneum becomes inflamed (e.g. secondary to an inflamed appendix), it has a somatic nerve supply, and therefore the pain becomes localised to the right iliac fossa at this point.

Appendicitis is such a common clinical condition that it is fair to expect it as a possible question area in viva exams. The above mechanism of pain is one such question.

Transpyloric plane of Addison (Figure 3.8)

This is located half way along a vertical line joining the suprasternal notch and the pubic symphysis. It is located at the same level as the L1 vertebra.

It is an important concept as it contains within it the following:

- L1 vertebra.
- Pylorus.
- D1 (first part of the duodenum).
- Origin of the SMA.
- Renal hilae.
- Splenic hilum.
- Splenic artery.
- Fundus of the gallbladder (GB).
- Head of the pancreas.
- Start of the portal vein.

Gallbladder

The gallbladder is a receptacle for bile located on the posterior surface of the liver. It receives bile from the liver's network of bile canaliculi, which converge to form the left and right bile ducts, and hence the common bile duct.

The cystic duct is a branch from the common bile duct before it reaches the sphincter of Oddi opening into the second part of the duodenum. The cystic duct leads to the gallbladder where bile is stored.

The gallbladder is stimulated to contract by gastric emptying (secretion of cholecystokinin [CCK] by the duodenal mucosa) and thus, bile is secreted into the duodenum to aid fat digestion.

Gallstones

This is the pathological crystallisation of bile salts or cholesterol in the gallbladder to form stones. Their presence can cause pain, flatulent dyspepsia (stomach ache and burping), predispose to cholecystitis, and occasionally cause obstructive symptoms.

While it is possible to treat some stones pharmacologically or by lithotripsy, the relapse (reformation of stones) rate approaches 100%.

Currently, the only permanently effective treatment for symptomatic gallstone disease is excision of the gallbladder (cholecystectomy). This is performed laparoscopically for the most part. Occasionally, there is a need to convert to open cholecystectomy due to the presence of adhesions which (when severe) make laparoscopic dissection impossible. Adhesions are a recognised sequela of cholecystitis, or previous local surgery.

Calot's triangle (Figure 3.9)

Calot's triangle locates the cystic artery between the following three areas:

- Common hepatic duct.
- Inferior border of liver.
- Cystic duct.

It is important to locate the cystic artery before proceeding to excise the gallbladder in a laparoscopic cholecystectomy.

The complications of laparoscopic cholecystectomy (see Chapter 4) relate to:

- The anaesthetic (MI/CVA/DVT/PE/atelectasis).
- The pneumoperitoneum (the insufflating needle can be malpositioned, e.g. into the aorta, bowel, or vena cava. The pneumoperitoneum can splint the diaphragm or cause a CO_2 embolism).

(a)

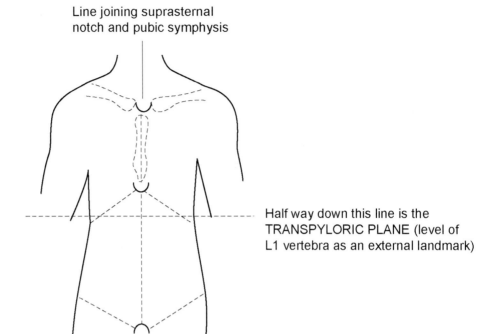

Line joining suprasternal
notch and pubic symphysis

Half way down this line is the
TRANSPYLORIC PLANE (level of
L1 vertebra as an external landmark)

(b)

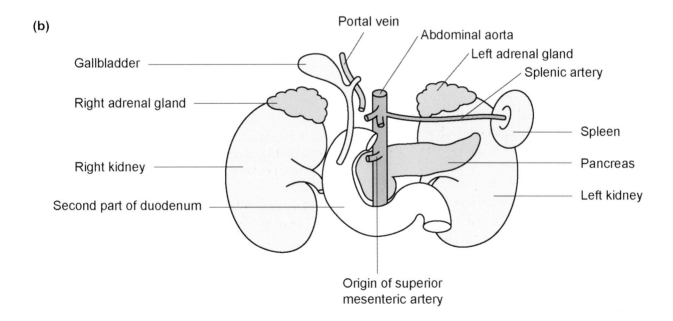

Portal vein

Abdominal aorta

Left adrenal gland

Splenic artery

Gallbladder

Right adrenal gland

Right kidney

Second part of duodenum

Spleen

Pancreas

Left kidney

Origin of superior
mesenteric artery

Figure 3.8. (a) The transpyloric plane and (b) the structures found within it.

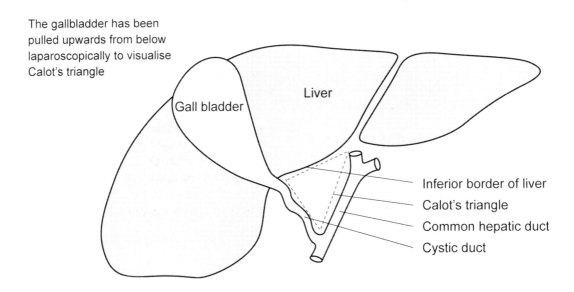

The gallbladder has been pulled upwards from below laparoscopically to visualise Calot's triangle

Gall bladder

Liver

Inferior border of liver

Calot's triangle

Common hepatic duct

Cystic duct

Figure 3.9. Calot's triangle.

- The area operated upon, the gallbladder, cystic duct, common bile duct, cystic artery - all can be damaged, leading to a bile leak/bleed.
- The port-site wounds (wound infection, hernia, port-site metastases).

Anatomy of the inguinal region

The inguinal canal runs from deep to superficial inguinal rings (lateral to medial). In males, the inguinal canal contains the spermatic cord and ilio-inguinal nerve. In females, the inguinal canal contains the round ligament of the uterus and the ilio-inguinal nerve.

The anatomic relations of the inguinal canal are:

- External oblique anteriorly.
- Inguinal ligament inferiorly.
- Internal oblique and transversus muscle form the roof.

- The inguinal ligament inserts the pubic tubercle medially as the conjoint tendon.
- The posterior wall is made up of the conjoint tendon medially (strong) and the transversalis fascia laterally (weak).

The spermatic cord, within the inguinal canal, is made up of cremasteric fascia and muscle surrounding the ductus deferens; it also contains the genitofemoral nerve.

It is important to remember that the 'canal' is not the same as the 'ligament'. The canal is the theoretical space between three sheets of muscle through which the testicle trailing the spermatic cord has passed.

The ligament is the convergence of all three muscle layers inferiorly. The conjoint tendon is further merging at the point of insertion into the pubic tubercle.

Femoral canal

The femoral sheath is made up of extraperitoneal fascia drawn from the transversalis fascia anteriorly and psoas fascia posteriorly.

The femoral canal lies medial to the femoral vein. It has two functions: providing dead space for the vein to expand during times of increased venous drainage and space for the lymphatic vessels.

The femoral ring is the abdominal opening of the femoral canal and comprises the following:

- Anteriorly - inguinal ligament (medial part).
- Medially - lacunar ligament.
- Posteriorly - pectineal ligament.

Repair of a femoral hernia

The peritoneal sac is first localised and then excised. The defect is repaired in the femoral canal by suturing the lacunar ligament and the pectineal ligament using J-sutures.

Surgical approaches:

- Inguinal/high (above and parallel to the inguinal ligament).

- Crural/low (in the groin crease, below and parallel to the inguinal ligament).
- Preperitoneal (McEvedy's incision, essentially a vertical incision parallel to the rectus abdominis fibres).

The anatomic relations of the femoral triangle (Figure 3.10) are as follows:

- Superior - inguinal ligament.
- Medial - medial border of the adductor longus (counter-intuitive).
- Lateral - medial border of sartorius.

The femoral nerve, artery and vein lie in the femoral triangle.

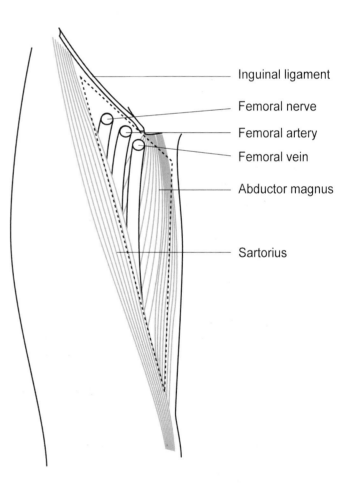

Inguinal ligament

Femoral nerve

Femoral artery

Femoral vein

Abductor magnus

Sartorius

Figure 3.10. Femoral triangle borders.

PELVIC ANATOMY

Pelvic anatomy (as it relates to general surgery)

Pelvis is latin for 'basin'. The average human pelvis is tilted anteriorly by 60°. It is broader in females for childbirth.

Identification of anatomical landmarks

In viva exams you may well be confronted with a prosection of the pelvic region, and all of the following may be covered:

- Sacral promontory.
- Anterior superior iliac spine.
- Anterior inferior iliac spine (origin of rectus femoris).
- Inguinal ligament.
- Lacunar ligament (joins the inguinal ligament to the pubic tubercle).
- Obturator fossa.
- Obturator membrane (origin of obturator internus and externus).
- Obturator groove. A small hole superiorly not covered by obturator membrane, through which the obturator nerve, artery and vein pass. (N.B. An obturator hernia passes through here, if present).
- Ischial tuberosity (insertion of sacrotuberous ligament).
- Ischial spine (insertion of sacrospinous ligament).
- Sacrotuberous and sacrospinous ligaments (these two ligaments bisect the sciatic foramen into the greater and lesser sciatic foramina).
- Piriformis muscle. Passes through the greater sciatic foramen, a very important landmark. Above it are the superior gluteal nerve, artery and vein, and beneath it are the inferior gluteal nerve, artery and vein, as well as the sciatic nerve and pudendal nerve, the nerve to quadratus and femoris, and the nerve to obturator internus.
- Sacrum.

Pelvic floor

This is a gutter-shaped sheet of muscle (also known as the pelvic diaphragm) surrounding the urogenital hiatus anteriorly and anal canal in the midline.

Levator ani and coccygeus are continuous, one with the other. Levator ani is made up of iliococcygeus and pubococcygeus. Levator ani meets itself in the midline in the anococcygeal ligament or raphe (slings around the anal canal from anterior to posterior. The raphe is posteriorly located).

Note

— The anococcygeal ligament joins the anus to the coccyx.

The order of muscles from posterior to anterior as they spread out to form the pelvic floor, is:

- Coccygeus (nerve supply is via the perineal branches of S4,5).
- Iliococcygeus (nerve supply is via the perineal nerve).
- Pubococcygeus (nerve supply is via the branches of S3,4).

Note

— There are also puborectalis and levator prostatae beneath pubococcygeus.

Actions of the pelvic floor

- Supports the pelvic viscera.
- Counteracts the rise in abdominal pressure during quiet inspiration.
- During defaecation it relaxes which straightens out the anorectal junction.
- During parturition the pelvic floor directs the fetal head down to the pelvic outlet.

Note

— The pelvic floor can be damaged in parturition, leading to stress incontinence and a prolapse of the vagina, rectum, and uterus, hence the need for an episiotomy on occasion.

Pelvic fascia

The pelvic fascia covers the walls of the pelvis (obturator internus and piriformis); it is tough and inextensible. The pelvic fascia covering the pelvic floor is totally different from that covering the walls, in that it is loose and extensible. It fills the 'dead space' between the viscera of the pelvis (e.g. around the bladder, rectum and vagina).

Note

— It provides a plane in which pelvic sepsis can rapidly spread.

There are sections that are tougher, e.g. condensations of pelvic fascia around the neurovascular bundles (iliac vessels, hypogastric plexus). These condensations of tissue also form the lateral ligaments of the bladder and uterus.

The rectum

Rectum is latin for 'straight' (this is of course a misnomer, as the rectum is not actually straight). It starts at the level of S3, where the sigmoid colon ends (this point is defined as being where the sigmoid mesocolon terminates as the rectum has no mesocolon). The rectum ends at the anal ring where levator ani slings round the anorectal junction.

Note

— The rectum has a continuous outer circular muscle layer which differentiates it from the rest of the colon as the tinae coli merge at the level of formation of the rectum.

The rectum has two curves to the right and one to the left (the middle). The upper third is covered anteriorly and laterally with peritoneum, but the middle third is covered anteriorly only with peritoneum (strangely, this apparently insignificant fact seems to be frequently asked in exams!).

The rest of the rectum is beneath the level of the peritoneum and is covered in Waldeyer's fascia between the rectum and bladder (the rectovesical pouch, in males), or the uterus (recto-uterine pouch of 'Douglas', in women).

The blood supply of the rectum is as follows:

♦ The superior rectal artery supplies the upper third, which is a direct continuation of the inferior mesenteric artery.
♦ The lower two thirds of the rectum are supplied by the middle and inferior rectal arteries (also from the median sacral arteries), which are branches of the internal iliac artery.

The anal region (Figure 3.11)

The anal canal is the last 4cm of the alimentary tract.

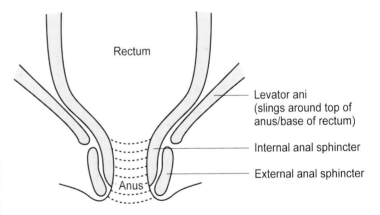

Figure 3.11. The anal region.

It is a tube of circular muscle fibres, with both internal and external anal sphincters: the internal anal sphincter is a visceral smooth involuntary muscle; the external anal sphincter is a skeletal voluntary muscle.

The junction of the anal canal is where the levator ani slings round the anus from anterior to posterior, forming the anococcygeal ligament which joins the anus to the coccyx.

Note

— Because it is a sling, the anterior quarter of the anus is deficient of levator ani muscle cover (the left and right sides and posterior border have a layer of levator ani muscle cover).

Internal anal sphincter

The internal anal sphincter is an involuntary visceral muscle which is a direct continuation of the inner circular layer of rectal muscle.

External anal sphincter

The external anal sphincter is in continuity with the levator ani muscle, except anteriorly where the levator ani is deficient, and continues to loop round to form a coherent circular layer. It is made up of voluntary skeletal muscle. The spaces between these two sphincters are fatty planes, which become relevant in peri-anal sepsis.

Blood supply, venous drainage, and the portosystemic anastomosis of the anus

The superior rectal artery supplies the superior anal canal. The middle rectal and median sacral arteries supply the middle anal canal. The inferior rectal artery supplies the inferior portion of the anal canal.

The veins correspond to the arteries forming a rectal venous plexus. The upper part of the rectal venous plexus drains into the portal circulation (via the superior rectal and inferior mesenteric veins), hence it is a site of portosystemic anastomosis. This is thought to be behind the 3/7/11 o'clock positions of the venous anal cushions becoming swollen as haemorrhoids. However, it has yet to be explained why there is no increase in the incidence of haemorrhoids in people with portal hypertension.

Ischio-anal (ischiorectal) fossae

These were previously termed ischiorectal, illogically, because, at no point do they come into contact with the rectum. These fossae are wedge-shaped spaces filled with fat, lateral to the anal canal. The anal canal and sloping levator ani thus make up the medial border of the ischio-anal fossae. The lateral borders are the ischial tuberosity and obturator internus. The apex is where the lateral and medial borders meet.

Note

— The anococcygeal body separates the two ischio-anal fossae low down, but they come into contact with each other above the anococcygeal body, i.e. leaving a 'horseshoe-shaped' tract for sepsis to travel.

Perineal body

The perineal body is also known as the central perineal tendon. It is a midline structure lying in front of the anal canal.

The perineal body provides the origin for the following muscles:

◆ External anal sphincter.
◆ Internal anal sphincter.
◆ Levator prostatae (pubovaginalis in the female).
◆ Levator ani.
◆ Bulbospongiosus.
◆ Superficial and deep transverse perineal muscles.

Fissure-in-ano

A longitudinal tear in the anoderm, almost always midline in males; 90% are posterior, 10% are anterior. In females, 80% are posterior, 20% are anterior. There is an equal sex ratio, and it is common in young adults. The aetiology is uncertain. Constipation has a 'chicken and egg' relationship, i.e. is it the cause of the problem, or the result?

Symptoms of fissure-in-ano

Pain on defaecation (and for 1-2 hours later), PR bleed (on paper), pruritis, watery discharge, and constipation.

Diagnosis is made by parting the anal margin, and inspecting the area affected.

Treatment of fissure-in-ano

Conservative

Soften stool with laxatives, topical GTN, topical 0.2% diltiazem.

Surgical

Lateral sphincterotomy or anal dilatation (which is now only very rarely performed).

Note

— The risk of incontinence is increased when performing an anal dilatation if the patient has already had obstetric sphincter damage.

Anorectal sepsis

The aetiology is development of an abscess in the anal glands, which normally drain mucus into the anus through the crypts of Morgagni.

This can result in the following:

◆ Simple peri-anal abscess. The treatment is to incise and drain it.
◆ Intersphincteric abscess. When the internal opening is found by a probe it must be laid open to release the infection and allow healing from the base upwards.
◆ Trans-sphincteric abscess. Surgical treatment is complicated involving the use of a seton (latin for bristle), as these abscesses cannot be laid open without causing faecal incontinence (the incision would have to cross the anal sphincter muscle).
◆ Ischio-anal (ischiorectal) or suprasphincteric abscess. Similar surgical management problems to trans-sphincteric abscesses.

Goodsall's rule

Posterior fistulae always drain into the midline and anterior fistulae drain radially to the corresponding region of the anteror anus.

Prostate, ductus deferens and seminal vesicles

Prostate

The prostate lies beneath the bladder and above the urogenital diaphragm and is the size of a walnut, 4cm × 3cm × 2cm. Laterally, levator prostatae (part of levator ani) is present. It provides 30% of the seminal fluid during ejaculation. The anterior surface is connected to the pubic bone by the puboprostatic ligaments (these are strong enough, that, during pelvic trauma, the prostate is held fixed, and the bladder can be torn away). It has a true and a false capsule. The ejaculatory ducts (seminal vesicles) insert posteriorly into the prostate, and open into the verumontanum, half way down the prostatic urethra.

The prostate is divided into anterior, middle, posterior and two lateral lobes. Blood supply is from the prostatic branch of the inferior vesical artery and some branches of the middle rectal and internal pudendal vessels.

Transurethral resection of the prostate (TURP) must not extend beyond the verumontanum to prevent urinary incontinence.

Ductus deferens (Figure 3.12)

The ductus deferens runs from the epididymis (from the testicle), going upwards and entering the abdomen through the deep inguinal ring, running along the side wall of the floor of the pelvis to meet the bladder. Throughout its course it is completely subperitoneal; nothing runs between it and the peritoneum.

Each ductus deferens dilates towards its end to form an ampulla, which is used for the storage of spermatozoa. It then enters the seminal vesicles, which are responsible for 60% of seminal volume secretion. It leaves the seminal vesicles as the

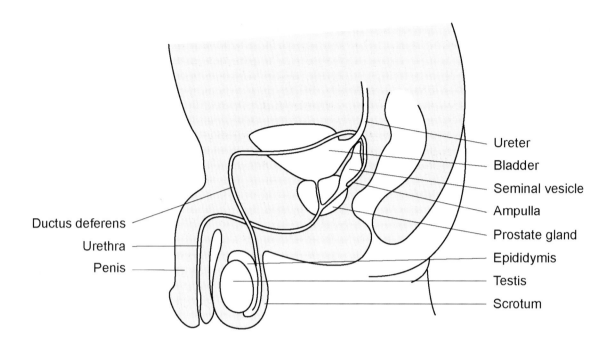

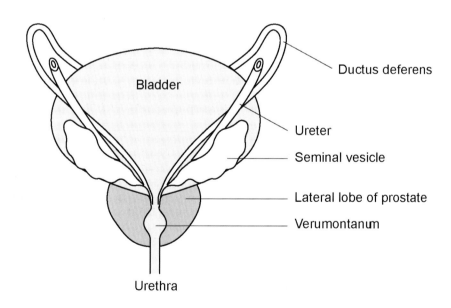

Figure 3.12. Ductus deferens.

ejaculatory duct, entering the prostate and opening into the prostatic urethra at the verumontanum.

Spermatic cord, epididymis and testis

Spermatic cord

This runs from the testis, via the superficial inguinal ring, through the inguinal canal, via the deep inguinal ring, down the lateral pelvic wall, under the bladder, into the seminal vesicles and prostate, and entering the prostatic urethra at the verumontanum.

It gains three coverings as it passes the inguinal canal:

- Internal spermatic fascia (from the transversalis fascia and deep inguinal ring).
- Cremasteric muscle (from the transversalis fascia and internal oblique).
- External spermatic fascia (from the external oblique muscle).

Note

- The coverings are gained in the opposite direction to the description above, because the covering tissues are acquired during the descent of the testicle from the abdomen, through deep, then superficial inguinal rings to the scrotum.

The constituents of the spermatic cord (Figure 3.13) are as follows:

- Ductus deferens.
- Testicular artery.
- Pampiniform plexus of veins.
- Lymphatics (drain to the para-aortic nodes, NOT the superficial inguinal nodes like the scrotal skin).
- Nerves (genital branch of the genitofemoral nerve).
- Processus vaginalis (if patent, leads to an indirect inguinal hernia).

Testis

The testis is covered by tunica vaginalis and on its posterolateral surface lies the epididymis (a tortuous store of spermatozoa for maturation). A hydrocoele of the testis is fluid collecting under the tunica vaginalis.

Note

- A hydrocoele always lies anterior to the testis.

The right and left testes are separated by the median scrotal septum. Blood supply is via the testicular artery branch of the abdominal aorta. Venous drainage is by the pampiniform plexus of veins, involved in heat exchange to keep the testes cool for spermatogenesis.

A varicocoele is a varicosity of the pampiniform plexus, more common on the left (not known why).

Note

- The seminal vesicles make 60% of the volume of seminal fluid, the prostate makes 30%, and the testes make the remaining 10%.
- Testes also contain Leydig cells that produce testosterone.

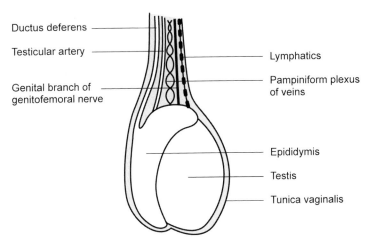

Figure 3.13. Constituents of the spermatic cord and testis.

Hydrocoele of the testis

Hydrocoele of the testis is a collection of fluid within the tunica or processus vaginalis.

Classification

- Primary:
  - congenital;
  - funicular;
  - hydrocoele of the cord;
  - vaginal.
- Secondary:
  - inflammatory;
  - malignancy;
  - parasitic;
  - postoperative.

Clinical findings

On examination there is a smooth cystic swelling, transillumination is positive, the testis is not felt separately, one can get above the swelling (as opposed to, for example, a varicocoele which extends up into the abdomen, and hence one cannot palpate above it), and it is usually not tender.

Investigation

If suspicious clinically, an ultrasound of the scrotum in adults should be performed to rule out a testicular neoplasm.

Treatment

A congenital hydrocoele requires a herniotomy as a hydrocoele is associated with a patent processus vaginalis.

Other treatment options are:

- Jaboulay's procedure.
- Lord's plication.
- Aspiration and instillation of sclerosant.

Undescended testis

The testis develops in the retroperitoneum and starts to descend into the scrotum. By the third month it is in the false pelvis and by the eighth month it is in the region of the deep inguinal ring. It descends into the scrotum by the ninth month.

Factors contributing to descent are:

- Testosterone.
- Gubernaculum testis.
- Intrinsic testicular defect.

Incidence:

- Premature infants - 30%.
- At term - 4%.
- At one year - 1%.

Clinical findings

An undescended testis has to be differentiated from a retractile testis. A retractile testis can be brought down to the scrotum which is usually fully developed.

Investigation

- Ultrasound is useful in identifying a testis in up to 15% of impalpable testis.
- MRI is useful in 60-80% of cases.
- Laparoscopy is the modality of choice as it can be used to both detect and repair at the same time.

Treatment

- Watchful waiting: wait up to the first birthday.
- Hormone therapy: in physiologic cryptorchidism, human chorionic gonadotrophin (HCG) 1500 units/week intramuscularly every other day or three times a week for a total of nine injections.
- Surgery:
  - one-stage procedure - orchidopexy;
  - a two-staged procedure is usually done for a high-lying testis in the retroperitoneum where the cord cannot be mobilised enough without compromising the blood supply.

THORACIC ANATOMY

Anatomy of the thoracic wall and diaphragm

Articulation of the ribs

Ribs articulate with the vertebral column in two ways:

- By their heads (joints of heads of ribs).
- By their tubercles (costotransverse joints).

Collectively, the above are known as the costovertebral joints.

Joints of heads of ribs

- Ribs have two articular facets.
- Each rib articulates (with its inferior facet) with its own vertebra (after which the rib is named) inferiorly. The rib also articulates (with its superior facet) with the rib superiorly; these are synovial joints.
- Note that the first rib articulates ONLY with T1, (not with C7). Also, ribs 11 and 12 articulate ONLY with their own vertebrae (T11 and T12, respectively).
- There is an intra-articular ligament (in three bands) holding the rib to its vertebra.

Costotransverse joints

- Join the tubercle of the rib to the vertebra.
- Are small synovial joints.
- Three ligaments are present: the superior costotransverse, lateral costotransverse and costotransverse.

Thoracic muscles

- External intercostals.
- Internal intercostals.
- Innermost intercostal muscle.

The diaphragm

- Its action is for inspiration.
- The right side is higher than the left.
- The crura are the tendons posteriorly from which the diaphragm originates (they themselves originate from the lumbar vertebral bodies, L1, 2 and 3).
- The diaphragm has a central tendon from which its muscle fibres radiate outwards.
- The median arcuate ligament is a loop at T12, in the crura, through which the aorta passes.
- An oesophageal orifice is found at the level of T10.
- A vena caval foramen at the level of T8 is found within the central tendon itself.

Valsalva's manoeuvre

This is forced exhalation against a closed glottis that has the effect of raising intra-abdominal pressure, or of opening up the Eustachian tubes from the oropharynx to the ear. The sequence is as follows:

- Closed glottis.
- Contraction of intercostal muscles (raising intrathoracic pressure).

♦ Contraction of the diaphragm and abdominal wall muscles (against the high pressure of the thorax).

All of these together act to raise intra-abdominal pressure.

Anatomy of the mediastinum

The mediastinum is divided anatomically into the superior and inferior mediastinum by a plane passing through the level of the manubriosternal joint (aka the Angle of Louis which corresponds to T4).

Note

— The relevance of the level T4 to surface anatomy is that the manubriosternal joint, the angle of Louis, the arch of the aorta, the carina (bifurcation) of the trachea, and the bifurcation of the pulmonary arteries are all located in the chest cavity here.

The inferior mediastinum is divided into anterior, middle and posterior sections.

Superior mediastinum

This comprises the thoracic inlet containing the great veins of the neck (on the right) which merge into the superior vena cava (SVC) from the right and left brachiocephalic veins. These in turn were formed from the internal jugular and subclavian veins. It also contains the great arteries, the ascending aorta (which is midline, arching posteriorly), then gives off the brachiocephalic trunk and left common carotid and left subclavian arteries from right to left.

The arch is directly behind the manubriosternal joint (T4). The mediastinum contains the oesophagus posteriorly, and the trachea before it bifurcates in the mediastinum, anterior to the oesophagus (starts at C6 level of the larynx). It also contains the ligamentum arteriosum, a remnant of ductus arteriosus (which was a shunt from the pulmonary artery to the aorta in the fetus).

Note

— The left recurrent laryngeal nerve loops round the ligamentum arteriosum and arch of the aorta.

The cardiac plexus of nerves is formed from the vagus (parasympathetic) and sympathetic trunk. It contains the phrenic nerves, which rest, on both sides, on the lateral-most extent of the mediastinum. The right phrenic nerve is in contact with veins throughout its length (right brachiocephalic, SVC, RA, IVC) before it reaches the right diaphragm (passes through the central tendon; the orifice in the diaphragm is named the vena caval foramen). The left phrenic nerve runs over the subclavian artery, common carotid artery, arch of the aorta and the left ventricle until it reaches the left diaphragm muscle (not the tendon, as with the right phrenic nerve).

The left and right vagus nerves are also found in the mediastinum. They can be visualised as always trying to reach the midline along their course. The right vagus is in contact with the lateral trachea. The left vagus is kept from the trachea by the left common carotid and left subclavian arteries. Both vagus nerves give off their recurrent laryngeal branches (the left branch looping round the ligamentum arteriosum and the aortic arch, and the right looping round the subclavian artery, before both track up the lateral aspects of the trachea).

Note

— The path of the left and right recurrent laryngeal nerves is a common question in the anatomy section of viva exams.

Anatomy of the heart

The four heart chambers (right and left atria, right and left ventricles)

The right atrium and ventricle lie anterior to the left atrium and ventricle. The right atrium contains openings from the SVC and the IVC, and the coronary sinus. Between the right atrium and ventricle lies the tricuspid valve. The right ventricle contains papillary muscles, the bundle of His, and the chordae tendinae which subdivide into three, one for each septum of the tricuspid valve, which prevents them from everting during systole. The left atrium contains four pulmonary vein openings in square formation, two left and two right, an auricle, and the mitral (bicuspid) valve. The left ventricle has muscular walls three times as thick as its right-hand partner. It contains two papillary muscles which link to chordae tendinae, one for each septum of the mitral valve, the bundle of His and, of course, the aortic (bicuspid) valve leading into the aorta.

Surface markings of the heart

The right sternal edge from the third intercostal space (ICS) to the sixth ICS marks the position of the heart. The left side of the heart is at the second ICS to the fifth ICS.

Note

- The ascending aorta contains right and left coronary sinuses, which form the right and left coronary arteries, respectively.
- The sino-atrial (SA) node is found in the right atrium, just below the SVC, and the atrioventricular (AV) node is found in the interatrial septum.

Anatomy of the coronary arteries

The left coronary artery runs anteriorly down the atrioventricular groove as the left anterior descending (LAD) artery, and gives off the circumflex branch early.

The right coronary artery runs down posteriorly to the heart in the atrioventricular groove, and gives off the marginal branch late.

Note

- Venous blood from the myocardium drains finally into the coronary sinus which empties into the right atrium (its tributaries are the great, middle and small cardiac veins).

Arch of the aorta

The anatomic relations of the aorta are as follows:

- The aorta originates from the ascending aorta (from the left ventricle), travels up, and arches posteriorly.
- The top of the arch is at the level of the manubriosternal junction/angle of Louis/T4.
- The left recurrent laryngeal nerve hooks around it.
- The aortic arch contains baroreceptors which regulate the HR in response to stretch and hence pressure.
- Aortic bodies (detect hypoxia).

Branches from the aorta are:

- The brachiocephalic trunk (becomes the right common carotid artery and right subclavian artery).
- The left common carotid artery.
- The left subclavian artery.
- The ligamentum arteriosum (remnant of ductus arteriosus).

Vena cava, phrenic and vagus nerves

Vena cava

The SVC is formed by the convergence of the left and right brachiocephalic veins, which are in turn each formed by the convergence of the internal jugular and subclavian veins. The SVC enters the right atrium superiorly; the superior mediastinum (serous and fibrous layers) originates from the SVC and passes downwards. The IVC passes vertically into the inferior area of the right atrium.

Note

- The vena cava overlies the aorta.

Phrenic nerve

Remember the rhyme: C3, 4, and 5, keep the diaphragm alive.

The right phrenic nerve is associated with venous structures in the anterior pericardium. The left phrenic nerve is associated with arterial structures in the anterior pericardium.

Vagus nerve

The vagus nerves (right and left) pass down the posterior pericardium in close approximation with the oesophagus which they supply, give off branches to the pulmonary plexuses, a right and a left recurrent laryngeal nerve (left hooks the ligamentum arteriosum, right hooks the right subclavian artery), and also give off a branch to the cardiac plexus.

Anatomy of the pulmonary tree

The trachea

Begins at the level of C6, and is attached to the cricoid cartilage by the cricothyroid ligament. It contains C-shaped rings, which are deficient posteriorly. The trachea is 10cm in length at rest, but 15cm long on deep inspiration.

The anatomical relations of the pulmonary tree are as follows:

- Posterior relations. The oesophagus and recurrent laryngeal nerve.
- Lateral relations. The carotid sheath and lobes of the thyroid gland (2nd-6th rings).
- Anterior relations. The isthmus of the thyroid (2nd-4th rings), the inferior thyroid vein and the thyroidea ima (if present). The trachea bifurcates at the level of T4 (manubriosternal joint, angle of Louis), which is the same level as the arch of the aorta and pulmonary artery bifurcation.

Pleural surface markings

This is a common question in surface anatomy in either clinical or viva exams. It is important that you have the difference between pleural surface markings and lung surface markings clear in your head. The apex of the pleura is 2cm above the clavicle. The left border

moves over the heart at the level of the 4th costal cartilage (CC). The right border moves laterally (over the right border of the heart) at the level of the 6th CC. It crosses the mid-claviclular line bilaterally at the 8th CC and crosses the mid-axillary line bilaterally at the 10th CC, reaching the lowest point posteriorly at the 12th CC.

Lung surface markings

These are exactly as for pleural markings, except they are two ribs higher for all of the above factors (with the obvious exception of the apex of the lung which is also located 2cm above the clavicle).

Lung fissures

The right lung has both oblique and horizontal fissures (therefore, the right lung is divided into upper, middle and lower lobes). The left lung only has oblique fissures (therefore, upper and lower lobes).

Note

— The left lung also has a lingular lobe.

Surface markings of lung fissures

Both oblique fissures trace a line from the body of T3 (posteriorly) to the 6th rib (anteriorly) or, put differently, can be said to be in line with the 5th rib. The horizontal fissure is at the level of the 4th rib (only the right lung has a horizontal fissure).

The arterial blood supply of the lungs (parenchyma) is via:

- The bronchial arteries found at the level of the hilum, two on the left and one on the right, which is paradoxical, as the right lung has three lobes.

The venous drainage of the lungs (parenchyma) is via:

- The pulmonary veins draining into the azygos vein on the right, and into the accessory azygos on the left. Both merge to drain into the left atrium, i.e. venous blood mixing with oxygenated blood (a shunt).

Lymph drainage of the lungs is via:

- The hilar lymph nodes, to the mediastinal lymph nodes, and then into the brachiocephalic veins.

The nerve supply of the lungs is via:

- The pulmonary plexus.
- A branch of the cardiac plexus (sympathetic).
- The vagus (parasympathetic).

Oesophagus

The blood supply of the oesophagus is as follows:

- Upper third - inferior thyroid artery.
- Mid third - branches from the aorta.
- Lower third - left gastric artery.

The anatomic relations of the oesophagus are as follows:

- The oesophagus starts at C6 level, entering the thoracic inlet at T1, crossing the diaphragm at T10 level.
- It lies posterior to the trachea and anterior to the prevertebral fascia.
- It is indented by the aorta, left main bronchus and diaphragm. If the left atrium is enlarged or mediastinal lymph nodes are enlarged, these can indent the oesophagus.

Note

- The oesophagus has a loose connection to the diaphragm. If this connection is loosened or lost it may result in a sliding-type hiatus hernia.

The nerve supply of the oesophagus is as follows:

- Upper third - recurrent laryngeal nerve and sympathetic fibres.

- Lower two thirds - vagus nerve.

Note

- The vagus is divided into anterior and posterior trunks. The anterior contains mostly left vagal fibres and the posterior contains mainly right vagal fibres. However, both contain a mixture of anterior and posterior.

Anatomically, the oesophagus contains an inner circular layer and an outer longitudinal layer.

The upper third of the oesophagus is skeletal muscle, i.e. under voluntary control. The lower two thirds are visceral muscle, i.e. automatically continues the swallowing process once initiated.

The lowest 5cm of the oesophagus acts as a physiological sphincter, although it is not thickened (i.e. not visible as a sphincter on endoscopy), compared with the rest of the oesophagus.

The normal swallow involves relaxation of the oesophagus preceding the bolus down the oesophagus (called receptive relaxation). Failure of receptive relaxation, especially at the lower oesophageal sphincter results in achalasia (the arrest of the food bolus in the oesophagus). Not only is this uncomfortable, but it results in aspiration of foodstuff into the trachea and a high incidence of pneumonia.

Note

- The above peristalsis is termed primary, but if the bolus is not in the stomach then there is a wave of secondary peristalsis, i.e. starts in the body of the oesophagus.

Tertiary waves are disordered contractions, indicative of a motility disorder. It is never normal to see tertiary waves.

Anatomy of the breast

The base of the breast extends from the 2nd to the 6th rib, overlying pectoralis major, serratus anterior and the rectus sheath with an external oblique belly. There are 15-20 lactiferous ducts converging to open in separate parts of the nipple. The breast has fibrous septae dividing lobules apart from each other.

The blood supply is via the lateral thoracic artery and some branches of the internal thoracic artery and thoraco-acromial artery. Venous drainage follows the above arteries.

Lymph drainage of the breast is very relevant to malignant disease. The lateral breast (upper and lower quadrants) drains to the axillary nodes. The medial breast (upper and lower quadrants) drains to the parasternal nodes through the intercostal spaces.

Note

—   Lymph can flow between the lateral and medial sides of the breast.

The nerve supply is via the intercostal nerves T4-T6.

Note

—   The breast is a modified sweat apocrine gland.

In studies, the left breast is usually (almost imperceptibly) larger than the right.

ORTHOPAEDIC ANATOMY

The humerus (Figure 3.14)

The humerus is involved in the shoulder (glenohumeral) and elbow joints.

It is important to remember that the shoulder joint is technically a ball and socket joint, although the head of the humerus and the curve of the glenoid fossa of the scapula are poor examples of this type.

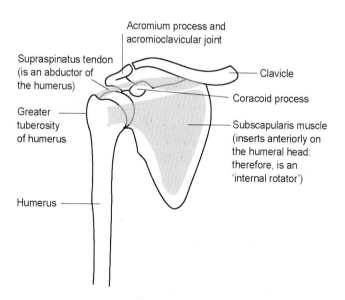

Anterior view of rotator cuff

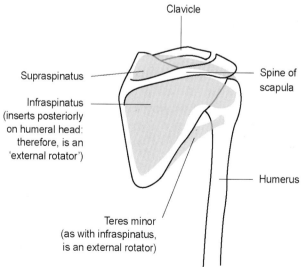

Posterior view of rotator cuff

Figure 3.14. The humerus: rotator cuff muscles.

The stability of the joint is helped by the glenoid labrum (lip), the joint capsule, but most importantly, the rotator cuff muscles.

The order of insertion of rotator cuff muscles to the humeral head from medial to lateral are:

- Subscapularis (medial to bicipital groove) (lesser tubercle).
- Supraspinatus (lateral to bicipital groove) (greater tubercle).
- Infraspinatus (lateral to bicipital groove) (greater tubercle).
- Teres minor (posterior aspect of humeral head).

Note

- One way of remembering the order of insertion, from medial to lateral of the rotator cuff tendons on the humeral head is 'SSIT', i.e. subscapularis, supraspinatus, infraspinatus, teres minor.

The radial nerve derives its name from its behaviour as it wraps itself around the humerus, along the radial groove.

The radial groove begins half way down the humerus and rotates laterally, ending up anterolaterally at the level of the elbow (in between the brachialis and brachioradialis bellies).

Distal humerus (Figure 3.15)

The elbow joint is not a simple hinge. It has components that allow flexion and extension (hinge activity), but also, a region (the capitulum) that allows a form of rotation (called pronation and supination) in the forearm. The capitulum is a part of a sphere, located laterally and articulates with the radial head. The trochlea is the articular surface for the ulna, located centrally, forming a hinge joint. The medial epicondyle is the common origin of all the flexor muscles of the forearm; posteriorly, it contains a groove for the ulnar nerve.

The lateral epicondyle is a common origin for all the extensor muscles of the forearm.

Nerves in the arm (Figure 3.16)

Musculocutaneous
Runs deep to biceps laterally and continues, after giving branches to biceps and brachialis, to become the lateral cutaneous nerve of the forearm (sensory to the lateral forearm).

Median
Runs deep to biceps medial to the musculo-cutaneous nerve and is closely associated with the brachial artery. Depending on the level affected, a palsy of the median nerve would present as either of the following:

- Carpal tunnel syndrome (CTS). Wasting of the thenar eminence, weakness of opposition of the thumb, and sensory loss over the lateral three and 1/2 fingers (not the palm as the palmar branch passes anterior to the carpal tunnel).
- Median nerve palsy. At a higher level than CTS. It is a palmar sensory loss and loss of power in flexor pollicis longus, i.e. weakness of flexion of the distal phalanx of the thumb.

Ulnar
Runs deep to biceps medial to the median nerve, it passes behind the medial intermuscular septum, closely associated with the basilic vein in the upper arm. A palsy that is commonly at the medial epicondyle results in claw hand, reduced sensation over the little and 1/2 ring fingers, reduced adduction of the little finger, reduced adduction of the thumb, and wasting of the hypothenar muscles. A reason for claw hand is the paralysis of intrinsic muscles of the hand, particularly of the little and ring fingers.

The 'ulnar paradox' is so called because the higher (more proximal) the lesion to the ulnar nerve, the less pronounced is the 'clawing'. The reason for this is the paralysis of the long flexors to the little and ring fingers, i.e. the ulnar side of the flexor digitorum profundus muscle, to which a branch of the ulnar nerve supplies innervation at the level of the elbow. Thus, a high lesion (above the level of the elbow) results in less clawing (less flexion of the fingers).

The exact position the fingers are held in claw hand is: extension at the metacarpophalangeal joints (MCPJ), and flexion at the proximal interphalangeal joints (PIPJ) and distal interphalangeal joints (DIPJ),

Anterior distal humerus

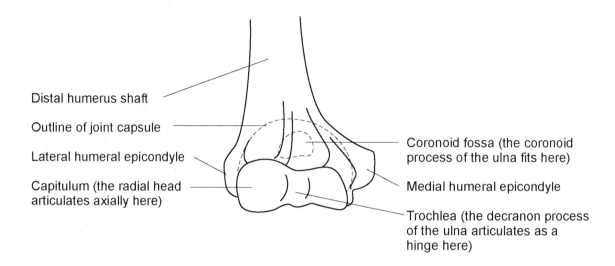

Distal humerus shaft

Outline of joint capsule

Lateral humeral epicondyle

Capitulum (the radial head articulates axially here)

Coronoid fossa (the coronoid process of the ulna fits here)

Medial humeral epicondyle

Trochlea (the decranon process of the ulna articulates as a hinge here)

Right lateral elbow

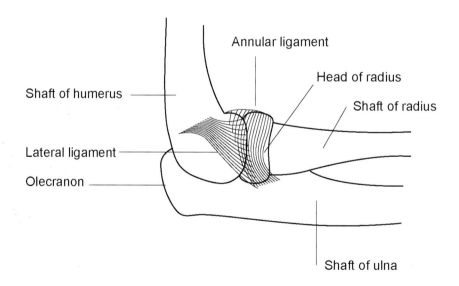

Annular ligament

Head of radius

Shaft of radius

Shaft of humerus

Lateral ligament

Olecranon

Shaft of ulna

Figure 3.15. Distal humerus.

MEDIAN
Carpal Tunnel Syndrome

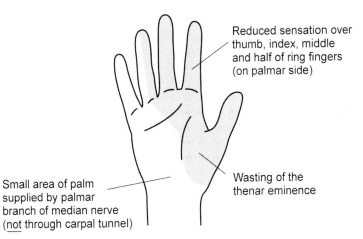

Reduced sensation over thumb, index, middle and half of ring fingers (on palmar side)

Small area of palm supplied by palmar branch of median nerve (not through carpal tunnel)

Wasting of the thenar eminence

Right hand (palmar)

ULNAR
Ulnar Nerve Palsy

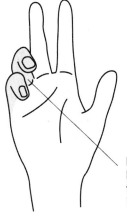

Reduced sensation over little and half of ring fingers and clawing of little and ring fingers

Right hand (palmar)

RADIAL
Radial Nerve Palsy

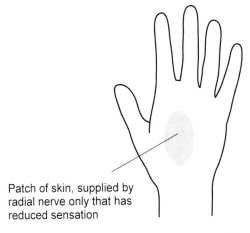

Patch of skin, supplied by radial nerve only that has reduced sensation

Right hand (dorsal)

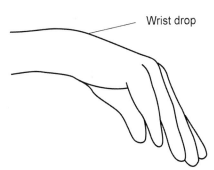

Wrist drop

Right wrist (lateral)

Figure 3.16. Nerve supply to the hand.

because the lumbricals and interossei are palsied in this case, and flexor digitorum profundus (FDP) and flexor digitorum superficialis (FDS) are not.

Radial

See above. It wraps radially around the humerus, ending up laterally at the level of the elbow.

Saturday night palsy (when one falls asleep intoxicated with one arm over the back of a chair) or Crutch palsy, are both types of radial nerve palsy, resulting in weak wrist and finger extension, and decreased sensation over the first webspace.

Anterior interosseous nerve palsy, a branch of the median nerve, results in weakness of FDP and flexor pollicis longus (FPL), thus weakness of flexion of the DIPJ of the thumb, index and middle fingers. There is no sensory loss (this is the key differentiating point between this lesion and that of radial nerve palsy).

Posterior interosseous nerve palsy, a branch of the radial nerve, results in weakness of extensor digitorum, thus weakness of finger extension (no wrist drop and no sensory loss).

The radius and ulna (Figure 3.17)

The radius and ulna are two bones found in the forearm. There are four joints in the forearm: from proximal to distal, the elbow (olecranon to trochlea, and radial head to capitulum), the proximal radio-ulnar joint, the distal radio-ulnar joint, and the wrist (radius to scaphoid and part of the lunate; the distal ulna has a small contribution to the joint).

The types of movement available at these joints are:

◆ Elbow - flexion extension (olecranon-trochlea).
◆ Pronation supination (radial head-capitulum).
◆ Proximal and distal radio-ulnar joints - pronation and supination.
◆ Wrist - flexion, extension, abduction, adduction, circumduction (circular combination of the previous movements).

The radius

The radius has a small articular surface at the elbow (cored out and partially spherical) and an annular ligament joining it to the ulna proximally.

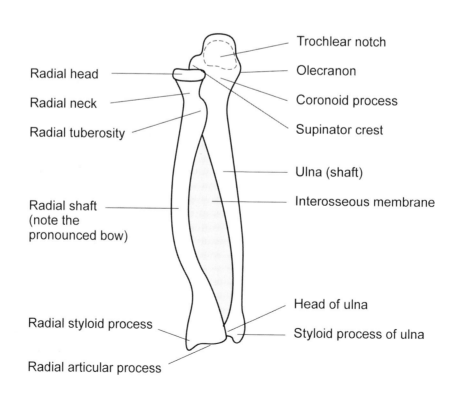

Figure 3.17. The radius and ulna.

The shaft is attached to the ulna by an intraosseous septum. Distally it has a large articular surface with the scaphoid at the wrist, and a styloid process laterally.

The ulna

There is an extensive articular surface at the elbow. The coronoid process is the anterior part of the hinge of the olecranon (its posterior equivalent is the olecranon process). The ulna also has the origin of the interosseous membrane along its length. At the wrist there is a small articular surface in contact with the lunate bone. The ulna ends in a styloid process.

Note

— The ulna is attached distally to the radius by the triangular fibrocartilaginous (distal radio-ulnar) ligament.

Anatomical snuffbox

The anatomical snuffbox is bounded on the ulnar side by the tendon of extensor pollicis longus (EPL), and on the radial side by extensor pollicis brevis (EPB) and abductor pollicis longus (APL).

Note

— The radial artery is found at the base of the anatomical snuffbox and the cephalic vein originates here. The scaphoid is (significantly) palpable, as are the trapezoid and radial styloid bones.

Antecubital fossa

The antecubital fossa contains the following structures:

- Biceps tendon.
- Brachial artery.
- Median nerve.

Note

— A simple way of remembering the order of structures from lateral to medial is TAN, i.e. tendon, artery, nerve.

It is a triangular area on the anterior elbow/forearm with the following boundaries:

- Pronator teres (medially).
- Brachioradialis (laterally).
- Theoretical line between both epicondyles of the humerus.
- The roof is the deep fascia of the forearm.
- The floor is the brachialis muscle.

Also in the region (but not within the boundaries) of the antecubital fossa are the median basilic vein, medial cutaneous nerve of the forearm, lateral cutaneous nerve of the forearm and median cephalic vein.

The hand

Thenar eminence

This is the pad on the palm immediately proximal to the thumb. The thenar eminence contains the following muscles:

- Abductor pollicis brevis.
- Flexor pollicis brevis.
- Opponens pollicis.

All are supplied by the median nerve, therefore they become weak and wasted in carpal tunnel syndrome (test movements of the thumb for evidence).

Note

— In carpal tunnel syndrome there is also a loss of sensation on 3 1/2 fingers on the thumb side of the hand, but there is no sensory loss on the palm, as the palmar branch does not pass through the carpal tunnel. Phalen's test is a palmar flex wrist for one minute, which exacerbates and/or brings on symptoms. It is useful in diagnosis, as are electromyography (EMG) studies.

Hypothenar eminence

This is the pad on the palm immediately proximal to the little finger. The muscles that make up the hypothenar eminence are:

- Abductor digiti minimi.
- Flexor digiti minimi brevis.
- Opponens digiti minimi.

All intrinsic muscles of the hand are supplied by the ulnar nerve, except the 'LOAF' group of muscles (lumbricals, opponens pollicis, abductor pollicis and flexor pollicis brevis), which are all supplied by the median nerve. The ulnar nerve also supplies sensation to the skin of the little and ulnar border of the ring fingers.

Superficial palmar arch (Figure 3.18)

This is an arterial arch formed by the radial and ulnar arteries in the palm. It is in direct contact with the palmar aponeurosis, i.e. superficial to all other hand structures. It is, in fact, a direct continuation of the ulnar artery, which anastomoses with the radial artery (but in 66% of the population it fails to anastomose as an arch and exists as a hockey stick-shaped structure), sending off the digital arteries on either side of each finger.

Deep palmar arch

This arch is formed by the terminal branch of the radial artery anastomosing with the ulnar artery (usually a complete arch, unlike the superficial arch).

(Left hand, palmar surface)

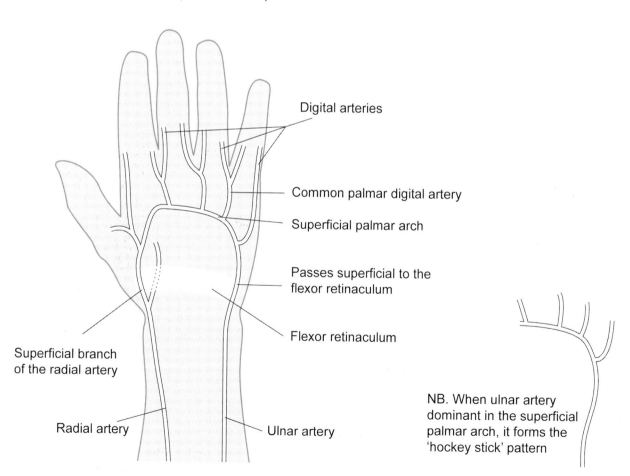

Digital arteries

Common palmar digital artery

Superficial palmar arch

Passes superficial to the flexor retinaculum

Flexor retinaculum

Superficial branch of the radial artery

Radial artery

Ulnar artery

NB. When ulnar artery dominant in the superficial palmar arch, it forms the 'hockey stick' pattern

Figure 3.18. Superficial palmar arch.

Fibrous flexor tendon sheaths

All five digit flexor tendons are encased in tough fibrous tendon sheaths from the metacarpal heads to the distal phalanges.

Note

— The thumb's sheath contains only the tendon of flexor pollicis longus.

Synovial flexor tendon sheaths

Flexor tendons passing through the carpal tunnel are invested in synovial sheaths.

Note

— Flexor digitorum superficialis and profundus both share the same sheath.

Digital attachment of the long flexor tendons (Figure 3.19)

The flexor digitorum profundus (FDP) tendon splits into two at the level of the PIPJ and inserts into the middle phalanx. The flexor digitorum superficialis (FDS) tendon passes through the split in the FDP tendon to insert the distal phalanx. When testing the flexor tendons in the hand, remember that the deeper (profundus) tendon goes further (distal phalanx).

Digital attachment of the extensor tendons (the extensor expansion) (Figure 3.19)

The extensor expansion is a common endpoint for all tendons causing extension in the digits. Extensor digitorum tendons join with the extensor expansion immediately beyond the MCPJ. The extensor expansion then splits into three at the level of the PIPJ, the middle branch inserts the middle phalanx (this is called the central slip), and the other two go round it to insert the distal phalanx.

Note

— The tendons from the interossei and lumbricals also insert the extensor expansion beyond the PIPJ.

(a)

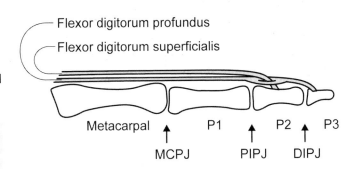

(b)

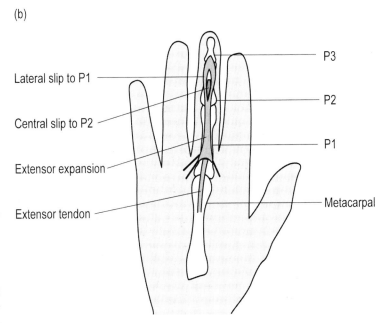

Figure 3.19. (a) Digital attachment of the long flexor tendons; (b) digital attachment of the extensor tendons (the extensor expansion).

Interossei

There are two groups of these little muscles:

◆   The palmar interossei.
◆   The dorsal interossei.

They originate between the metacarpal bones (hence 'interossei'). The palmar interossei are more superficial, and the dorsal interossei are deeper.

A useful mnemonic for remembering the actions of these muscles is:

◆   PAD, i.e. the palmar interossei ADDuct.
◆   DAB, i.e. the dorsal interossei ABDuct.

Lumbricals

There are complex functions ascribed to these little muscles arising from the tendons of the FDP. They are thought to have synergistic and proprioceptive function in fine movements of the hand.

Important exceptions to remember

◆   The extensor indicis tendon inserts onto the ulnar side of the common extensor expansion of the index finger (relevant to tendon transfer operations).
◆   In cases where tendon is needed for reconstruction of deficiency, a spare tendon can be derived from the tendon of extensor digiti minimi which splits into two as it passes over the dorsum of the hand (one can be used without adverse motor consequence).

The clavicle

There are two ends to the clavicle: the sternal and acromial. The sternal end has a fibrocartilaginous joint with a fibrocartilaginous disc between the manubrium and clavicle.

The anatomic relations of the clavicle are:

◆   Sternohyoid (superior).
◆   Brachial plexus (posterior).

◆   Subclavian artery and vein (posterior/inferior).
◆   Trapezius (superior).
◆   Deltoid (lateral).
◆   Sternocleidomastoid (superior).
◆   Interclavicular ligament (medial).
◆   Costoclavicular ligament (medial).
◆   Subclavius muscle (inferior).
◆   Manubrium sterni (medial).
◆   Acromium (lateral).
◆   Coracoclavicular ligament (lateral).

The popliteal fossa

This is an important anatomical landmark as it contains the major neurovascular structures travelling past the knee to the leg (see below). It is a diamond-shaped space in the posterior knee.

The anatomic relations of the popliteal fossa are:

◆   Upper lateral - biceps femoris.
◆   Upper medial - semimembranosus and semitendinosus.
◆   Lower medial and lateral - medial and lateral heads of gastrocnemius.
◆   Roof - fascia lata.
◆   Floor - popliteal surface of the posterior femur.

Structures found within the politeal fossa are (Figure 3.20):

◆   Lateral - the common peroneal nerve.
◆   Centrally - the tibial nerve.
◆   Superficially - the popliteal vein (the small saphenous vein pierces the fascia lata at the level of the popiteal fossa).
◆   Deep - the popliteal artery.
◆   Lymph nodes.

Note

–   Baker's cyst is a herniation of the posterior part of the synovial capsule of the knee joint, which can rupture and/or mimic a popliteal aneurysm.
–   The sciatic nerve is the major nerve passing posteriorly down the thigh, which splits to form the common peroneal nerve and tibial nerve, both of which are found in the popliteal fossa.

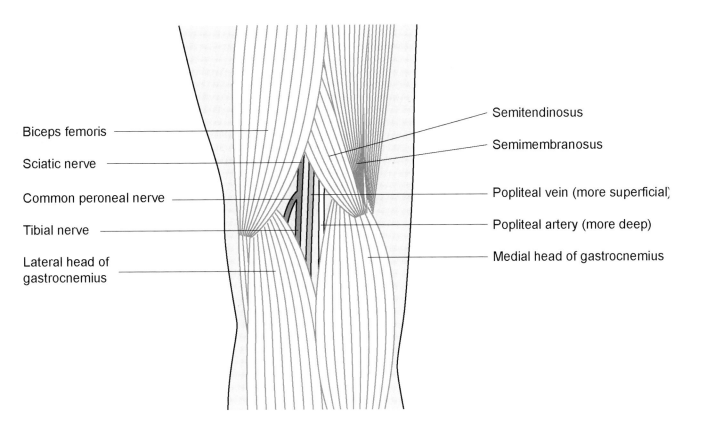

Biceps femoris

Sciatic nerve

Common peroneal nerve

Tibial nerve

Lateral head of
gastrocnemius

Semitendinosus

Semimembranosus

Popliteal vein (more superficial)

Popliteal artery (more deep)

Medial head of gastrocnemius

Figure 3.20. The popliteal fossa (lying posterior to the knee).

The gluteal region and hip joint

The gluteal region

The gluteal region lies behind the pelvis, an area from the iliac crest to the gluteal fold (which is the posterior horizontal crease of the hip joint) (Figure 3.21).

The muscles of the gluteal region are:

- Gluteus maximus/medius/minimus.
- Piriformis.
- Quadratus femoris.
- Obturator internus.
- Inferior and superior gemellus.

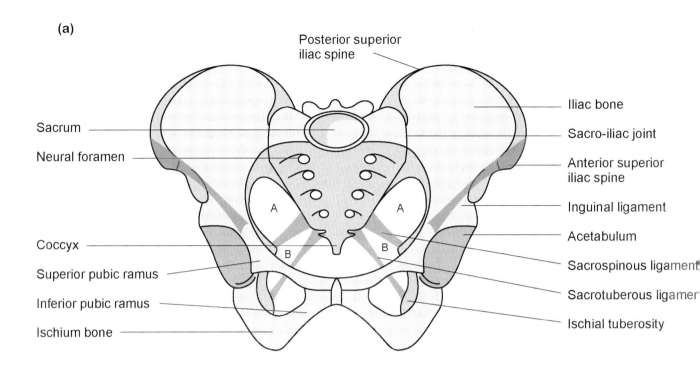

Figure 3.21. The gluteal region and hip joints: (a) AP view of the pelvis including its ligaments (A = greater sciatic foramen; B = lesser sciatic foramen). (b) View of the inner surface of the pelvis and sacrum after it has been split down the sagittal plane, from a lateral viewpoint.

The greater sciatic foramen is bounded by the bony contour of the sciatic notch posteriorly and the sacrospinous ligament anteriorly. The lesser sciatic foramen is formed from the lesser sciatic notch bounded by the sacrotuberous and sacrospinous ligaments.

Note

– The gluteal fold is NOT formed by the base of gluteus maximus; instead it is the horizontal skin crease of the posterior hip joint.

Cutaneous innervation of the gluteal region

Rami from the spinal levels L1 to S5 supply sensation to the gluteal region.

Muscles of the gluteal region (Figure 3.22)

Gluteus maximus

♦ Largest and most superficial.
♦ Runs at 45° to vertical.
♦ Three bursae lie beneath the muscle body of gluteus maximus:
  • ischial tuberosity;
  • hamstring origin;
  • greater trochanter.
♦ Originates from the gluteal fold of the ilium and inserts into the gluteal tuberosity of the femur.
♦ Action covers extension and lateral rotation of the hip joint.
♦ Nerve supply is via the inferior gluteal nerve (L5, S1, S2).
♦ Blood supply is via the superior and inferior gluteal arteries.

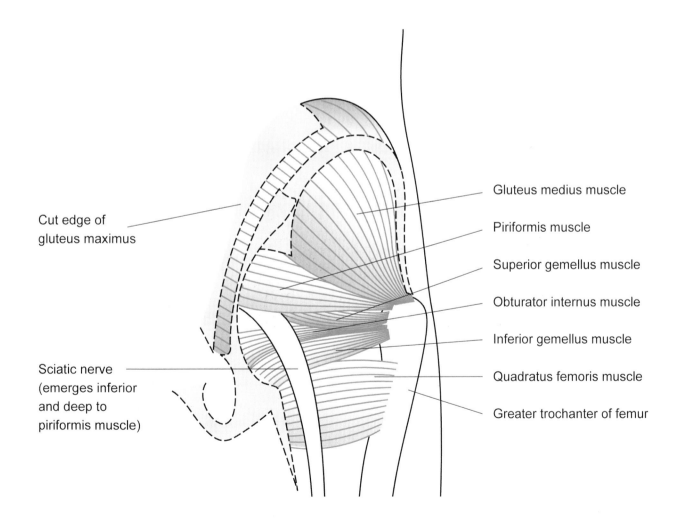

Cut edge of gluteus maximus

Sciatic nerve (emerges inferior and deep to piriformis muscle)

Gluteus medius muscle

Piriformis muscle

Superior gemellus muscle

Obturator internus muscle

Inferior gemellus muscle

Quadratus femoris muscle

Greater trochanter of femur

Figure 3.22. Muscles of the gluteal region: posterior view of the buttock with gluteus maximus removed, showing the passage of the sciatic nerve in the buttock before it progresses down the leg posteriorly.

Gluteus medius

- Originates in the gluteal fold of the ilium.
- Inserts into the greater trochanter of the femur.

Gluteus minimus

- The origin is under cover of the gluteus medius from the gluteal fold of the ilium.
- Inserts into the greater trochanter of the femur.

Nerve supply to gluteus medius and minimus is via the superior gluteal nerve (L4, 5, S1). The superior gluteal nerve emerges from the greater sciatic foramen, supplying both gluteus medius and minimis. Actions of both gluteus medius and minimus are as abductors of the hip, but more accurately they prevent adduction of the hip during walking (tested for by the Trendelenberg test).

Note

- The Trendelenberg test is positive when the patient tries to raise one leg from the ground to stand on one foot only, and when the abductors of the hip on the contralateral side to the leg raised are weak, the patient will lean heavily to one side to maintain balance (lean to the side of the weak abductors as an overcompensation).

Piriformis muscle

- Very important and a favourite of examiners, for the relations it forms in the gluteal region.
- Origin is from the middle three fused vertebrae of the sacrum.
- Inserts into the greater trochanter of the femur.
- Passes through the greater sciatic foramen (fills it).
- Therefore, everything else emerging from the greater sciatic foramen must either be above or below it (above are the superior gluteal artery, vein, nerve; below are the inferior gluteal artery, vein, nerve, pudendal nerve, nerve to quadratus femoris, nerve to obturator internus, and the sciatic nerve).
- Nerve supply is via S1 and S2.

Obturator internus and gemelli

- Stabilise the hip joint during walking.

Quadratus femoris

- Stabilises the hip joint during walking.

Trochanteric anastomosis

- Source of blood supply for the head of the femur, via the capsule.
- Anastomosis of the superior gluteal artery, and the medial and lateral circumflex femoral arteries. The superior gluteal artery emerges from the pelvis above the piriformis muscle, supplying all three gluteal muscles and continues to form the trochanteric anastomosis (which supplies the femoral head, via the capsule).

Note

- Gluteal intramuscular injections must be in the upper outer quadrant to avoid the sciatic nerve.

Hip joint (Figure 3.23)

The hip joint has a good range of movement and stability (rare to have both in a joint). It is a synovial joint with an extremely strong capsule. The head of the femur sits in the acetabulum (made from the three hip bones, the pubis, ilium and ischium with a Y-shaped cut-off between them). The acetabulum has a C-shaped hyaline cartilage lining, which continues as a labrum (lip), deepening the joint, and contains the haversian fat pad in its non-articular section. The head of the femur also has a hyaline cartilage covering, and ligamentum teres in its centre attaching it to the acetabulum.

The capsule of the hip joint is attached to the intertrochanteric line anteriorly and to half way along the neck of the femur posteriorly. It also contains the retinacular fibres in which the trochanteric anastomosis inserts its arterial supply to the head of the femur.

The ligaments of the hip joint are:

- Iliofemoral ligament (of Bigelow). This is V- not Y-shaped, anterior and is very strong.
- Pubofemoral ligament.
- Ischiofemoral ligament.

(a)

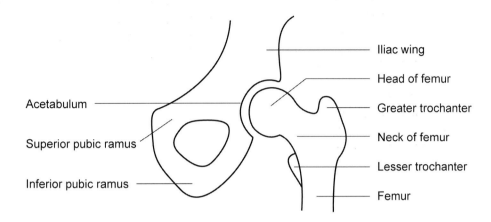

Acetabulum

Superior pubic ramus

Inferior pubic ramus

Iliac wing

Head of femur

Greater trochanter

Neck of femur

Lesser trochanter

Femur

(b)

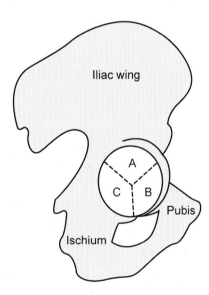

Iliac wing

A

C   B

Pubis

Ischium

Figure 3.23. The hip joint. (a) AP view of the hip joint (with left hemi-pelvis). (b) Lateral view of the acetabulum of the right hip (A = portion of acetabulum from ilium; B = portion of acetabulum from pubic bone; C = portion of acetabulum from ischium.

The blood supply of the head of the femur is as follows:

- Trochanteric anastomosis via the capsule.
- Ligamentum teres (atrophies after seven years of age).
- Nutrient arteries of the neck of the femur.

Note

— This blood supply is, of course, crucial to the orthopaedic management of neck of femur fractures. The fundamental principle is that if the capsule of the hip joint is damaged by an intracapsular fracture, i.e. proximal neck of the femur and hence the blood supply to the head of the femur is potentially compromised, it should be removed entirely at surgery, necessitating a hemi-arthroplasty (half a hip replacement, literally). Furthermore, if the fracture is distal to the capsule of the hip joint, it is considered to be extracapsular (i.e. basicervical or inter-trochanteric fractures) and hence the head of the femur is not at risk and can be preserved in surgical fixation (the dynamic hip screw).

Disturbance to the blood supply to the head of the femur will necessarily result in avascular necrosis of the head.

Surgical approaches to the hip joint (see Chapter 4)

- Anterior: between sartorius and tensor fascia lata (TFL). Detach TFL, rectus femoris and the anterior parts of gluteus medius and minimus; the joint capsule can then be reached.
- Lateral (anterolateral): undermines gluteus medius from the anterior femoral neck. The joint capsule lies underneath the muscle bellies of gluteus medius and minimus.
- Posterior: split the middle of gluteus maximus (in line with fibres). Detach piriformis, obturator internus and gemelli from their femoral attachments to expose the capsule. The sciatic nerve needs to be identified in this approach and preserved.

The tibia

This is the larger of the two bones of the lower leg (the other is the fibula), with a large upper end and a small lower end. It is mostly a subcutaneous bone. The periosteum of the tibia over its medial portion is subcutaneous; this is the reason a direct blow to the shin is so painful, as periosteal pain is particularly unpleasant in character. The superior articular surface is the tibial plateau, divided into medial and lateral tibial condyles. It articulates with the femoral condyles and is covered with cartilage menisci (medial is oval and lateral is circular). Between the tibial condyles is the intercondylar eminence (tibial spine). Anterior to the intercondylar eminence is the origin of the anterior cruciate ligament (ACL), and posterior to the intercondylar eminence is the posterior cruciate ligament (PCL). This is relevant to ACL injuries (seen more commonly in children) as, on X-ray, an avulsion fracture of the tibial spine occurs as a result of the ACL having pulled the portion of bone, here, with it, as the result of an injury.

The knee joint

This is a synovial joint and therefore has a capsule. The capsule is attached to the circumference of the tibial plateau in continuity, except for two places:

- Laterally where the tendon of the popliteus passes through it.
- Posteriorly where it attaches below the PCL origin.

The tibia also articulates with the fibula superiorly, a synovial joint with a capsule, the superior tibiofibular joint.

Note

— The tibia has an anterior tuberosity above which the patella inserts.

The shaft of the tibia is triangular but as it travels down it becomes rectangular to then form the medial malleolus, part of the ankle joint, which is a synovial joint with a capsule.

The ankle

The ankle is a hinge joint (not 100%, but the amount of rotation is very small). It is a synovial joint with the capsule in contact with all three bones in the joint (the tibia, fibula and talus). The joint is stabilised by both medial and lateral malleoli. Most of the articulation is between the tibia and talus. The medial ligament is the deltoid, which has two components: deep and superficial (deltoid is triangular), that join the tibia to the talus. The lateral ligament is the talofibular which has two components: anterior and posterior.

Blood supply of the capsule and ligaments is via the anterior and posterior tibial arteries and peroneal artery. Nerve supply is via the deep peroneal and tibial nerves. Plantar flexion results from contraction of gastrocnemius and soleus. Dorsiflexion results from contraction of tibialis anterior and peroneus tertius.

The fascial compartments of the leg

Fascial leg compartments are especially relevant in the clinical setting, as they provide inextensible boundaries that are responsible for the entity called compartment syndrome (Figure 3.24). This entity will

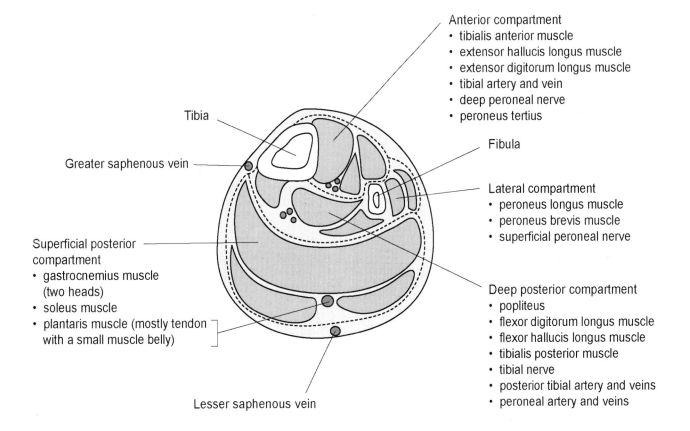

Anterior compartment
- tibialis anterior muscle
- extensor hallucis longus muscle
- extensor digitorum longus muscle
- tibial artery and vein
- deep peroneal nerve
- peroneus tertius

Tibia

Fibula

Greater saphenous vein

Lateral compartment
- peroneus longus muscle
- peroneus brevis muscle
- superficial peroneal nerve

Superficial posterior compartment
- gastrocnemius muscle (two heads)
- soleus muscle
- plantaris muscle (mostly tendon with a small muscle belly)

Deep posterior compartment
- popliteus
- flexor digitorum longus muscle
- flexor hallucis longus muscle
- tibialis posterior muscle
- tibial nerve
- posterior tibial artery and veins
- peroneal artery and veins

Lesser saphenous vein

Figure 3.24. Compartment syndrome of the leg (axial section through the right leg, viewed from above).

most commonly be seen in the trauma setting, after a tibial fracture (or a circumferential leg burn). Haematoma and soft-tissue swelling raise the pressure in the compartment affected; a vicious cycle then ensues. When the pressure has risen beyond that of the venous blood flow, venous return is impeded, forcing pressure in the compartment higher. The pressure will then exceed arterial and impede the flow of arterial blood. Ischaemic damage follows to the compartmental structures and the distal foot. The patient is in tremendous pain, and this characteristically cannot be relieved by even opiate analgesics. This ischaemic damage rapidly becomes permanent, i.e. the ischaemia turns to necrosis. This myonecrosis results in joint contractures (termed Volkman's ischaemic contracture). The end result is a painful, useless limb.

The fascial compartment's inelasticity is the problem, which is solved by a fasciotomy (vertical incision through skin and fascia along the length of the leg).

There is a common trick question in clinical and viva exams pertaining to an imaginary attractive, young female (or male!) patient, who has compartment syndrome: would you perhaps consider making a small skin incision, and performing a fasciotomy using a tendon stripper subcutaneously? The argument for this approach is that the scar left behind will be more cosmetically acceptable, and that the skin is extensible over the cut fascia so that the compartment will have been decompressed anyway. Do not be tempted by the subtle logic of this question, as clinicians who have tried this technique have frequently fallen foul of not cutting enough fascia and as a consequence have left an even more cosmetically unacceptable result of contracture (with a poor functional component). The answer should always be to perform a full fasciotomy.

The four compartments of the leg

- Extensor.
- Lateral.
- Superficial posterior.
- Deep posterior.

Extensor compartment of the leg

Bounded by the deep fascia of the leg and the interosseous membrane, medially by the tibia, and laterally by the fibula, and by the anterior intermuscular septum of the leg.

This compartment contains four muscles:

- Tibialis anterior.
- Extensor hallucis longus.
- Extensor digitorum longus.
- Peroneus tertius.

Motor innervation of all four muscles is supplied by the deep peroneal nerve (from the bifurcation of the common peroneal nerve), which also supplies sensation to the anterior tibial and fibular periosteum.

Muscles of the extensor compartment are responsible for extension of the ankle and toes.

Tendons pass under superior and inferior extensor retinacula, except for tibialis anterior which pierces the superior extensor retinaculum, but is slung under the inferior flexor retinaculum.

Blood supply is from the anterior tibial artery, which arises from the popliteal artery. Tibialis anterior is to be found medial to the anterior tibial artery, and extensor digitorum longus and peroneus tertius are to be found lateral to the anterior tibial artery.

Lateral compartment of the leg

Bounded by the deep fascia of the leg, the fibula, and the anterior and posterior intermuscular septae of the leg.

This compartment contains two muscles:

- Peroneus longus.
- Peroneus brevis.

These are both evertors of the ankle.

The lateral compartment also contains the superficial peroneal nerve.

Blood supply is from branches of the peroneal artery. Venous drainage is into the small saphenous vein.

Posterior compartment of the leg

This compartment contains deep and superficial muscle groups, and is commonly called the calf. It is bounded posteriorly, laterally and medially by the deep fascia of the leg, and anteriorly by the tibia, fibula and interosseous septum.

Note

— The deep fascia of the leg is continuous with the subcutaneous tibia, flexor retinaculum, and tendo-achilles inferiorly.

Superficial muscle group

Gastrocnemius, soleus and plantaris all converge into a common tendon (tendo-achilles); these muscles are major plantar flexors of the ankle and foot.

Deep muscle group

Popliteus, flexor digitorum longus, flexor hallucis longus and tibialis posterior all pass under the flexor retinaculum to the sole of the foot (for inversion of the foot).

The nerve supply of the posterior compartment of the leg is the tibial nerve, a continuation of the sciatic nerve (runs deep to soleus).

Blood supply of the posterior compartment of the leg is via the posterior tibial artery, a branch of the popliteal artery and its peroneal branch.

Cutaneous sensation of the lower leg is derived from numerous nerves, including the posterior femoral cutaneous, sural, peroneal, tibial, common peroneal and saphenous nerves.

The foot

The sensory nerve supply to the foot is predominantly from the superficial peroneal nerve (covering the majority of the dorsum), but also from the sural nerve (lateral border), saphenous nerve (medial border), and a small contribution from the deep peroneal nerve (first web space, i.e. between the great and index toes).

The veins form into a dorsal venous arch and drain into the great and small saphenous veins medially and laterally, respectively.

The only muscle of the dorsum of the foot is the extensor digitorum brevis which is supplied by the deep peroneal nerve in common with all the other foot extensors.

Note

— The extensor digitorum brevis muscle is visible as a bulge on the lateral aspect of the foot when the toes are extended. Its absence is a positive clinical sign on an L5-S1 prolapsed intervertebral disc.

The arterial supply of the dorsum of the foot is via the anterior tibial artery, which then becomes the dorsalis pedis artery; this dives deep towards the sole (from the first intermetatarsal space) to form the plantar arch, with the lateral plantar artery.

Bones of the foot (Figure 3.25)

◆ Talus. Lies on top of the calcaneus, supported by the sustentaculum tali and bears the weight of the entire body.
◆ Calcaneum. The heel bone, in contact with the ground, has the sustentaculum tali as part of it.
◆ Navicular. Articulates with the talus posteriorly in the medial foot, and with the medial cuneiform laterally.

Note

— Navicular means 'boat like', and is the foot equivalent of the scaphoid (which also, interestingly, means 'boat like'). Both are located proximal to the first metacarpal/tarsal, i.e. on the same side of the hand as the thumb, and the same side of the foot as the great toe.

◆ Cuneiforms (medial, intermediate and lateral, articulate with the metatarsals).

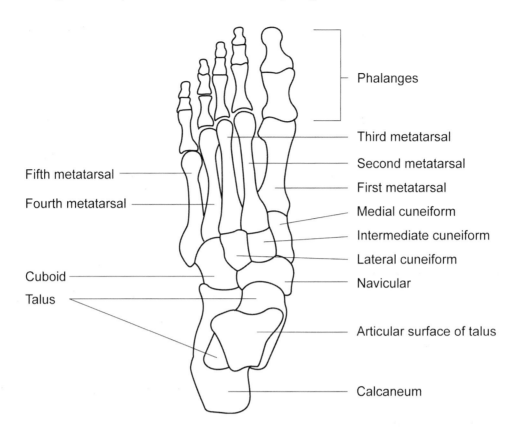

Figure 3.25. Bones of the foot (dorsal surface).

◆ Cuboid (lateral bone also articulates with the metatarsals).
◆ Metatarsals (five).
◆ Phalanges (of which there are 12 in the lesser toes and two in the great toe, making a total of 14).

Arches of the foot

◆ Medial longitudinal arch.
◆ Lateral longitudinal arch.
◆ Transverse arch (this arch is only complete when both feet are placed together; the above two arches are complete entities on individual feet).

Note

— Arches are maintained by bony architecture, ligaments and tendons.

Propulsive mechanism of the foot

The foot is not simply a rigid structure. Its bony, ligamentous, tendinous and muscular architecture combine to make an efficient composite for mobilisation. (This is much less efficient than the feet of many animals, however, as most of them have the benefit of four limbs for balance and propulsion, and have not had to make sacrifices for bipedal locomotion, freeing up their upper limbs for manipulation).

The major propulsive muscles are gastrocnemius and soleus. The propulsive action is enhanced by arching of the foot and flexion of the toes.

The sequence of events of walking is:

◆ Heel strike.
◆ Support phase.

◆ Toe off.
◆ Swing phase.

Note

— In running, the heel remains off the ground.

The weight of the foot, in walking, is taken successively by heel, lateral border, and ball of the foot. The last part to leave the ground is the medial longitudinal arch.

The cervical spine (Figure 3.26)

There are seven cervical vertebrae:

◆ C1 and 2 are specialised.
◆ C1 is known as the atlas (holds the world on its back).
◆ C2 is known as the axis (allows rotation and has an odontoid peg projecting into C1).
◆ C3-6 are typical cervical vertebrae, because they all have similar anatomical properties.
◆ C7 is atypical, the so-called vertebra prominens (it is prominent posteriorly, visible in slim people, protruding at the base of the neck).
◆ The cervical spine has a characteristic lordosis in the normal individual.

The thoracic spine (Figure 3.27)

There are 12 thoracic vertebrae. They differ from the cervical vertebrae by having longer pedicles. They have a smaller vertebral foramen (the circular space framed by pedicles and laminae through which the spinal cord passes), as the cord (having given off cervical branches) is less large at this level and there are longer spinous processes than the typical cervical vertebra (with the possible exception of the vertebra prominens, C7). There are no vertebral artery foraminae and they have more pronounced transverse processes. One specialised adaptation of thoracic vertebrae is their articulations with the ribs with facets on both the vertebral body and transverse process. The thoracic spine has a characteristic kyphosis in the normal individual.

The lumbar spine (Figure 3.28)

There are five lumbar vertebrae. They differ from thoracic vertebrae by having a larger, and wider, vertebral body. They have more posteriorly oriented transverse processes. Obviously, there are no ribs (nor corresponding articular surfaces). The vertebral foramen is more triangular. The lumbar spine has a characteristic lordosis in the normal individual. The fifth lumbar vertebra articulates with the sacrum beneath it.

VASCULAR ANATOMY

Major branches of the abdominal aorta (Figure 3.29)

◆ Coeliac trunk.
◆ Superior mesenteric artery.
◆ Inferior mesenteric artery (behind the third part of the duodenum).
◆ Adrenal arteries (split into smaller branches before entering the adrenal glands).
◆ Renal arteries (level of L2 vertebra).

Note

— The left renal artery gives off an adrenal branch, but the right adrenal artery actually branches directly from the aorta. Each renal artery gives off a ureteric branch.

◆ Gonadal arteries. There is a similar origin and course in both sexes: it is the testicular artery in men, and the ovarian artery in women. The ovarian artery enters the suspensory ligament to serve the ovary and tube. The testicular artery runs along the pelvic brim and then enters the inguinal canal travelling with the spermatic cord to the testis.
◆ Inferior phrenic arteries.
◆ Lumbar arteries, of which there are four, at the level of their corresponding lumbar vertebra; there is none at L5 - its place is taken by the iliolumbar artery.

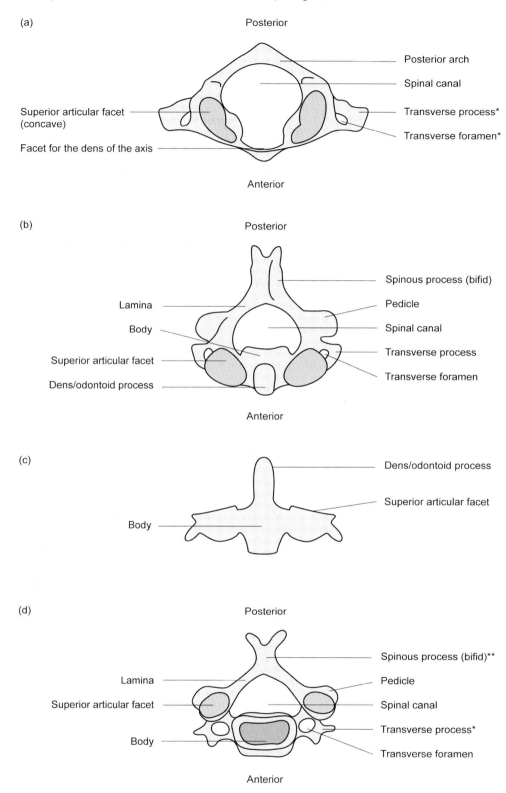

Figure 3.26. The cervical spine: (a) atlas viewed from top. * = nothing goes through the foramen. The vertebral artery passes posterior to it, leaving a characteristic groove in the bone; (b) axis viewed from top; (c) axis viewed from the front; (d) 'typical' vertebra (C3-6). * = The vertebral artery passes through these foramina; ** = The major difference between a typical vertebra and C7 (vertebra prominens) is that the spinous process is non-bifid and much longer.

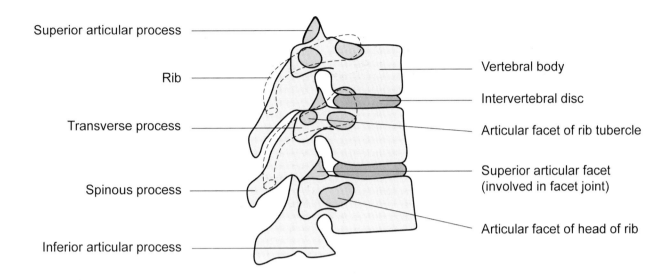

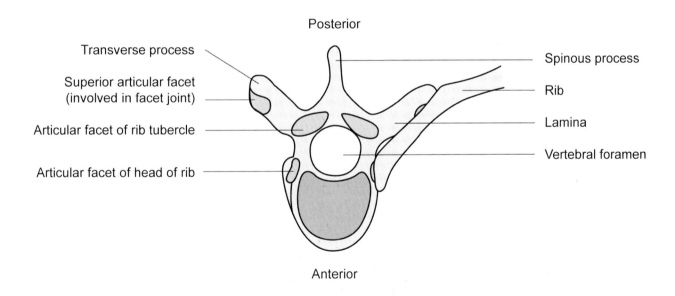

Figure 3.27. Thoracic spine.

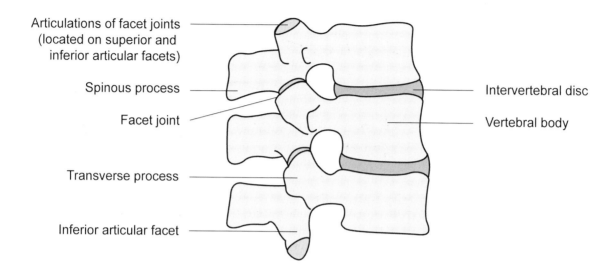

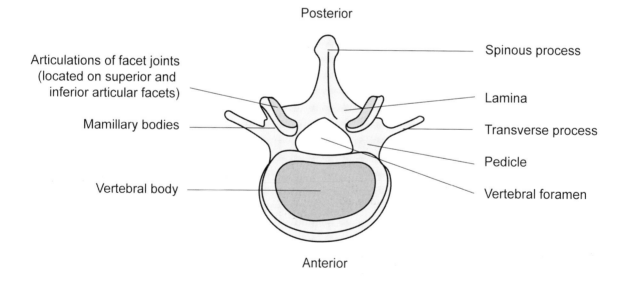

Figure 3.28. Lumbar spine.

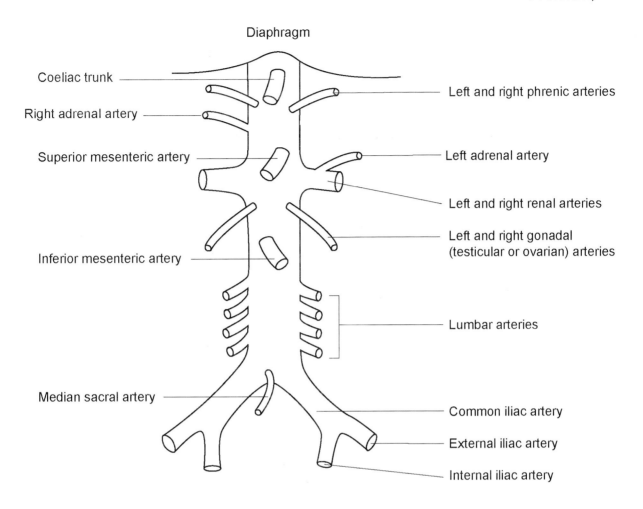

Diaphragm

Coeliac trunk

Right adrenal artery

Superior mesenteric artery

Inferior mesenteric artery

Median sacral artery

Left and right phrenic arteries

Left adrenal artery

Left and right renal arteries

Left and right gonadal
(testicular or ovarian) arteries

Lumbar arteries

Common iliac artery

External iliac artery

Internal iliac artery

Figure 3.29. Major branches of the abdominal aorta.

◆ Common iliac arteries, L4, which further subdivide into the internal and external iliac arteries.

The external iliac artery enters the femoral sheath, becoming the femoral artery. The internal iliac artery enters the pelvis.

The inferior vena cava (Figure 3.30)

The inferior vena cava (IVC) is formed by the convergence of the common iliac veins at the level of the L5 vertebra. It then runs upwards and to the right of the aorta.

It pierces the central tendon of the diaphragm at the level of T8, having invaginated the posterior liver (called the bare area).

Note

— The branches of the IVC do not match the aorta because of the drainage into the portal circulation.

Branches from the common iliac veins onwards are the 4th and 3rd lumbar veins (bilaterally), right gonadal vein, both renal veins, right lumbar azygos vein, right adrenal vein, and both inferior phrenic veins.

Diaphragm

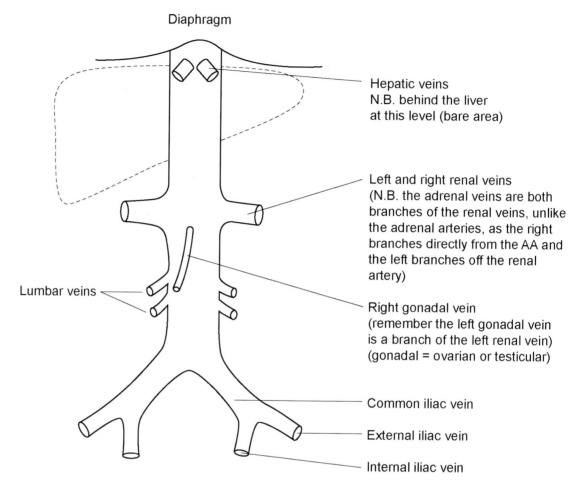

Hepatic veins
N.B. behind the liver
at this level (bare area)

Left and right renal veins
(N.B. the adrenal veins are both
branches of the renal veins, unlike
the adrenal arteries, as the right
branches directly from the AA and
the left branches off the renal
artery)

Lumbar veins

Right gonadal vein
(remember the left gonadal vein
is a branch of the left renal vein)
(gonadal = ovarian or testicular)

Common iliac vein

External iliac vein

Internal iliac vein

Figure 3.30. The inferior vena cava.

Lymph nodes

The alimentary tract, liver, pancreas, biliary tract and spleen are drained by the pre-aortic nodes. The lower limb drains into the deep inguinal nodes along the external iliac vessels into the para-aortic nodes.

Both aortic groups join the cysterna chyli, which becomes continuous with the thoracic duct and empties into the confluence of the left internal jugular and subclavian vein.

Upper limb vascular anatomy

The brachial artery is a continuation of the axillary artery, which is itself a continuation of the subclavian artery (Figure 3.31). It splits into radial (more

Note

- The subclavian artery becomes the axillary artery beyond the first rib, then the brachial artery (Figure 3.32) beyond the teres major muscle. It is the only major artery in the upper arm, which then goes on to divide beyond the elbow joint.
- The brachial artery divides within the antecubital fossa (see the section on 'The radius and ulna' for boundaries of the antecubital fossa).

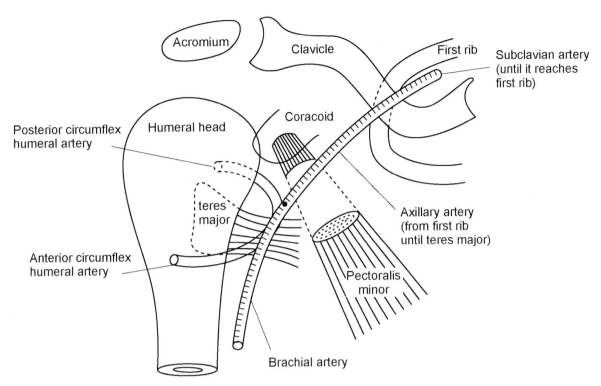

Figure 3.31. Axillary artery.

Anterior view of rotator cuff

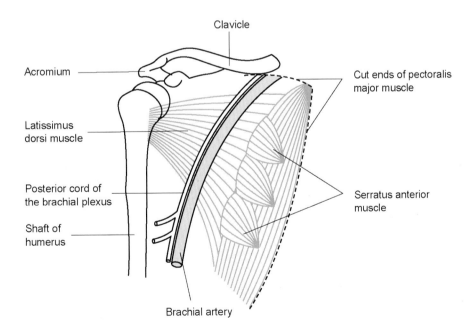

NB. Lies anterior to latissimus dorsi, on its belly.
Starts as subclavian artery when it is behind the clavicle,
then becomes axillary artery as it passes the teres
major muscle, thereafter, is known as the brachial artery.

Figure 3.32. Brachial artery.

superficial and lateral) and ulnar (deeper and more medial) arteries. The radial artery has a recurrent radial branch laterally.

The ulnar artery has an ulnar recurrent branch and a common interosseous branch (splits to form anterior and posterior interosseous arteries) (Figure 3.33).

Note

— Both radial and ulnar arteries anastomose in the palm to form a superficial and deep palmar arch which gives off the digital arteries supplying each digit with radial and ulnar collateral arteries as part of their neurovascular bundles (Figure 3.34).

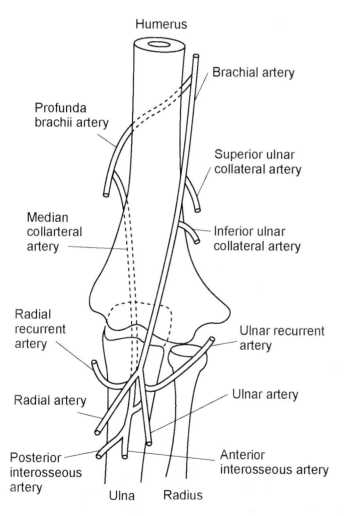

Figure 3.33. Brachial, radial and ulnar arteries in the elbow.

Axillary lymph nodes

The axillary lymph nodes are divided into different groups anatomically. This is particularly relevant in breast surgery when performing an axillary clearance or node sampling. The groups are:

♦ Anterior (pectoral).
♦ Posterior (subscapular).
♦ Lateral.
♦ Central.
♦ Apical.

Lower limb vascular anatomy

Femoral artery (Figure 3.35)

The femoral artery is a direct continuation of the external iliac artery. It enters the femoral triangle at the mid-inguinal point. This is a favourite question of examiners in clinical exams, which is often followed up with a question as to the landmarks used in locating it. It is located at exactly half the distance between the anterior superior iliac spine and pubic symphysis.

Branches of the femoral artery are:

♦ Profunda femoris. Arises laterally, supplying all the muscles of the thigh.
♦ Lateral circumflex femoral artery. Ascending, transverse and descending branches. (N.B. The ascending branch takes part in the trochanteric anastomosis, supplying the retinacular fibres in the capsule of the hip joint to the femoral head).
♦ Medial circumflex femoral artery.
♦ Perforating arteries. There are four of these, which supply the adductor muscles and the hamstrings.

Femoral vein (Figure 3.36)

The femoral vein receives the great saphenous vein as its tributary on the anteromedial side in the femoral triangle. It then travels proximally to become the external iliac vein.

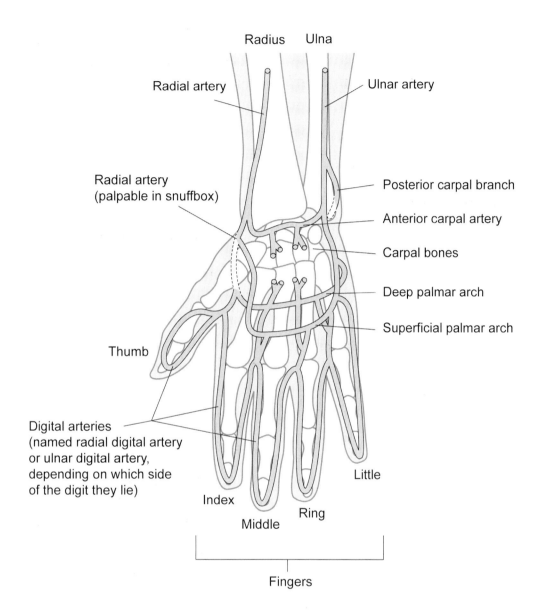

Radius   Ulna

Radial artery

Ulnar artery

Radial artery
(palpable in snuffbox)

Posterior carpal branch

Anterior carpal artery

Carpal bones

Deep palmar arch

Superficial palmar arch

Thumb

Digital arteries
(named radial digital artery
or ulnar digital artery,
depending on which side
of the digit they lie)

Little

Index

Ring

Middle

Fingers

Figure 3.34. Radial and ulnar arteries as they become deep and superficial palmar arches in the hand.

The femoral and saphenous veins are distinguished by the fact that the femoral vein receives only one tributary in the triangle. However, the great saphenous vein receives other tributaries (a useful fact in 'high tie' varicose vein surgery, so that the correct vein is tied ensuring success of the operation).

Femoral nerve (Figure 3.37)

The femoral nerve is a nerve of the extensor compartment of the thigh and is derived from L2, 3 and 4. It enters the thigh by passing deep to the inguinal ligament at the lateral edge of the femoral sheath (which separates it from the artery).

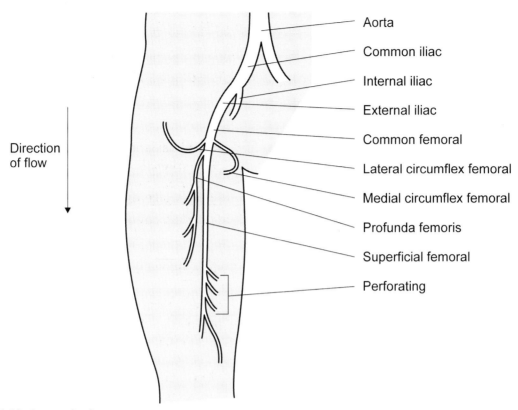

Aorta

Common iliac

Internal iliac

External iliac

Common femoral

Lateral circumflex femoral

Medial circumflex femoral

Profunda femoris

Superficial femoral

Perforating

Direction of flow

Figure 3.35. Femoral artery.

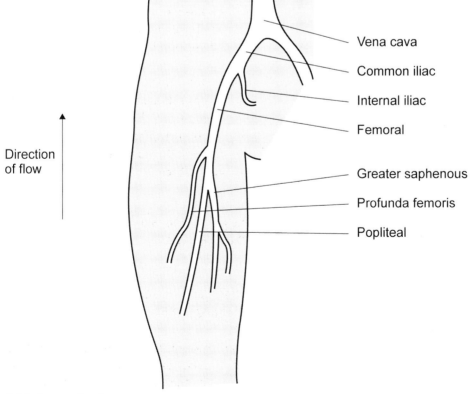

Vena cava

Common iliac

Internal iliac

Femoral

Greater saphenous

Profunda femoris

Popliteal

Direction of flow

Figure 3.36. Femoral vein.

Adductor canal (aka subsartorial or Hunter's canal)

The adductor canal lies between the sartorius muscle (roof) and adductor longus (floor).

Contents:

◆ Superficial femoral artery.
◆ Femoral vein.
◆ Saphenous nerve.
◆ Subsartorial plexus (also nerve to vastus medialis in upper part of canal).

Compartments of the thigh

Anterior (extensor) compartment

◆ Muscles (vastus medius, intermedius, lateralis and rectus femoris).
◆ Nerve supply (femoral nerve L3, 4).
◆ Separated from the posterior (hamstring) compartment by lateral and medial intermuscular septae.

Medial (adductor) compartment

◆ Muscles (adductor magnus, longus and brevis, gracilis, obturator externus).
◆ Nerve supply (obturator nerve).

Posterior (hamstring) compartment

◆ Muscles (semimembranosus, semitendinosus, biceps femoris).
◆ Nerve supply (sciatic nerve).
◆ Separated from the anterior (extensor) compartment by the lateral intermuscular septum.

Popliteal fossa

See page 128.

Vascular anatomy below the knee (Figure 3.38)

The popliteal artery gives off the anterior tibial artery, leaving the tibioperoneal trunk to continue vertically for 1cm. This divides into the posterior tibial artery and peroneal artery. This is referred to as the

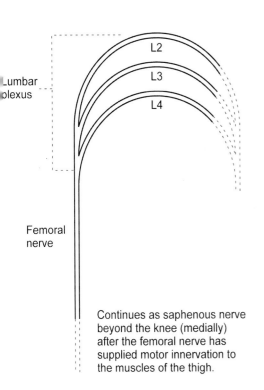

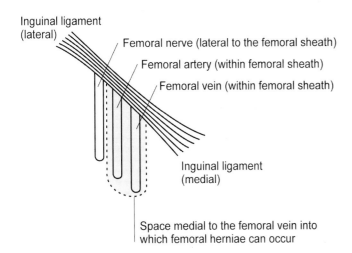

Figure 3.37. Femoral nerve.

Left-figure labels:

Lumbar plexus

L2
L3
L4

Femoral nerve

Continues as saphenous nerve beyond the knee (medially) after the femoral nerve has supplied motor innervation to the muscles of the thigh.

Inguinal ligament (lateral)

Femoral nerve (lateral to the femoral sheath)

Femoral artery (within femoral sheath)

Femoral vein (within femoral sheath)

Inguinal ligament (medial)

Space medial to the femoral vein into which femoral herniae can occur

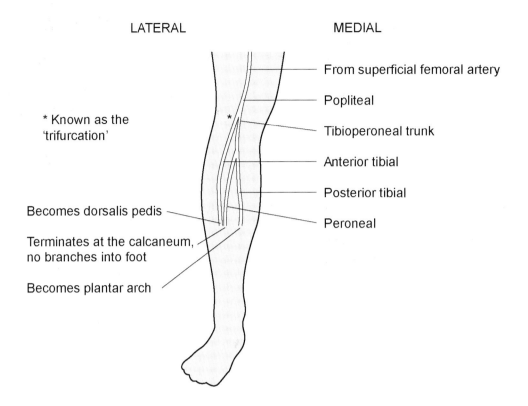

LATERAL   MEDIAL

From superficial femoral artery

Popliteal

* Known as the 'trifurcation'

Tibioperoneal trunk

Anterior tibial

Posterior tibial

Becomes dorsalis pedis

Peroneal

Terminates at the calcaneum, no branches into foot

Becomes plantar arch

Figure 3.38. Vascular anatomy of the lower leg.

'trifurcation', even though it is two divisions of a single artery in rapid succession.

The anterior tibial artery becomes the dorsalis pedis artery in the foot, and the posterior tibial artery becomes the plantar arch vessels inferior to the metatarsals of the foot.

HEAD AND NECK ANATOMY

Anatomy of the meninges

Knowing which form of vascular structure is found within each meningeal layer is the basis from which an understanding of the type of intracranial haemorrhages can originate.

The meningeal layers are (Figure 3.39):

◆ Dura mata. Adherent to the periosteum.

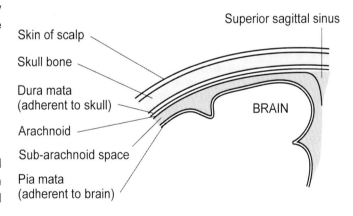

Skin of scalp

Skull bone

Dura mata (adherent to skull)

Arachnoid

Sub-arachnoid space

Pia mata (adherent to brain)

Superior sagittal sinus

BRAIN

Figure 3.39. The three meningeal layers.

- Arachnoid mata. Lies between the dura mata (to which it is adherent) and the pia mata.
- Pia mata. The surface lining of the brain.

Anatomical spaces (relating to intracranial bleeds) are (Figure 3.40):

- Extradural - between the periosteum and dura, containing the middle meningeal artery.
- Subdural - between the dura and arachnoid, containing bridging veins which drain to the venous sinuses.
- Subarachnoid - between the arachnoid and pia mata, containing CSF and the arteries of the circle of Willis and cerebral arteries.

Anatomy of the scalp

Layers of SCALP (from superficial to deep)

A mnemonic for SCALP is Skin, Connective tissue, Aponeurosis, Loose areolar tissue, Pericranium.

Note

— All mnemonics seem to have at least one 'contrived' portion. In this case it is clearly the 'Loose areolar tissue'. But such a contrivance actually helps the reader to remember the mnemonic.

Extradural haematoma (appearance on CT)

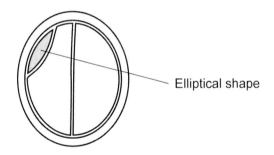

Elliptical shape

Subdural haematoma (appearance on CT)

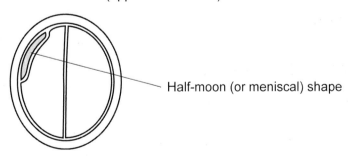

Half-moon (or meniscal) shape

Figure 3.40. Types of intracranial bleed.

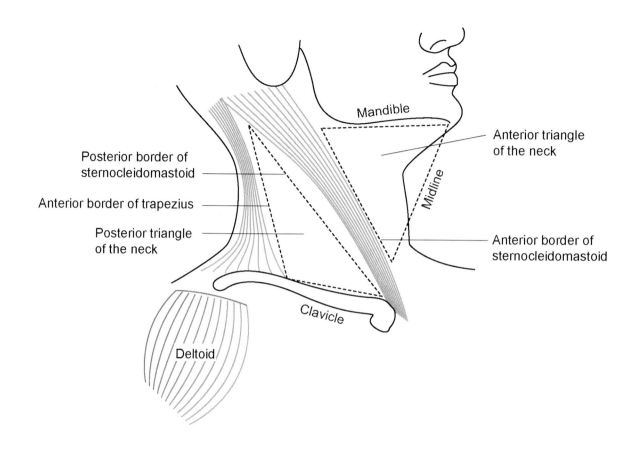

Figure 3.41. Triangles of the neck

Triangles of the neck

Posterior triangle (Figure 3.41)

The anatomic relations of the posterior triangle are:

- Trapezius.
- Sternocleidomastoid (SCM).
- Clavicle.

The contents of the posterior triangle are:

- Accessory nerve (from one third down the SCM to one third up trapezius).
- Cervical plexus.

Note

— This contains the nerves C1, 2, 3, 4.

- Brachial plexus (trunks), although technically they are deep to the prevertebral fascia which is the floor of the posterior triangle.
- Lymph nodes.
- A small part of the subclavian artery.
- External jugular vein (as it heads towards the subclavian vein).
- Transverse cervical artery and vein.

Anterior triangle

The anatomic relations of the anterior triangle are:

◆ Anterior border of SCM.
◆ Midline.
◆ Mandible.

The structures found within the anterior triangle are:

◆ Hyoid bone.
◆ Suprahyoid muscles (mylohyoid, digastric, stylohyoid, geniohyoid).
◆ Infrahyoid muscles (omohyoid, thyrohyoid, sternothyroid, sternohyoid).
◆ Thyroid gland.
◆ Thyroid cartilage.
◆ Cricoid cartilage.
◆ Submandibular gland.
◆ Lymph nodes.

Note

– The common carotid artery lies deep to the SCM.

Neck lymph nodes

◆ Occipital and pre-auricular - drain scalp.
◆ Submental - drains lips and tongue tip.
◆ Submandibular - drains mouth and tongue.
◆ Prelaryngeal - drains larynx.
◆ Supraclavicular - drains breast, lung, viscera.
◆ Deep cervical nodes are in receipt of lymph from ALL channels from the head and neck.
◆ Pretracheal - drains trachea.

Note

– Lymphadenopathy is not necessarily due to drainage from an anatomical position. It can be due to systemic disease, e.g. HIV, TB, toxoplasmosis, leukaemia, lymphoma, etc.

The thoracic outlet

The thoracic outlet is the surgical name for what anatomists call the thoracic inlet (the two are the same). It contains the major structures going to and from the trunk and head, as detailed in the next sections.

The arch of the aorta (Figure 3.42)

The aorta ascends from the left ventricle and arches to the left, wraps around the left main bronchus, and becomes the thoracic aorta.

The arch has three main branches:

◆ Brachiocephalic artery, which gives off the right common carotid artery and the right subclavian artery.
◆ Left common carotid artery.
◆ Left subclavian artery.

Associated structures of the aortic arch include the ligamentum arteriosum (remnant of the ductus arteriosum, the connection from the aortic arch to the left pulmonary artery that bypasses the pulmonary circulation in the foetus), left recurrent laryngeal nerve, left vagus nerve, cardiac plexus and the pulmonary trunk (bifurcates into the left and right pulmonary arteries inferior to the arch).

Organs of the aortic arch:

◆ Aortic baroreceptors. Vagus innervated and responsible for reflex control of heart rate.
◆ Aortic bodies. Vagus innervated and responsible for reflex control of respiratory rate; they are a kind of chemoreceptor.

Great vessels of the head and neck

This is an important subject. You must be aware of the anatomy of these great vessels for the following reasons: central access, trauma, operations such as carotid endarterectomy and other head and neck surgery, and the living anatomy section of viva exams (you will be asked for very specific landmarks on the surface to help identify these structures).

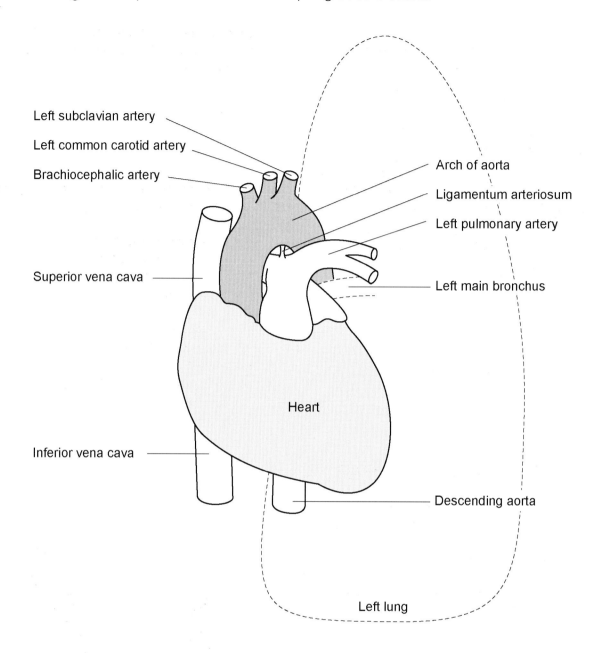

Figure 3.42. The arch of the aorta.

Carotid sheath contents (Figure 3.43)

- Common carotid artery (which has no branches before the bifurcation at the level of C3/4).
- Internal jugular vein.

- Vagus nerve.
- Ansa cervicalis. A cervical nerve plexus embedded in the anterior wall of the carotid sheath, but considered to be one of its contents.

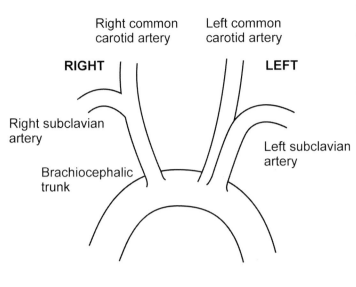

Figure 3.43. Carotid sheath contents.

endarterectomy' in Chapter 4) is from behind the upper SCM muscle, before it enters the parotid gland. The carotid sheath is then incised.

Note

— Beware of the hypoglossal nerve at this level.

The branches of the external carotid artery (before entering the parotid) are:

- ◆ Three anterior branches:
  - superior thyroid artery;
  - lingual artery;
  - facial artery.
- ◆ Posterior branches:
  - occipital artery;
  - posterior auricular artery.
- ◆ One medial branch:
  - ascending pharyngeal artery.

Note

— The sympathetic trunk is NOT (strictly speaking) one of the carotid sheath contents.
— The left common carotid artery is derived from the aortic arch directly. It passes behind the subclavian artery.
— The right common carotid artery is derived from the brachiocephalic trunk, which branches into this and the right subclavian artery.

External carotid artery (Figure 3.44)

Commences at the bifurcation of the common carotid artery, at the level of the hyoid bone, and travels upwards, giving off six branches before entering the parotid gland, where it divides into two: the maxillary and superficial temporal arteries.

For surgery, surface marking of the external carotid artery is between the angle of the mandible and the tragus of the ear. The surgical approach (see 'Carotid

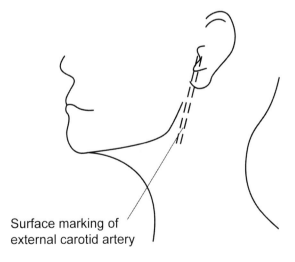

Figure 3.44. External carotid artery.

Note

– There is a small maxillary artery arising from the bifurcation itself.

Internal carotid artery

The internal carotid artery arises at the bifurcation of the common carotid artery (it is distinguished from the external carotid artery by virtue of it having no branches arising from it whatsoever), at the level of the hyoid bone. It has the carotid sinus at its origin and contains baroreceptors for blood pressure control.

At a similar level is the carotid body, a chemoreceptor and also the organ that, interestingly, has the greatest blood flow relative to its size in the body.

The internal carotid artery travels up lateral to the pharynx to the carotid canal at the base of the skull.

Surface marking of the internal carotid artery is in a line between the lateral horn of the hyoid and the head of the mandible. The surgical approach of the internal carotid artery (see 'Carotid endarterectomy' in Chapter 4) is by retracting the upper part of SCM and incising the carotid sheath.

Internal jugular vein (Figure 3.45)

The internal jugular vein emerges from the jugular foramen of the skull. The first tributary is the inferior petrosal sinus. It enters the carotid sheath and travels down with the carotid artery and vagus nerve. Termination of the vein is between the heads of SCM; then it joins the subclavian vein to become the brachiocephalic vein. Tributaries to the internal jugular vein are the inferior petrosal sinus, pharyngeal plexus, facial vein, lingual vein, and the superior and inferior thyroid veins.

Surface marking of the internal jugular vein is in a line from the lobule of the ear to the sternal end of SCM.

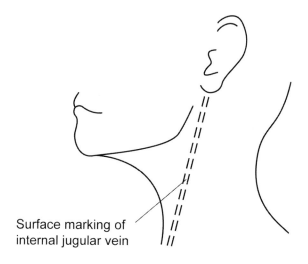

Surface marking of internal jugular vein

Figure 3.45. Internal jugular vein.

Anatomy of the oropharynx

The oropharynx extends from the soft palate to the epiglottis. The fauces at the back of the orpharynx are called palatopharyngeal and palatoglossal arches. The tonsils are, strictly speaking, called the palatine tonsils (to differentiate them from the lingual tonsils). The blood supply is via the palatine branch of the facial artery. Venous drainage is in the form of a plexus, but there is a large vein called the palatine vein, which can bleed a great deal post-tonsillectomy. Nerve supply is via a tonsillar branch of the glossopharyngeal nerve. Lymph drainage is to the deep cervical nodes.

The larynx

Functionally, the larynx is a protective sphincter for the lungs, adapted to provide speech. The larynx extends from the 3rd to the 6th vertebra.

The laryngeal framework (Figure 3.46) comprises the hyoid bone, thyroid cartilage, cricoid cartilage, epiglottic cartilage and arytenoid cartilage. The larynx lies between the epiglottis and the cricoid ring. Surgically, the larynx is subdivided into supraglottic, glottic and infraglottic components (this is useful in the TNM classification of laryngeal cancer).

Extrinsic muscles of the larynx are subdivided into elevators and depressors of the larynx (swallowing involves elevation of the larynx so that the glottis closes and food tracks over lateral channels).

Intrinsic muscles of the larynx are sudivided into abductors and adductors of the vocal cords.

Nerve supply of the larynx is from the vagus. This branches to form the superior laryngeal nerve, which supplies sensation, as well as motor fibres to the cricothyroid muscle, which is an adductor muscle of the vocal cords.

Also, the recurrent laryngeal nerve (left and right) supplies motor fibres to all muscles, except the cricothyroid muscle, which is supplied by the superior laryngeal nerve.

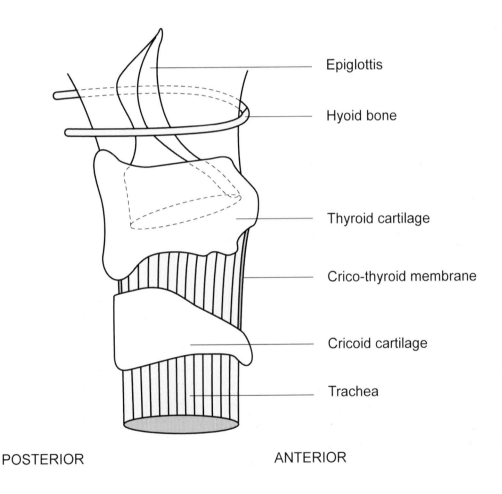

POSTERIOR   ANTERIOR

Figure 3.46. The larynx.

Note

- The left recurrent laryngeal nerve loops under the arch of the aorta and ligamentum arteriosus. The right recurrent laryngeal nerve loops under the subclavian artery.

Stridor

Stridor is an abnormal wheezing upper airway noise from turbulence of airflow in conditions of upper airway obstruction. Stridor has mural and extramural causes.

Mural causes

Laryngeal web, laryngomalacia, subglottic stenosis, angioedema, Wegener's granulomatosis, trauma (e.g. intubation), epiglottitis, polyps, laryngotracheo-bronchitis and malignancy.

Extramural causes

Trauma (e.g. bleeding following thyroidectomy), malignancy (e.g. bronchial, oesophageal, thyroid, lymphadenopathy) and neuropathy.

Note

- Heimlich's manoeuvre is used for a laryngeal foreign body or cricothyroidotomy.
- Epiglottitis is caused by *Haemophilus influenzae*.

Laryngeal nerve palsies

Unilateral recurrent laryngeal nerve palsy results in a hoarse voice. Bilateral recurrent laryngeal nerve palsy results in stridor.

Causes of recurrent laryngeal nerve palsy are:

- Post-thyroidectomy.
- Secondary to bronchial carcinoma.
- Secondary to aortic aneurysm.
- Right-sided recurrent laryngeal nerve palsy can be idiopathic.

Trachea

The trachea is joined to the cricoid cartilage by the tracheal ligament and is positioned in front of the oesophagus. It starts at the level of C6 and has a total length of 10cm (15cm on deep inspiration). Incomplete rings of cartilage are present, which are deficient posteriorly. The recurrent laryngeal nerve tracks between the oesophagus and trachea. The thyroid is anterior to the trachea.

The tongue (Figure 3.47)

The main subdivisions are the dorsum, tip, inferior surface and root. The mucous membrane of the pharyngeal and oral part are of different origins and function: the oral part is for gripping of food and chewing, and the pharyngeal part is for swallowing. A lingual tonsil is located on the posterior third of the tongue.

The muscles of the tongue are:

- Genioglossus.
- Hyoglossus.
- Palatoglossus.
- Styloglossus.

Each one is paired, joining in the middle at the septum.

Blood supply is via the lingual artery. Venous drainage is via venous tributaries converging to make the lingual vein.

Nerve supply is via the:

- Hypoglossal nerve.
- Chorda tympani (facial).
- Glossopharyngeal nerve.

Lymph drainage is to the submandibular nodes and deep cervical nodes.

Note

- In cancer of the tongue, there can be spread across the midline (not restricted to one side or the other).
- The tongue tip drains to the submental nodes.

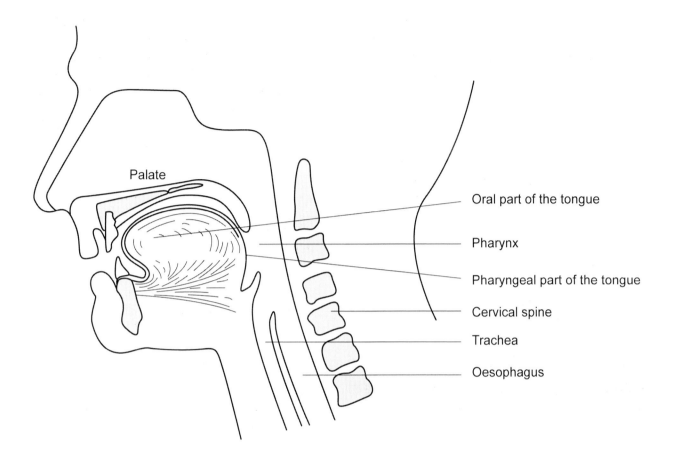

Palate

Oral part of the tongue

Pharynx

Pharyngeal part of the tongue

Cervical spine

Trachea

Oesophagus

Figure 3.47. The tongue.

Anatomy of the thyroid gland

The thyroid gland comprises two symmetrical lobes, united in front of the second, third and fourth tracheal rings. A capsule formed by the pretracheal fascia envelopes it completely. Lateral lobes are covered by the infrahyoid strap muscles:

♦ Sternohyoid.
♦ Sternothyroid.

The posterior surface overlaps the carotid sheath (common carotid artery, internal jugular vein, vagus nerve); this is where the parathyroid glands are usually located.

Note

— The recurrent laryngeal nerve enters the larynx posteriorly and runs posterior to the thyroid but always behind the pretracheal fascia.

The isthmus of the thyroid gland joins the lateral lobes together and is firmly adherent to the second, third and fourth tracheal rings. A pyramidal lobe projects upwards from the isthmus in the midline.

One of the unique properties of the thyroid gland is that it comprises 'follicles', meaning walled off colloid droplets of T3 and T4, not contained in the cells that actually secrete them. The thyroid gland also contains C cells, which are 'parafollicular' and are responsible for secreting calcitonin.

Blood supply is via the:

- Superior thyroid artery. This is the first branch of the external carotid artery, and pierces the pretracheal fascia before branching in the superior pole of the lateral lobe of the thyroid.
- Inferior thyroid artery. This is a branch of the thyrocervical trunk (from the subclavian artery; other branches being the suprascapular and transverse cervical arteries), and pierces the pretracheal fascia after having branched into 4-5 branches beneath the inferior pole of the thyroid gland.

Note

— In 3% of individuals there is a thyroidea IMA artery that enters the isthmus of the gland.

Venous drainage is via the superior and middle thyroid veins which drain into the internal jugular, and the inferior thyroid vein which drains into the brachiocephalic vein.

Lymph drainage is via the deep cervical lymph nodes. (N.B. These lie behind the SCM muscle).

NEURO-ANATOMY

Overall organisation of the nervous system

The nervous system is the means by which the brain interacts with its external environment, i.e. it senses the world around it and effects motor information into actions. A loop forms along the lines of sensation, information processing (brain) and motor (action). Then it loops around to sensation again in a cycle of self-awareness. The nervous system is divided into central (CNS) and peripheral (PNS) components. The basic element of the nervous system is the neurone and the means by which neurones transmit information is the synapse. The chemical means by which this communication is effected is the neurotransmitter.

The neurone

The cell body contains the nucleus and specialised organelles. The dendrite is a projection (of which there are usually many) from the cell body that contains neurofilaments and microfilaments, which are capable of chemical transport along their length. The axon is a specialised form of dendrite which is recognisable (from dendrites) by its greater length. Axons can be remarkably long, considering they are part of one cell only, for example, over a metre in length in some axons in the sciatic nerve. Axons are encased in Schwann cells in the PNS, a significant proportion of which are myelinated, i.e. coated in a substance, derived from Schwann cells, that markedly increases the conduction velocity of the nerve impulse, but there is no Schwann cell casing in the CNS nerves. The glial cells take on this function to some exent, regulating the chemical and physical environment of the CNS neurones.

The synapse

The synapse is the site of communication between two neurones, which can be from an axon to a dendrite (axodendritic synapse), but other types include:

- Axosomatic (axon to muscle).
- Axoaxonal (axon to axon).
- Dendrodendritic (dendrite to dendrite).

The axosomatic synapse at the end of a motor neurone is termed the neuromuscular junction (also known as the motor end plate).

The central nervous system (CNS)

The human brain contains 10^{12} neurones (there are ten times more glial, supportive cells of the neurones, present). It is bathed in cerebrospinal fluid (CSF) and lined by the meninges (see p.256, 'Head injury', for greater detail on the meninges).

The brain, fundamentally, has two main components: the forebrain and hindbrain. The forebrain is comprised of the:

- Frontal lobe.
- Parietal lobe.
- Temporal lobe.
- Occipital lobe.
- Thalamus.
- Hypothalamus.

The forebrain is often also referred to as the cerebrum.

The hindbrain is comprised of the:

- Midbrain.
- Pons.
- Medulla.
- Cerebellum.

As a direct continuation of the fore and hindbrains is the spinal cord. It is named by the vertebral level, i.e. cervical, thoracic, lumbar. However, beyond L2 the spinal cord ends (the conus) and divides into numerous branches, spinal nerves, called the cauda equina (because it is said to resemble a horse's tail). This continues, giving off branches at each vertebral level, until the base of the sacrum.

The spinal cord, when looked at in cross-section, contains both grey matter (central, in a 'bat's wing' shape, and grey because it contains the cell bodies and dendrites) and white matter (which surrounds the grey and is white because it is composed entirely of axons).

The spinal cord gives off branches, two for each vertebral level, called spinal roots. Spinal roots contain both neurones that are bringing sensory information in from the PNS (afferent), as well as neurones that are carrying motor (and other) information from the CNS to the PNS (efferent).

The equivalent to spinal roots in the head are the cranial nerves, numbered I-XII, (see p.383, 'Examination of the cranial nerves' for greater detail). Each spinal root is formed from two roots itself: a ventral and dorsal root. The dorsal root has a ganglion (a swelling in the substance of the root where neurones synapse, i.e. contains neurone cell bodies, dendrites, axons and synapses), and is composed of sensory neurones only. The ventral root has no ganglion and is composed of motor fibres (and some autonomic fibres).

The spinal cord is fundamentally divided as per the dorsal and ventral roots, i.e. for the most part the dorsal columns contain only sensory nerves, and the ventral columns for the most part contain motor nerves.

The peripheral nerve system (PNS)

The PNS is the system of branches from (and to) the CNS that send (and receive) information to (and from) the brain, that encompass the entirety of the human body's organs.

It is organised into:

- Sensory neurones.
- Motor neurones.
- Autonomic neurones (which are themselves divided into sympathetic and parasympathetic neurones).
- Enteric neurones.

Sensory neurones

Sensory neurones receive information from sensory receptors (these can be mechanoreceptors, i.e. detect mechanical stimuli, such as pressure, or stretch), thermoreceptors (temperature), or nociceptors (pain).

Note

— There are also specialised sensory receptors (special senses):
  • hearing;
  • taste (chemoreceptor);
  • vision (photoreceptor);
  • balance (vestibular).

The most important of the ascending somatosensory pathways, i.e. transmitting information from the 'soma' or 'body', are the dorsal column and spinothalamic tract.

The different modalities of sensation are:

◆ Touch/presssure.
◆ Vibration.
◆ Proprioception (position sense and joint movement).
◆ Thermal sense.
◆ Pain.
◆ Visceral distension.
◆ And the aforementioned special senses.

Nociceptors

Nociceptors are defined as receptors responding to painful stimuli causing actual or potential tissue damage.

There are two basic types:

◆ A-Delta nociceptors. Fast transmission, myelinated and respond to mechanical pain stimuli, e.g. sharp, pressure, crush.
◆ C nociceptors. Slow transmission, unmyelinated and respond to mechanical, thermal and chemical pain stimuli.

Dermatome

A dermatome is an anatomical region of the body corresponding to the distribution of a single spinal nerve root (Figure 3.48). This is determined embryologically.

Myotome

A myotome is a group of muscles all supplied from the distribution of a single nerve root.

Motor system

The motor system is made up of neurones that lead to skeletal muscle. They co-ordinate voluntary movement, posture, co-ordination and reflexes.

The basic element of the motor system is the motor unit, i.e. one 'alpha neurone', and the group of muscle fibres (within the substance of a single muscle) that it supplies.

Muscle fibres contain stretch receptors; these are called muscle spindles. Tendons also contain stretch receptors; these are the Golgi tendon organs.

Stretch receptors are (obviously) sensory neurones and not motor neurones, but their importance in this context is in their role in the reflex arc. The reflex arc comes from the definition of a reflex, which is a simple motor response to a defined sensory input.

The classic example is the knee jerk, also known as the quadriceps stretch reflex:

◆ The gamma neurone transmits stretch information from the quadriceps muscle, after the strike of the tendon hammer to the patellar tendon to the spinal cord (it is not, however, the tendon's stretch involved in this arc).
◆ A monosynaptic excitatory connection with an alpha neurone travels to the quadriceps muscle, stimulating muscle contraction (knee extension).
◆ There is also a di-synaptic inhibitory pathway along a group IA neurone which inhibits the knee flexor (e.g. semitendinosus), i.e. overall, there is reflex extension of the knee, and reflex inhibition of flexion of the knee - a knee jerk.

Autonomic nervous system

The autonomic nervous system (ANS) is defined as a motor system for regulation of smooth and cardiac muscle, and glands. It is not under direct voluntary control. It is largely responsible for homeostasis: keeping the body's internal environment optimised, despite the changing external environment of the world around the body.

It is made up of three main groups:

◆ Sympathetic.
◆ Parasympathetic.

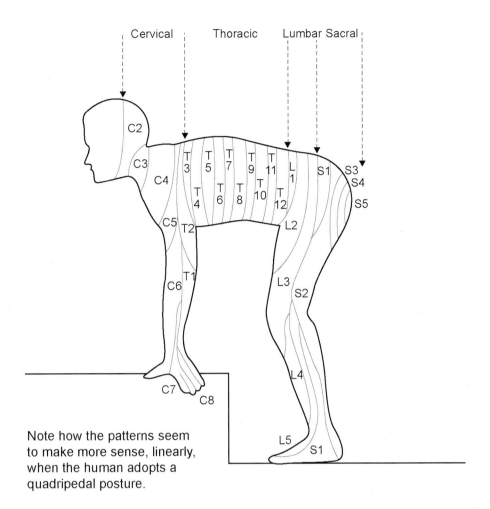

Note how the patterns seem to make more sense, linearly, when the human adopts a quadripedal posture.

Figure 3.48. The dermatomes.

♦ Enteric (a peripheral, reflex network located within the walls of the GI tract, e.g. Meissner's and Auerbach's plexuses). Although enteric neurones are truly autonomic, questions relating to the autonomic nervous system are generally referring to sympathetic and parasympathetic systems. This is something to bear in mind when questioned in exams.

Sympathetic

This is a very widely distributed nerve system throughout the body. It supplies the smooth muscle of vessels (vasoconstriction), sweat glands (stimulates sweating), heart (increased rate and force of contraction), lungs, and the abdominal visceral organs.

It also has effects in the head, pupillary dilation, eyelid elevation, sweat glands to the skin, and others.

The organisation of the sympathetic nervous system is as follows. Preganglionic sympathetic nerves (located in the white matter of the spinal cord) exit the spinal cord at the level of each spinal root. Then they either:

♦ Enter the sympathetic chain (a nerve complex, lateral to the spinal cord, that contains sympathetic nerves travelling either caudally [down] or rostrally [up], to synapse with a post-ganglionic nerve in a ganglion); or

◆ Synapse, in the ganglion, at the level they exit the spinal cord, and then go on to their organ of destination; or

◆ Enter the splenic nerve and then synapse nearer their organ of destination.

Pre-ganglionic sympathetic nerves use acetylcholine as their neurotransmitter when they synapse with post-ganglionic nerves.

Post-ganglionic sympathetic nerves supply the intrathoracic organs directly and the intra-abdominal organs, travelling first via the splenic nerve and then branching out. There are some branches from the sacral nerve plexus that branch directly out to the organs of destination as well. The branches to vessels and skin, and sweat glands peripherally, are direct branches, independent of the splenic nerve.

Post-ganglionic sympathetic nerves use noradrenaline as their neurotransmitter (except those to sweat glands and vasodilatory nerves to vessels, which use acetylcholine instead).

Note

— Pre-ganglionic sympathetic nerves directly innervate the adrenal gland, where instead of synapsing with post-ganglionic sympathetic nerves, they synapse with the adrenal chromaffin cells (related structures), which release adrenaline and noradrenaline into the blood stream as hormones.

— Horner's syndrome is a clinical example you may be asked to explain in terms of autonomic neurology. It is an interruption to the sympathetic chain (e.g. apical lung tumour causing local compression) as it transmits information rostrally (to the head). Thus, one sees a unilateral ptosis (no motor supply to the superior tarsal muscle of the eyelid), unilateral miosis (pupillary constriction due to the unopposed pupil dilatory effects of the parasympathetic nerve supply), and unilateral anhydrosis (decreased sweating, interruption to the nerve supply of the sweat glands).

Parasympathetic

This nerve system is not as widely distributed as the sympathetic. Pre-ganglionic parasympathetic nerves are located in cranial nerve nuclei and in the sacral parasympathetic nucleus. They synapse outside of the cranial nerve nuclei (and sacral parasympathetic nucleus) in the cranial ganglia (and in separate ganglia near their abdominal organs of destination) to post-ganglionic parasympathetic nerves. Both the pre- and post-ganglionic parasympathetic nerves use acetylcholine as a neurotransmitter.

The parasympathetic nerves that supply the abdominal organs all initially travel via the vagus nerve (cranial nerve X). This supplies parasympathetic information to the heart (decreased heart rate and power of contraction), lungs, abdominal organs and intestine as far distally as the splenic flexure of the colon. From the splenic flexure of the colon onwards (distally), parasympathetic nerves take their origin from the sacral parasympathetic nucleus (S2-4) with direct branches.

The parasympathetic nerves that supply the head travel through the oculomotor nerve (dilates pupil), facial nerve (to salivary glands), and glossopharyngeal nerve (to the parotid gland).

SURFACE ANATOMY

Surface anatomy is difficult to find in textbooks and is gleaned usually from various sources, and yet it is tested fairly rigorously in postgraduate clinical exams. This section outlines the landmarks necessary to identify the various anatomical structures relevant to a surgeon.

Thorax

◆ T2 - superior angle of the scapula.
◆ T2/3 - suprasternal notch.
◆ T3 - spine of the scapula.
◆ T4/5 - angle of Louis, junction of middle and superior mediastinum.
◆ T8 - inferior angle of scapula.

- T9 - xiphisternal joint.
- L3 - 10th rib (lowest part of costal margin).
- Angle of Louis - corresponds to the 2nd rib and is, therefore, a constant landmark for counting ribs.
- Male nipple - ~4th intercostal space.
- Apex beat - ~5th intercostal space, in the mid-clavicular line.

Trachea

- C6 - trachea commences at the lower border of the cricoid cartilage.
- T6 - trachea bifurcates (subject in erect position at full inspiration).

Pleura

Superiorly

A curved line between the sternoclavicular joint and the junction of the medial and middle third of the clavicle (the apex of the curved line extends ~2.5cm above the clavicle).

Reflections

From the medial extremity of the line described above to the midline at the angle of Louis. In the right lung this line continues vertically downwards until the 6th costal cartilage, crosses the 8th rib in the midclavicular line, crosses the 10th rib in the midaxillary line, then crosses the 12th rib at the lateral border of the erector spinae. The left lung pleural reflections only differ when the line arches laterally at the 4th costal cartilage, then travels vertically down parasternally and crosses the ribs at the same levels.

Lungs

- The apex of the lung is closely applied to the pleural reflection described.
- The anterior border of the right lung follows the pleura.
- The anterior border of the left lung has the cardiac notch behind the 5/6th costal cartilages.

- In the neutral position (halfway between inspiration and expiration), the lower borders of both lungs cross the 6th rib in the midclavicular line, cross the 8th rib in the midaxillary line and then cross the 10th rib adjacent to the vertebral column posteriorly.
- The oblique fissure can be approximated to the line of the medial border of the scapula when the subject places a hand on the top of his head.
- The horizontal fissure is in a horizontal line passing through the 4th costal cartilage.

Heart

The region is defined by lines joining the 3rd rib at the right sternal edge, 2nd rib at the left sternal edge, 5th intercostal space in the midclavicular line and along the 6th rib back up to the first point.

Breast

- From the 2nd to the 6th rib at its thoracic origin in the vertical plane.
- From the sternal border to the anterior wall of the axilla in the horizontal plane.
- It lies on pectoralis major, serratus anterior and external oblique.

Abdomen

- T9 - xiphoid.
- L1 - transpyloric plane (of Addison). Halfway between the suprasternal notch and the pubis.
- L3 - subcostal plane. The inferior margin of the 10th rib corresponds to the lowest position of the thoracic cage.
- L4 - plane of the iliac crests. Aortic bifurcation. (A safe level for lumbar puncture.)
- L3/4 - umbilicus (variable).

Structures in the transpyloric plane (of Addison) are: the lower border of L1, pylorus, gallbladder fundus, termination of the spinal cord, neck of the pancreas, second part of the duodenum (D2), attachment of the transverse mesocolon, origin of the superior mesenteric artery, confluence of the splenic vein and superior mesenteric vein forming the portal vein, hilum of both kidneys and the hilum of the spleen.

Liver

Superiorly - horizontal line connecting just below the right and left nipple; inferiorly - oblique line from the left nipple to the top of the 10th rib.

Spleen

Underlies the 9th/10th/11th ribs posteriorly on the left side commencing ~5cm from the midline.

Gallbladder

The fundus is where the lateral border of the rectus abdominis meets the costal margin. It corresponds to the tip of the 9th costal cartilage (the palpable step in the costal margin).

Pancreas

The neck is in the transpyloric plane of Addison in the midline. The head extends inferiorly and to the right; the body and tail pass upwards and to the left.

Aorta

Bifurcates to the left of the midline in the plane of the iliac crests (level of L4).

Kidney

The hilum is in the transpyloric plane of Addison, four fingerbreadths from the midline. Posteriorly, the upper pole lies deep to the 12th rib.

Note

— The right kidney is usually 2.5cm lower than the left. This is because it is displaced inferiorly by the liver.

Upper limb

Bones

Acromium
The bony edge at the lateral extremity of the scapular spine.

Coracoid process
Immediately below and at the junction of the middle and outer third of the clavicle.

Pisiform
At the base of the hypothenar eminence.

Hook of hamate
Deep palpation just distal to the pisiform.

Scaphoid
At the base of the thenar eminence and within the anatomical snuffbox.

Muscles/tendons

The anterior fold of the axilla is formed by pectoralis major. The posterior fold of the axilla is formed by teres major and latissimus dorsi. The anatomical snuffbox laterally consists of abductor pollicis longus, extensor pollicis brevis and medially, extensor pollicis longus.

Blood vessels

Brachial artery
Can be palpated in the antecubital fossa immediately medial to the biceps tendon.

Radial artery
Can be palpated on the volar surface of the radius at the level of the wrist.

Ulnar artery

Can be palpated on the volar surface of the ulna at the level of the wrist.

Nerves

Supraclavicular nerves

Can be rolled under the fingers as they cross the clavicle.

Brachial plexus

Palpable against the humeral head when the arm is abducted.

Axillary nerve

Close to the neck of the humerus ~5cm below the acromium.

Radial nerve

Crosses the posterior aspect of the humerus at its midpoint.

Posterior interosseous nerve (PIN)

Henry's method is three fingers placed along the proximal radius (with the first finger just proximal to the radial head); the PIN will be under the third finger.

Median nerve

Lies in the median plane of the forearm.

Ulnar nerve

Immediately medial to the ulnar pulse. Lies radial to the pisiform on the hook of the hamate.

Lower limb

Bones

Head of talus

Block of bone immediately in front of the malleoli.

Tuberosity of the navicular bone

2.5cm in front of the medial malleolus (insertion of tibialis posterior).

Base of 5th metatarsal

Palpable on lateral foot (insertion of peroneus brevis).

Nelaton's line

From the anterior superior iliac spine (ASIS) to the ischial tuberosity (indicates presence of femoral head/femoral neck pathology, if the greater trochanter is not below this line).

Bryant's triangle (performed with the patient supine on a bed)

- ♦ A. Straight line connecting the greater trochanter of the femur with the anterior superior iliac spine.
- ♦ B. Vertical line down from the ASIS towards the bed.
- ♦ C. Horizontal line starting at the greater trochanter, and meeting side B. The length of C is gauged on each side and the sides compared. The pathology of the femoral head or neck which displaces the greater trochanter will tend to shorten this side of the triangle, e.g. fracture of the neck of the femur (NOF), coxa vara, slipped upper femoral epiphysis (SUFE), or a congenitally dislocated hip.

Muscles/tendons

Behind the lateral malleolus are peroneus longus and brevis. Behind the medial malleolus are tibialis posterior, flexor digitorum longus and flexor hallucis longus. Remember the mnemonic (medial to lateral) of Tom, Dick and Harry (tibialis, digitorum and hallucis). The tibial artery and nerve pass between Dick and Harry.

Blood vessels

Femoral artery

Its course is described by the proximal two thirds of a line drawn from the midinguinal point (half way between the ASIS and pubic symphysis) to the adductor tubercle (located on the medial aspect of the medial femoral condyle at the knee).

Dorsalis pedis artery

Palpable between the tendons of extensor hallucis longus and extensor digitorum on the dorsum of the foot.

Posterior tibial artery

One fingerbreadth below and behind the medial malleolus.

Short saphenous vein

Commences as a continuation of the veins on the lateral dorsum of the foot and continues to run behind the lateral malleolus, terminating by draining into the popliteal vein behind the knee.

Great saphenous vein

Commences as a continuation of the veins on the medial dorsum of the foot and continues to run 2cm in front of the medial malleolus and runs a hand's breadth posterior to the medial border of the patella. It terminates by draining into the femoral vein at the groin ~2.5cm below the inguinal ligament immediately medial to the femoral pulse.

Nerves

Femoral nerve

Emerges under the inguinal ligament just lateral to the femoral pulse, then continues for ~5cm before dividing into its terminal branches.

Sciatic nerve

Commences at the midpoint of the posterior superior iliac spine and ischial tuberosity, then curves outwards and downwards through a point between the greater trochanter and ischial tuberosity. It continues downwards in the median plane in the posterior thigh and divides into the tibial and common peroneal nerves at variable levels.

Common peroneal nerve

Can be rolled under the finger against the neck of the fibula, posterior to it.

Head and neck

- C3 - hyoid bone.
- C4 - notch of the thyroid and carotid bifurcation.
- C6 - cricoid cartilage, junction of the larynx and trachea, junction of the pharynx and oesophagus. The carotid pulse is palpable against the transverse process of C6. The inferior thyroid artery enters the thyroid; the middle thyroid vein leaves the thyroid.
- T2/3 - suprasternal notch.

Carotid sheath

A line joining (1) the midpoint of the mastoid process and angle of the jaw to (2), the sternoclavicular joint.

Spinal accessory nerve

A line from (1) one third of the way down the SCM to (2) two fingerbreadths above the clavicle on the anterior border of the trapezius.

Parotid duct

Middle third of a line joining the subtragic notch to the midpoint of the philtrum. The orifice is seen at the level of the upper second molar tooth.

Jugal point

Junction of the zygomatic bone and zygomatic process of the frontal bone (surface marking for the middle meningeal artery).

Chapter 4

Operative surgery

The following chapter contains a series of common surgical techniques, including indications and complications. It is not intended as an exhaustive list of all operative procedures, but rather to outline the more common procedures to be aware of for postgraduate exams.

GENERAL SURGERY PROCEDURES

Excision of skin lesions ('the minor ops list')

Langer's lines

The first element required in the planning of excision of skin lesions is the classic diagram of Langer's lines, also known as the lines of tension (Figure 4.1). The reason for this is that scars along these lines heal well, but those at right angles to these lines heal poorly.

The minor ops list

The tradition of minor ops lists for junior doctors seems to be less common than it once was, so the knowledge and experience derived from them may not be available to you to draw upon when asked about it, particularly in the clinical part of exams. Here, then, are some of the main points to be aware of.

Lesions are excised as ellipses (Figure 4.2). The reason for this is that when elliptical wound edges are sutured together they form a straight scar. Obviously, with a circular incision around a lesion, the resulting sutured wound would have a more 'rucked up' appearance.

The length of the ellipse from apex to apex should be three times the length of the lesion in this axis. The axis of the ellipse should be parallel to Langer's lines in the relevant part of the body.

The margin around the lesion for the incision should be chosen based on the likely histological nature of the lesion (see below for a guide on malignant lesions).

Lumps and bumps on the face frequently arise in clinical exams, and a common follow-up question on how to excise them asks what local anatomical structures should care be taken to avoid, e.g. facial nerve anterior to the ear, lacrimal duct/gland near the eye, etc.

You should also be prepared to answer questions on choice of suture material and size. A common question is whether you would insert dermal sutures deep to the skin sutures, using an absorbable suture material (e.g. Maxon) to provide strength to the wound during and beyond the time the skin sutures are left in.

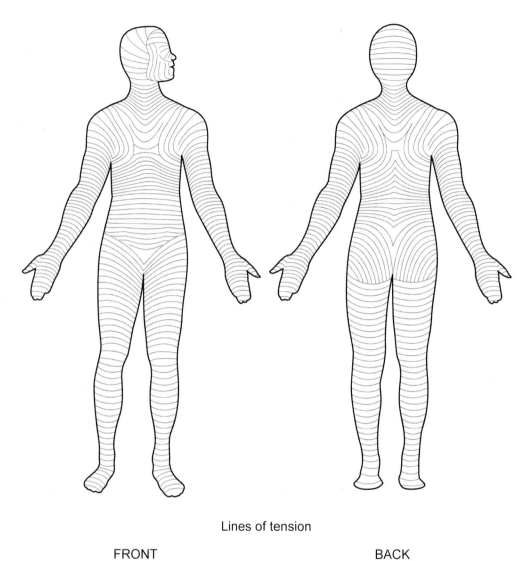

Lines of tension

FRONT   BACK

Figure 4.1. Excision of skin lesions: Langer's lines.

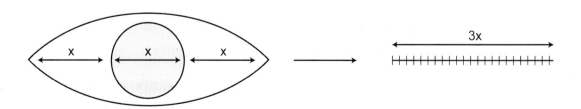

Total length of ellipse = 3x

Figure 4.2. Elliptical incision around a lesion.

Surgical technique

If you have no experience in performing these minor ops, the following is a helpful guide to answering the above questions.

Make an elliptical incision around the lesion with an appropriate margin in Langer's lines. Excise the full thickness of the lesion (usually down to fat is deep enough, but be guided by your findings at the time of surgery) and send it off for histological analysis. Mark the superior margin of the lesion with a suture, i.e. at 12 o'clock (to help the histologist orientate the sample as part of their microscopic analysis). Use a fine suture (size 5-0) for facial lesions and hand lesions, a slightly wider suture (size 4-0) for limb lesions where the wound is not particularly large or under much tension, and larger yet (size 3-0) for trunk lesions or pre-tibial lesions, or wounds where the skin edges are under tension due to the size of the excision.

Always put in dermal sutures with a buried knot for wound strength (absorbable material, e.g. Maxon), followed by interrupted sutures or continuous sutures using a non-absorbable material, e.g. Ethilon or nylon to close the skin. Apply steri-strips and cover with a water-resistant dressing, e.g. Tegaderm.

The recommended margins for excision of common malignant skin lesions are:

◆ Basal cell carcinoma (BCC): 0.3cm for a small lesion; 1cm for a large lesion.
◆ Squamous cell carcinoma (SCC): 0.5-1cm.
◆ Malignant melanoma (MM): depends on depth of the lesion (see table below).

Margin for excision for MM.

Depth	Excision margin required
In situ MM	<5mm
Up to 1mm	1cm
1-2mm	<2cm
2-4mm	2cm
>4mm	2-3cm

Note

— The above are the current UK guidelines published in the *British Journal of Plastic Surgery* in December 2001.

Types of biopsy technique

Biopsies are useful adjuncts to patient management. One should always, however, question whether this investigation will alter the management or simply delay it.

One limitation of biopsies is that they must hit that part of the lesion that contains malignant cells in order to see these cells under the microscope. The hit rate is not always 100%, irrespective of biopsy technique.

Brush cytology

Provides cytology results only.

Fine needle aspiration (FNA)

Twelve passes should be made through the lesion with a green needle. This provides cytology results only.

Excision biopsy

This is removal of the entire lesion which provides histology results including the status of margins of the lesion.

Incision biopsy

This is removal of part of the lesion, an intralesional biopsy, which provides histology results, but no information about margins or invasion.

Endoscopic biopsy

Provides histology results.

Core biopsy

This is done using a very wide-bore needle that 'cores' out tissue for biopsy, which provides histology results.

Note

—   The advantage of histological results over cytological is that it provides information on the structure and type of tissue invaded and margins of the lesion, whereas cytology only provides information on the cell type found in the biopsy sample.

Hartmann's procedure

Hartmann's procedure is a colostomy with a rectal stump.

Indications

◆   Obstructing carcinoma at the rectosigmoid junction.
◆   Perforated diverticulum with inflamed adjacent colon (including faecal peritonitis).
◆   First stage of treatment of faecal volvulus.

Surgical technique

◆   The incision is made in the midline or the left paramedian.
◆   Mobilise the sigmoid colon dividing and ligating the inferior mesenteric vessels to the sigmoid colon.
◆   Divide the peritoneal reflection of the sigmoid mesentery to mobilise the upper one third of the rectum (beware the left ureter).
◆   Clamp the lesion using crushing bowel clamps placed within 2cm of soft bowel clamps.
◆   Cut the specimen flush with the crushing bowel clamps and remove it.
◆   Close the rectal stump in two layers.
◆   A drain may be needed if there is gross contamination.

◆   A colostomy will need to be fashioned with 8-10 interrupted sutures (usually sited as a 3cm hole midway between the ASIS and umbilicus).

Complications

◆   Stoma complications.
◆   Pelvic abscess.
◆   Wound infection.
◆   Septicaemia.

Nissen fundoplication

This is surgical folding of the fundus of the stomach around the junction of the oesophagus and upper stomach to treat gastric reflux disease in the presence of hiatus hernia.

Indications

◆   Treatment of symptomatic hiatus hernia.

Surgical technique

◆   The incision is in the upper midline or via a laparoscopic approach.
◆   Retract the liver and mobilise the gastric fundus by ligating and dividing the short gastric arteries and the upper branches of the left gastric artery.
◆   Divide the peritoneum overlying the lower oesophagus (beware of damage to the spleen).
◆   Reduce a hiatus hernia if present.
◆   Draw the fundus around the oesophagus and perform fundoplication by suturing its apex loosely to the anterior lower oesophagus with several non-absorbable sutures.
◆   Repair any hiatal defect with several non-absorbable sutures.
◆   Close in layers.

Complications

Early
◆   Acute gastric dilatation.
◆   Reactionary haemorrhage.

- Gastric fistula.
- Dysphagia.

Late
- Recurrent gastro-oesophageal reflux.

Note

— This is commonly performed laparoscopically.

Ramstedt's pyloromyotomy

This is an operation that opens up a tight (hypertrophic) gastric pylorus.

Indications

- Pyloric stenosis (congenital, or secondary to scarring from ulcer disease).

Surgical technique

- Perform a transverse, muscle splitting, upper abdominal laparotomy incision.
- Deliver the hypertrophic pylorus into the incision.
- Perform the pyloromyotomy by incision of the peritoneum over the length of the pylorus and split both the longitudinal and circular muscles down to the submucosa only (beware of opening the mucosa; this is suspected if any bubbles of gastric juice and air escape). If damaged, repair with fine absorbable sutures.
- Close in layers.

Complications

Early
- Peritonitis due to unrecognised submucosal perforation and an inadequate pyloromyotomy with persistent vomiting.

Late
- Recurrent pyloric stenosis (rare).

Cholecystectomy

This is excision of the gallbladder.

Indications

- Symptomatic gallstone disease.
- Cholecystitis.
- Open cholecystectomy is indicated in cases of multiple previous abdominal operations, due to the presence of adhesions that complicate attempts at laparoscopic surgery.

Surgical technique

- There are several incision options: Kocher's (right subcostal), right paramedian, right upper transverse, and laparoscopic using port sites at the:
  - umbilicus;
  - midline epigastrium;
  - right subcostal in the mid-clavicular line.

Open

- Display the gallbladder by packing off the small bowel, retracting the stomach and duodenum downwards and retracting the liver upwards.
- Retract the gallbladder (GB) laterally (using sponge-holding or Moynihan's forceps).
- Incise the peritoneum over the right free border of the lesser omentum.
- Then follow the instructions laid out in laparoscopic cholecystectomy (see below) as, after the approach, the excision of the GB proceeds along identical lines.

Laparoscopic

- Grasp and retract the GB laterally.
- Dissect out Calot's triangle. Ligate, clip and divide the cystic artery.
- Cannulate the cystic duct and aspirate bile for microbiology. Most surgeons perform an intra-operative cholangiogram.
- Clip the cystic duct to within 1cm of the common bile duct (CBD).
- Divide the peritoneal reflection between the GB and liver to dissect the GB out of its hepatic bed.

◆ Achieve haemostasis of the GB bed, then remove the GB. It is usually placed in a bag (or glove) and removed via the umbilical port.
◆ Close in layers (in open surgery, otherwise single sutures for laparoscopic wounds).

Complications

Early
◆ Biliary leak.
◆ Ileus.
◆ Wound infection.
◆ Jaundice with retained stones.
◆ Septicaemia.
◆ Pancreatitis.

Late
◆ Cholangitis.
◆ Biliary stricture.

Appendicectomy

This is excision of the appendix.

Indications

◆ Acute appendicitis (urgent).

Surgical technique

◆ The incision is a Gridiron (right iliac fossa, over MacBurney's point) or Lanz (transverse incision following skin-tension lines, beginning 1-2cm medial to the ASIS).
◆ Deepen the incision by splitting muscles in the direction of their fibres (external and internal obliques, and transversalis abdominis).
◆ Pick up the peritoneum with two forceps and make a nick in the peritoneum with the scalpel, and enlarge using scissors.
◆ Remove a sample of peritoneal fluid and send for microbiology.
◆ Locate and deliver the appendix.
◆ Place a clip over the mesoappendix and divide it, ligating the vessels.

◆ Some surgeons may place a purse string around the taenia coli 2cm from the appendix base at this point.
◆ Place a crushing clamp just distal to the base of the appendix.
◆ Ligate the base of the appendix just proximal to the clamp with an absorbable ligature.
◆ Remove the appendix flush with the caecal side of the crushing clamp and send for histology.
◆ At this point those surgeons who may have placed the purse string would invaginate the appendix and tie the suture; others may simply diathermy the lumen.
◆ Some surgeons may perform peritoneal toilet or simply extend a swab-on-a-stick into the right pelvis to check for any collection.

Complications

Normal appendix (there may be another pathology).

Early
◆ Infection: peritonitis, septicaemia, wound, pelvic abscess, subphrenic abscess, portal pyaemia, fistula.

Late
◆ Small bowel obstruction.
◆ Fallopian tube obstruction.

Ileostomy

This is surgically bringing out a stoma from a loop of ileum.

Indications

◆ Total colectomy.
◆ Defunctioning of the bowel to protect an ileo-anal anastomosis.
◆ Defunctioning of the bowel in severe colitis.

Surgical technique

◆ Ensure the ileum is viable, then clear off several centimetres of mesentery.

- Incise a 3cm circle of skin at a preselected position (often chosen in conjuction with the stoma nurse, for best access for stoma bag application), and continue a circular incision through the layers including the peritoneum (beware of the inferior epigastric vessels).
- Place tissue forceps through the hole and deliver the ileum ensuring there is no twisting of the bowel.
- Suture the ileal serosa and mesentery to the anterior abdominal wall ensuring that a length of 6-8cm remains external to the skin to fashion a spout.
- Wash out the peritoneal cavity leaving a suction drain close to the abdominal wall.
- Place eight evenly spaced sutures anchoring the ileum to the external oblique to prevent stomal prolapse. Then approximate the skin and bowel wall with interrupted absorbable sutures, thereby forming an everted spout.

Complications

- Skin excoriation.
- Retraction.
- Prolapse.
- Small bowel obstruction secondary to adhesions.

Colostomy

This is surgically bringing out a stoma from a loop of colon.

Indications

- In the elective setting, for defunctioning of the colon and rectum.
- In the emergency setting, for the first stage of treatment of distal colonic obstruction.

Surgical technique

- Make a 10cm transverse incision in the right upper quadrant (RUQ). Locate and withdraw the transverse colon.

- Locate a point proximal to the middle colic artery and detach the omentum at this point.
- Open a window in an avascular point in the mesocolon and, if performing a loop colostomy, place a plastic bridge through the window. Close the wound in layers around the prepared colon.
- Open the colon along the taenia and suture the mucosa of the colon to the skin edges with interrupted absorbable sutures.
- Place a colostomy bag.
- The loop colostomy's bridge can be removed in approximately four days.

Complications

- Retraction (of the colostomy back into the abdomen).
- Prolapse (of the stoma).
- Parastomal herniation.
- Ischaemia of the colostomy.
- Stomal stenosis.
- Stomal ulceration.
- Stomal obstruction.

Haemorrhoid surgery

Indications and treatment

First degree
There is no prolapse but bleeding and discharge causes pruritis ani. Treat by submucosal injection using a Gabriel's needle of 5ml 5% phenol in almond oil immediately above the haemorrhoid, i.e. above the dentate line, as there are pain fibres below it.

Second degree
There is a prolapse but the haemorrhoid withdraws spontaneously. Treatment is with banding. The haemorrhoid is withdrawn via the proctoscope with grasping forceps passed through the band applicator. Apply the band ensuring that the constriction is above the dentate line, again because there are pain fibres below it.

Third degree
This is a permanent prolapse of the haemorrhoids. Surgery is indicated.

Surgical technique

- The haemorrhoid is first injected with 1:100,000 adrenalin submucosally.
- A Parke's speculum is inserted and the haemorrhoid grasped and incised at its base using a v-shaped incision using scissors.
- The base of the pedicle is then transfixed and ligated with a silk suture.
- Finally, a paraffin-soaked pack is inserted into the anal canal and held in place with a T-shaped bandage.

Complications

Early
- Haemorrhage.
- Urinary retention.
- Constipation.

Late
- Anal stenosis.
- Fissure.
- Skin tag.
- Recurrent haemorrhoids.
- Incontinence (sphincter damage).

Splenectomy

This is surgical excision of the spleen.

Indications

Trauma
- Trauma (splenic laceration/rupture).
- Hypersplenism (idiopathic thrombocytopaenic purpurae [ITP]).
- Massive splenomegaly.
- Lymphoma (Hodgkin's and non-Hodgkin's).
- Splenic torsion.
- Primary or secondary tumours of the spleen.

Medical
- The medical indications for splenectomy are more often than not decided by haematologists, who request a general surgeon to perform the splenectomy.

Surgical technique

- The preferred approach is the vertical midline laparotomy incision, although it is possible to perform splenectomy through a left subcostal or a thoraco-abdominal incision (gives better access, at the expense of extending into the chest wall, e.g. for massive splenectomy).
- Once into the peritoneal cavity, pass a hand over the spleen (between the spleen and ribs), and pull it gently towards the incision. This puts the lienorenal ligament under tension (this structure joins the pancreas and kidney to the spleen and contains the splenic artery and vein).
- Incise the lienorenal ligament (where it lies next to the spleen, not more proximally) with dissecting scissors, and complete the incision of the ligament (avoiding cutting the vessels), thus exposing the artery and vein.
- Ligate the splenic artery first (if you do not, the spleen congests and this causes bleeding), followed by the splenic vein, at their insertion into the spleen. Then divide them both.
- Divide the gastrosplenic ligament (joins the stomach to the spleen).
- The spleen should now be free, and can be removed.
- Close the wound over a suction drain.

Note

- All splenectomy patients should have a nasogastric (NG) tube passed to prevent postoperative gastric dilatation.

Complications

- Left shoulder tip pain (diaphragmatic irritation).
- Left lung mild effusion and/or basal collapse.
- Gastric dilatation.
- Leukocytosis and thrombocytosis for 1-2 weeks after the operation.
- Wound infection.
- Subphrenic abscess.
- Pancreatic fistula (the tail of the pancreas is very close to the site of division of the lienorenal ligament).

Gastrectomy

This is surgical excision of the stomach in full (gastrectomy) or in part (partial gastrectomy).

Indications

◆ Malignancy. Carcinoma of the stomach.
◆ Bleeding. Gastric ulcer disease (emergency for life-threatening bleeds or, elective for a persistent ulcer despite medical treatment).

Surgical technique

Prior to surgery, the patient must be optimised as much as possible (with carcinoma, they may have dehydration, poor nutritional status, gastric dilatation) and an NG tube must be passed.

◆ The incision is made via an upper midline laparotomy, i.e. an incision from the xiphisternum to the umbilicus through the linea alba and into the peritoneal cavity. It is also possible to perform the operation through a thoraco-abdominal incision for greater access (e.g. in the case of a total gastrectomy), which is a paramedian type of upper abdominal incision with an extension into the thorax prising apart two ribs.
◆ The stomach has two omental attachments, the greater omentum (gastrocolic) and lesser omentum (joining the liver to the stomach). Mobilise these from the stomach to enable access to the stomach.
◆ Incise the greater omentum along the greater curvature (inferior surface) of the stomach. This contains arcades of vessels, all of which require tying off as part of the mobilisation. This is done from right to left, ending with the gastroduodenal artery at its insertion into the pylorus/duodenum.
◆ Ligate the right duodenal artery from the superior border of the duodenum.
◆ Mobilise the lesser omentum from the lesser curvature of the stomach (superior surface).
◆ The stomach is now exposed and the type of gastrectomy (partial or complete) can now be performed as follows.

Partial gastrectomy

This is suitable for cancers arising in the distal stomach, i.e. pre-pyloric region (the majority of tumours).

◆ Excise the pylorus, antrum and lesser curvature of the stomach.
◆ Sew up the lesser curvature.
◆ Anastomose the remaining open portion of the distal stomach to a loop of jejunum as an end-to-side anastomosis (end of stomach to side of jejunum).
◆ Close the duodenal stump.

This is a Bilroth II (Polya partial gastrectomy and reconstruction).

Note

— The 'Roux-en-Y' is a variation on the enterostomy loop mentioned. It is a procedure designed to avoid the complication of bilious vomiting. It differs from the above only in the addition of the division of the proximal jejunum, anastomosing a proximal loop to a more distal loop of jejunum, and having the gastrojejunal anastomosis as an end-to-end anastomosis (instead of an end-to-side). This results in a much greater distance that the bile would have to travel retrogradely to produce bilious vomiting and hence considerably reduces its incidence.

Total gastrectomy

Total gastrectomy is indicated if the tumour is more proximal, i.e. lesser curve or the body of the stomach.

◆ Excise the entire stomach leaving a duodenal and oesophageal stump.
◆ Anastomose the oesophageal stump to a mobilised loop of jejunum.
◆ Close the duodenal stump.

Oesophageal anastomoses are (to put it mildly) temperamental; they are at risk of leak/anastomotic breakdown. It is common practice to pass an NG tube beyond the anastomosis into the jejunum in an attempt to protect it.

Note

–   It is sometimes necessary to perform the operation through a thoraco-abdominal approach, particularly in total gastrectomy, if exposure is insufficient in the abdominal approach.

Postoperative care

Small amounts of fluid (approximately 30ml) are permitted by mouth. IV fluids should be given. The NG tube should regularly be aspirated to prevent gastric dilatation, and minimise gastric fluid present at the anastomosis. On return of bowel sounds (usually 2-4 days later), oral fluids can be incrementally increased, IV fluids incrementaly decreased, and eventually a light diet can be recommenced.

Complications

General complications
◆   Wound infection.
◆   Dehiscence.
◆   Bleeding.
◆   Haematoma.
◆   Chest infection.
◆   Basal atelectasis.
◆   DVT.
◆   PE.
◆   Incisional hernia.

Specific complications
◆   Bilious vomiting.
◆   Anastomotic dehiscence.
◆   Early dumping.
◆   Late dumping.
◆   Diarrhoea.

Bilious vomiting occurs characteristically 15-30 minutes post-meal, and is more common soon after surgery but tends to resolve. The problem can be solved, if it persists, by the aforementioned Roux-en-Y anastomosis (it can also be prevented by performing it as part of the original procedure).

Dumping can be early or late. Early dumping is due to rapid emptying of the stomach. A high osmotic load thus enters the small intestine, increasing splanchnic blood flow and hence a fluid shift from the systemic circulation to the intestinal circulation. Symptoms are sweating, flushing, tachycardia, palpitations, nausea, vomiting and diarrhoea. Late dumping is a reactive hypoglycaemia in response to the large insulin secretion following the earlier hyperglycaemia secondary to the sudden load of gastric contents into the small intestine. The symptoms are similar to those of early dumping, but delayed. Early dumping occurs immediately post-meal; late dumping occurs within 1-2 hours post-meal.

Right hemicolectomy

This is surgical excision of the right (ascending) hemi-colon.

Indications

◆   Carcinoma of the caecum or ascending colon.
◆   Carcinoid of the appendix (or the rare primary adenocarcinoma of the appendix).
◆   Crohn's disease (when it is refractory to medical treatment).
◆   Trauma, when damaged beyond repair.

Surgical technique

◆   The patient should be prepared such that the colon is empty prior to surgery. Different surgical units have differerent techniques for achieving this. Administering 'Kleen Prep' overnight, with IV fluids to prevent dehydration, is a common practice.
◆   Make a right paramedian laparotomy incision from the level of the xiphisternum to that of the ASIS.
◆   Enter the peritoneal cavity and perform an examination of the contents of the abdomen and pelvis (particularly important in the malignant context, e.g. looking for liver metastases, peritoneal metastases, lymph node involvement or fixity of the tumour in the

colon to local structures such as the duodenum or kidney, which can make the tumour unresectable).

◆ The ascending colon is retroperitoneal. The ileum is a peritoneal organ that inserts into the anterior portion of the caecum (which is also intraperitoneal, and has its own piece of mesentery). The transverse colon is intraperitoneal, with its own mesentery. Thus, to excise the ascending colon one must first dissect away its peritoneal covering. This is done from its left side (paracolic gutter) first.

◆ Then, ligate the pedicles of the right colic artery and the superior mesenteric arteries, as well as that of the ileocolic and superior mesenteric arteries.

◆ Finally, mobilise the hepatic flexure of the ascending colon from its greater (gastrocolic) omental attachments, remembering that there are arterial arcades located within that will require ligation.

◆ In malignant disease, the lymph nodes are located in the mesenteric attachment of the portion of colon being removed. The mesentery is, therefore, preferably removed as proximal to its posterior peritoneal insertion as possible (thus the excised tissue contains those lymph nodes, which can then be used to stage the disease).

◆ The cut end of the ileum must then be anastomosed to the cut end of the transverse colon. It is said that an end-to-end anastomosis is preferable to end-to-side, even with the obvious discrepency between luminal diameters of the ileum and transverse colon. This can be simply achieved by making an oblique cut across the end of the ileum, increasing its apparent diameter.

◆ The anastomosis is performed either with interrupted sutures (fine absorbable sutures in two layers), or an anastomotic stapling device.

◆ In addition, suture the gap between the resected margins of the mesenteries.

◆ Place a drain through a separate stab incision. This is particularly useful in monitoring for anastomotic dehiscence postoperatively (where the drainage would suddenly increase, as well as contain faecal material, along with a deterioration in the patient's clinical condition).

Postoperative care

Continue IV fuids until there are audible bowel sounds and passage of flatus, allowing incrementally increasing amounts of clear fluids by mouth until the patient has sufficient intake to warrant ceasing the IV fluid.

Complications

Early
◆ Haemorrhage.
◆ Wound infection.
◆ Wound dehiscence.
◆ Anastomotic leakage and, hence, peritonitis.
◆ Possible abscess formation (can result from an anastomotic leak).

Remember that after major abdominal surgery that coughing is painful, as well as difficult. Thus, chest infection and basal atelectasis are possible complications, as well as the classic DVT or PE.

Late
◆ Loose stools (less colon left behind).
◆ Disease recurrence (Crohn's disease or tumour).
◆ Incisional hernia.
◆ Macrocytic anaemia, due to the variable length of ileum being resected, from which vitamin B12 is normally absorbed.

Death
There is a significant mortality associated with right hemicolectomy, markedly increased in the emergency situation in the presence of peritonitis.

Left hemicolectomy

This is surgical excision of the left (descending) hemi-colon.

Indications

Most commonly performed for carcinoma of the colon, but other indications are:

◆ Diverticular disease.
◆ Inflammatory bowel disease.

- Trauma.
- Radiotherapy.

Surgical technique

- As for right hemicolectomy, the bowel must be prepped, i.e. it should preferably be empty of faecal matter. Kleen Prep 24 hours prior to surgery and IV fluids to prevent dehydration should be suitable.
- A left paramedian laparotomy incision is performed, from the xiphisternum, as far as the pubis (if necessary).
- Enter the peritoneal cavity, and perform an examination of the contents of the abdomen and pelvis (particularly important in the malignant context, e.g. looking for liver metastases, peritoneal metastases, lymph node involvement or fixity of the tumour in the colon to local structures such as the duodenum or kidney, which can make the tumour unresectable).
- Exteriorise the small bowel, not under tension, and protect with moist swabs. This enables a better, and less crowded, view of the abdominal contents. Dissect out the splenic flexure of the descending colon. This is done by dissecting the greater (gastrocolic) omentum off the greater curvature of the stomach, spleen, and transverse colon as far as its mid-point.
- The descending colon is then mobilised from its retroperitoneal attachments, starting on its lateral edge, using a combination of dissecting scissors and traction. The major underlying structure involved in this part of the procedure is the perinephric fat of the left kidney.
- This undermining of the descending colon is continued distally along its full length, then completed by passing a finger gently, up at the level of the splenic flexure, under and medially, until it pokes out on the medial border through the peritoneal covering. This allows incremental clamping and ligation of the greater omentum and peritoneum down its medial border. This can only be performed as far as half the length of the descending colon, mobilising the upper half.
- The lower half of the descending colon and the sigmoid colon are found by picking up the

sigmoid colon, placing it under tension, and dividing its attachment to the peritoneum.

- At this point, the common iliac artery and vein are found (at the base of the sigmoid mesocolon), as is the left ureter. And as the aide memoire states "the bridge travels over water", thus the arteries lie over the ureter (urine, in this aide memoire, is the water). Just lateral to this crossing, the testicular artery in men, or the ovarian artery in women, is located.
- From this point incise the peritoneum of the medial border of the descending colon upwards to its mid level, completing the peritoneal mobilisation.
- Ligate the blood vessels and divide the mesentery. In the case of malignant disease (the most common indication for this operation), the principle that the lymphatics follow the course of the arteries is highly useful. It means that ligating the arteries at their most proximal anatomical point and taking the excised tissue *en bloc* affords you the greatest chance of a curative resection. It also enables the histologist the greatest amount of tissue to accurately stage the disease. The arteries involved at this level are the inferior mesenteric artery and, if the transverse colon is involved, branches of the middle colic artery. Another useful point with reference to malignant disease, is that the tumour has been shown to very rarely extend into bowel wall more than 2cm beyond its palpable edge. It is generally recommended to excise 5cm in either direction if possible. If anatomic constraints exist, slightly less is permissable. Do not forget, also, that descending colon tumours are multiple in approximately 3% of cases, so you must feel to see if there are any other tumours before completing the operation.
- Isolate the length of colon to be excised in packs from the other abdominal contents and wound edges, and use a crushing clamp followed by sharp dissection to excise the length of bowel.
- Finally, perform an anastomosis of the two cut ends of colon. As in the right hemicolectomy, any disparity in the luminal size of the two cut ends can be compensated for by making a more oblique cut across the narrower of the

two lumens, increasing its apparent circumference.

♦ The anastomosis can then be performed using interrupted narrow diameter sutures, or a stapling device.

♦ A drain should be placed, which is brought out laterally. This is near the point of the anastomosis, and is intended to drain any blood, but more importantly to show any presence of faecal material indicative of an anastomotic leak in the first 3-5 days postoperatively. This would require re-operation to prevent (or mitigate) peritonitis, most likely performing a protective colostomy, which could be reversed at a later date.

♦ The abdominal incision is closed en masse (e.g. with a looped PDS) and a buried subcutaneous suture to the skin.

Postoperative care

Continue IV fuids until there are audible bowel sounds and the passage of flatus, allowing incrementally increasing amounts of clear fluids by mouth until the patient has had sufficient intake to warrant ceasing the IVs.

Complications

Early
♦ Haemorrhage.
♦ Wound infection.
♦ Wound dehiscence.
♦ Anastomotic leakage and, hence, peritonitis.
♦ Possible abscess formation (can result from an anastomotic leak).

Remember that after major abdominal surgery that coughing is painful, as well as difficult. Thus, chest infection and basal atelectasis are possible complications, as well as the classic DVT or PE.

Late
♦ Loose stools (less colon left behind).
♦ Disease recurrence (Crohn's disease or tumour).
♦ Incisional hernia.

Death
There is a significant mortality associated with left hemicolectomy.

Thyroidectomy

This is surgical excision of the entire thyroid (thyroidectomy) or part of it (partial or subtotal thyroidectomy).

Indications

♦ Suspected or diagnosed thyroid cancer.
♦ A recurrent thyroid cyst post-aspiration.
♦ Obstructive symptoms, i.e. airway/voice/ swallowing difficulties.
♦ Hyperthyroidism.
♦ Aesthetic, e.g. unsightly goitre; this is a relative indication.

Surgical technique

♦ Make a transverse incision 2.5cm above the jugular notch through subcutaneous fat and the platysma.
♦ Push aside the infrahyoid strap muscles (sternohyoid and sternothyroid) to reveal the lateral lobes of the thyroid.
♦ Ligate the vessels of each lobe (left and right superior and inferior thyroid arteries, and left and right superior, middle and inferior thyroid veins).
♦ Leave the recurrent laryngeal nerve and parathyroid glands intact.

Complications

♦ Recurrent laryngeal nerve (RLN) damage. RLN palsy may result in voice change and varying degrees of airway obstruction.

Note

– The RLN supplies motor innervation to all laryngeal muscles, except the cricothyroid.

◆ Haemorrhage can cause laryngeal oedema and airway obstruction. If this is severe and the neck is swollen (haemorrhage), remove the sutures or clips and summon immediate senior assistance to protect the airway. Cricothyroidotomy may be necessary to save the patient's life.

Note

— Superior laryngeal nerve palsy affects people who use their voice professionally, causing fatiguability and weakness of voice.

◆ Hypocalcaemia (parathyroid insufficiency due to local trauma or excision). This hypocalcaemia can present with peripheral paraesthesiae, carpopedal spasm and eventually leads to laryngeal spasm, which is potentially fatal. To prevent this, oral calcium and vitamin D, or IV calcium gluconate, is administered.
◆ Wound sepsis.
◆ Scar hypertrophy.
◆ Thyroid storm (rare because patients should be euthyroid pre-operatively).

Parathyroidectomy

This is excision of one or all of the parathyroid gland(s). The parathyroid glands are variable in number and position. Usually there are four (in 90% of cases), found posterior to the upper and lower poles of the thyroid (two up, two down).

Embryologically, the upper two are derived from the 4th branchial arch, and the lower two are derived from the 3rd branchial arch, i.e. have travelled further downwards, and therefore are more variable in position. They are sometimes identified by the presence of a branch of the inferior thyroid artery pointing to them.

Indications

◆ Primary hyperparathyroidism.
◆ Symptomatic secondary or tertiary hyperparathyroidism.

Surgical technique

As for thyroidectomy, but the lateral lobes are reflected so that the posterior surface is exposed and the parathyroids are located.

Complications

As for thyroidectomy above.

Inguinal hernia repair

This is the reduction of a hernia and surgical repair of the defect through which the hernia occurred.

Indications

The presence of an inguinal hernia, alone, does not necessarily constitute an indication for surgery. There is a risk of strangulation of the hernia, but generally this is low. Thus, the relative risks of strangulation versus operative repair need to be weighed up whenever deciding to operate or not.

Hernias can be symptomatic or asymptomatic, and patients can be fit or have serious comorbidities. Hernia repair is a short and relatively safe procedure, frequently performed as a day-case procedure. As a result, a large proportion of patients who develop an inguinal hernia present to their surgeon complaining of pain on effort and cosmetic deformity. So long as the risks of surgery are explained, and the patient understands them, as well as the finite, but nonetheless real, risk of hernia strangulation, then surgery can be offered.

Obviously, in the acute setting of strangulation, surgery is also indicated. This carries considerably greater risk than elective hernia repair, however.

Surgical technique in adults

This procedure can be done under local anaesthetic in the compliant patient, but more typically it is done under general anaesthesia. The groin should be prepped and draped in elective cases and the entire abdomen from nipple to knee in emergency cases.

The incision should be approximately 3cm above and parallel to the medial two thirds of the inguinal ligament (in the groin crease). Ligate and divide the superficial epigastric vein; then locate the spermatic cord at the external ring. Divide the external oblique muscle along the length of its fibres to expose the inguinal canal.

The surgical technique varies for the differing types of inguinal hernia along the following lines:

- Indirect hernias. Dissect the cremaster muscle layer off the hernia sac; then dissect the sac off the cord. Open the sac, explore and reduce its contents. Transfix the sac at the deep ring; then excise the rest of the sac.
- Direct hernias. Reduce the sac en masse. There should be no need to open the sac, transfix and excise.
- Strangulated hernias. Open the sac and inspect the contents. If it has already spontaneously reduced then it is probably viable, so this should be managed as for an indirect hernia. If not, then assess the colour, sheen, contractility and pulsatile mesenteric vessels. If the contents are potentially viable, dilate the neck with two fingers and wrap the bowel in warm saline-soaked swabs for 5-10 minutes. If the contents are non-viable, then a resection and primary end-to-end anastomosis is required. In either case careful postoperative assessment for signs of obstruction or peritonitis is essential.

Herniorrhaphy (actual repair procedure to prevent recurrence)

- Shouldice. Reconstitute the transversalis fascia and internal oblique/conjoint tendon in layers using nylon in a double-breasting suture technique.
- Lichtenstein. Close any direct defect using a non-absorbable suture. Then suture a polypropylene mesh in place using a non-absorbable suture or staples. The mesh must extend from the pubic tubercle to the lateral deep ring. The two 'tails' of the mesh should pass above and below the deep ring. Further non-absorbable sutures (or clips) should fix the mesh inferiorly to the length of the inguinal ligament and superiorly to the conjoint tendon. Close in layers.

Inguinal hernias in children

These are always indirect, as the external ring usually overlies the internal ring. These should be repaired via a herniotomy, i.e. open sac, reduce, transfix sac and excise remnant. A herniorrhaphy should not be performed.

Complications

- Infection.
- Recurrence.
- Bleeding.
- Haematoma.
- Scrotal swelling.
- Painful surgical site.
- Groin numbness.

Femoral hernia repair

This is the reduction of a femoral hernia and closure of the femoral canal.

Indications

- The risk of incarceration and obstruction is greater in femoral hernias than inguinal hernias. Therefore, the relative indication is greater in femoral than inguinal hernias.
- A painful hernia impeding lifestyle.
- A large mass with a narrow neck.

Surgical technique

- This should be carried out under general anaesthesia in the supine position, with the abdomen prepped and draped from nipple to knee.
- There are three classically described approaches:
  - inguinal/high (above and parallel to the inguinal ligament);
  - crural/low (in the groin crease, below and parallel to the inguinal ligament);
  - pre-peritoneal (McEvedy's; essentially a vertical incision parallel to the rectus abdominis fibres).

- In the low approach for elective surgery, the incision should proceed down through the superficial fascia in the line of the incision, taking care to protect the femoral vein and long saphenous vein.
- Identify the sac as it descends through the femoral canal medial to the femoral vein. Open the sac at its apex, reduce the contents and transfix the neck of the sac. Excise the remnant.
- Repair the femoral canal with three nylon sutures from the pectineal ligament to the inguinal ligament.
- In a strangulated emergency case, the sac is opened as for the elective procedure and any fluid sent for microbiology. The contents are then inspected.
- Gently dilate the femoral canal with a finger.
- If possible the bowel may be drawn out for inspection. If it is viable it can be returned to the abdomen and continue as before; if it is potentially viable, then it should be wrapped in warm saline swabs and re-inspected in 5-10 minutes. If it is non-viable and can be drawn out, it should be resected with a primary anastomosis; if it cannot be drawn out, then a low laparotomy should be performed for resection and hernia repair.
- Close in layers without drains.

Complications

- Infection.
- Recurrence.
- Bleeding.
- Haematoma.
- Scrotal swelling.
- Painful surgical site.
- Groin numbness.

ORTHOPAEDIC PROCEDURES

Dynamic hip screw (DHS)

This is the application of a pin-and-plate to the proximal femur which has a screw up the femoral neck and plate on the lateral femur.

Indications

- Fractures of the proximal femur that are intertrochanteric, or basi-cervical (at the base of the femoral neck, and hence extracapsular).

Surgical technique

This procedure requires a traction table and image intensifier.

- The patient is placed supine on the table. Both feet are placed in traction boots, with velband padding to prevent damage to elderly patients' delicate skin.
- The leg to be operated upon is kept straight. The other leg is flexed up and abducted out of the way to allow the image intensifier to come in between the legs to take AP and lateral X-rays of the operated hip.
- Using the image intensifier, apply traction and rotation of the leg to reduce the ends of the fractured bone into anatomical position.
- The proximal femur is approached by an incision along the lateral aspect of the thigh, from 1-2cm distal to the greater trochanter, extending distally some 15cm.
- Incise through skin, fat, then the fascia lata. This exposes the bulk of the vastus lateralis muscle.
- Incise the epimysium of vastus lateralis in line with your skin incision.
- Use a blunt instrument to push through the muscle fibres down to bone (the lateral cortex of the proximal femur). Pull the instrument distally along the length of the wound, splitting the fibres as you go. This, rather than using the knife, exposes the femur with minimal bleeding from the intramuscular vessels.
- Use the periosteal elevator to expose a good area of the bone (to which to apply the plate later).
- Slide an unmounted guidewire over the greater trochanter anteriorly in the direction of the femoral head. Use the image intensifier to superimpose the tip of the wire in the middle of the femoral head on the screen. This gives an idea of the anteversion of the femoral neck for aiming the guidewire up the femoral neck itself.
- Mount the guidewire on the power drill, and use the 135° guide to apply it to the lateral

cortex of the femur. Then, using the image intensifier, guide the wire up the femoral neck into the inferior 50% of the femoral head on the AP view (there is less risk of cut-out in this region), and the middle of the femoral head on the lateral view.

- Stop driving the wire in when it reaches the subchondral bone of the femoral head (the 'horizon' on the image intensifier).
- Use the measuring device on the protruding portion of the wire, and subtract 10mm from the measured value (this will give you a screw that stops 10mm short of the subchondral bone of the femoral head).
- Attach the reamer to the power drill. Set it to the calculated amount above. Ream along the guidewire.
- You must insert a lag screw of the calculated length along the guidewire (after removing the reamer). Use the image intensifier to ensure you stop screwing 10mm short of the subchondral bone of the femoral head.
- The screwdriver has a 'T' handle, and the handle must rest horizontally when you finish screwing. This ensures the flat sides of the lag screw are parallel to the plane the plate will be applied to the bone (otherwise the plate will be rotated relative to the bone).
- Apply the plate (generally a 135°, four-hole plate) over the screw and guidewire combination. Tap it down to the bone.
- Drill through the four holes using the drill guide. Measure the length of the screws needed with the measuring device on the set and pass the screws (some sets have self-tapping screws; if not, you must 'tap' the holes which involves screwing in an instrument that has sharp screw threads on its outer surface, providing spiral grooves for the screw to pass along).
- Use the image intensifier to ensure the plate and lag screw are ideally positioned in AP and lateral views.
- Close the epimysium with a continuous 1 vicryl, then the fascia lata.
- Use 2.0 vicryl to the subcutaeous fat and clips to skin.
- A drain is not (usually) necessary.

The patient is now safe to fully weight bear from the point of view of the solidity of the plate. They will, however, require the help of physiotherapists to do so, in view of the recent soft tissue trauma associated with both the fracture and surgical insult.

Complications

Non-union
Non-union can occur but it is uncommon as the lag screw is designed to slide through the barrel (dynamisation, hence the name dynamic hip screw) of the plate, achieving compression at the fracture site; this stability predisposes to good union rates.

Wound infection
Due to the age and morbidity of the population in whom these fractures occur, there is a considerable one-year mortality (30-40% in some series).

Hemi-arthroplasty of the hip

This is excision of the femoral head (usually for femoral neck fracture) and replacement with a monoblock stem and head, which can be either cemented or uncemented.

Indications

- Displaced intracapsular fracture of the neck of the femur (see Chapter 6, 'Proximal femoral fractures' for a more detailed discussion on the breakdown of indications for surgical intervention in this difficult patient group).

Surgical technique

- Generally, the patient is placed laterally on the operating table with a bolster anterior and posterior to the pelvis (holding them steady in position). The anterolateral approach (as opposed to posterior) is the most common approach in the setting of fractures.
- Ensure a gel pad is placed under the ankle of the leg against the bed and that the upper body and arms are well positioned to avoid injury during the procedure.
- The incision is based upon the landmark of the greater trochanter (GT). Incise linearly some 20cm, with the GT in the centre of your wound.

- Incise through skin, subcutaneous fat, then through the fascia lata. This exposes the common tendon attachment on the GT of the vastus lateralis (which extends distally down the femur) and gluteus medius (which extends proximally up to its insertion on the iliac blade).
- Using cutting diathermy make a cut into this common tendon origin (white tissue on either side of your cut, thus leaving a 'cuff' of tissue to suture back at the end of the procedure, because attempting to suture muscle back to tendon is unrewarding) from the tip of the GT down into the bulk of the vastus lateralis.
- This cut must extend directly down to bone, and then be extended anteriorly along the surface of the bone. This will naturally lead along the anterior surface of the femoral neck into the hip capsule.
- Where your incision started at the tip of the GT continue it along the line of the fibres of gluteus medius (approximately 135° to the lateral surface of the femoral shaft) directly down through the gluteus medius tendon and hip capsule as far as the rim of the acetabulum.
- Once both these dissections have been performed, a flap of musculo-tendinous tissue will be seen to be raised of the entire anterior hip joint.
- The fracture in the femoral neck is now apparent, and the leg can now be depended (into an anteriorly placed 'leg bag') in the position of flexion and adduction, and external rotation, such that the tibia is vertical with respect to the ground. This fully exposes the femoral neck and enables you to make your femoral neck osteotomy.
- There are two choices at this stage (these will already have been made prior to surgery, but it is at this stage that the surgical technique for each ceases to be identical). If you are performing a cemented hemi-arthroplasty (e.g. Thompson's prosthesis), your femoral neck osteotomy is a line from the piriformis fossa (base of the GT) to the lesser trochanter. If, however, you are performing an uncemented hemi-arthroplasty (e.g. Austin Moore), your femoral neck osteotomy is from the piriformis fossa to a point 1cm proximal to the lesser trochanter. As both the Austin Moore and Thompson's prostheses

- have collars that rest on the medial femoral neck (the 'calcar'), this difference in osteotomy site is necessary for the respective designs to have the appropriate 'offset' (distance from the GT to the centre of the femoral head, horizontally), for the patient to have appropriately anatomical articulation at the hip joint.
- With the femoral neck cut made, the fractured end of the femoral head is more visible. Remove the femoral head by passing a 'corkscrew' into the femoral head and levering it out.
- Measure the diameter of the native femoral head, and make a note of this number for later in the procedure.
- In the case of the uncemented Austin Moore, at this stage, you should use a box chisel to enter the femoral shaft more laterally than your initial neck cut would have allowed. Then pass the small rasp through this lateral entry point, and tap it down until the rasped portion of the rasp is no longer visible. If it is tight at this point, select the narrow shaft Austin Moore prosthesis of the measured femoral head size, and impact it into position. If the rasp is not tight, choose the standard rasp and tap it down completely, then select the standard shaft Austin Moore prosthesis of the measured femoral head size and impact it into position.
- In the case of the cemented Thompson's prosthesis, use the box chisel as for the Austin Moore and both rasps. Pass a universal (one size fits all) cement restrictor to a distance 2cm greater than that of your prosthesis into the femoral canal. Wash out with saline. Insert bone cement (preferably antibiotic-impregnated) into the canal retrogradely (from distal to proximal using a cement gun). Pressurise it with an obturator attachment on your gun. Then insert the prosthesis until its collar is flush with the cut femoral neck.
- Now, on both cemented (after the cement has set), and uncemented prostheses, you may relocate the hip. Test the stability of the joint by putting it through a range of movement. Close in layers.
- Use 1 vicryl to the cut in the hip capsule, also to the two ends of the cuff of the conjoined tendon of gluteus medius and vastus lateralis (interrupted), and the fascia lata (continuous).

- Use 2.0 vicryl to fat and clips to skin. Drains are not (usually) needed.
- The patient, as with DHS, can safely fully weight bear on the prosthesis from the point of view of stability of the prosthesis, but may need help from the physiotherapist to do so.

Complications

- Persistent thigh pain. May occur in uncemented hemi-arthroplasties, more commonly than the cemented versions.
- Dislocation. Can occur and seems to be a poor prognostic indicator for the patient (there is, in some series, a mortality of 50% in patients with dislocation of hemi-arthroplasty).
- Sciatic nerve damage. Very unusual in the anterolateral approach.
- Wound infection. Treatment is with washout and subsequent antibiotics, after taking samples for microscopy, culture and sensitivity (MC+S).

Total hip replacement

This is the replacement of both articulating surfaces of the hip (acetabulum and femoral head), hence the term total in this context.

Indications

- The most common indication, by far, is symptomatic osteoarthritis of the hip (resistant to analgesia, activity modulation, use of a stick and physiotherapy).

Other indications can be:

- Displaced intracapsular fracture of the neck of the femur.
- Metastatic bone deposit in the femoral neck or head (causing pain or pathological fracture).
- Rheumatoid arthritis of the hip.
- Post-traumatic arthritis of the hip.
- Avascular necrosis of the femoral head.

Surgical technique

The two main approaches to the hip are anterolateral and posterior. The anterolateral approach has been described in hemi-arthroplasty of the hip above. Both approaches have postulated advantages and disadvantages. Briefly, the posterior approach is thought to have a higher hip dislocation rate; the anterolateral approach has a higher rate of limp (Trendelenberg gait).

The posterior approach to the hip is as follows:

- Place the patient laterally on the operating table with a bolster anterior to and posterior to the pelvis (holding them steady in position).
- Ensure that a gel pad is placed under the ankle of the leg against the bed and that the upper body and arms are well positioned to avoid injury during the procedure.
- The incision is based on the landmark of the greater trochanter (GT). As with the anterolateral approach it is in the centre of the wound. However, the proximal half of the wound must curve posteriorly, whereas the distal half remains the same (as for the anterolateral approach), i.e. parallel to the shaft of the femur.
- The incision is continued through fat, then through the fascia lata (contiguous with the undersurface of the fascia lata at this level is the muscle belly of gluteus maximus, the fibres of which must be parted with those of the fascia lata, exposing the GT).
- Posterior to the GT lie the short external rotators of the hip (piriformis, gemellus inferior and superior, and quadratus femoris). To expose the hip joint posteriorly, these must then be peeled off the posterior proximal femur.
- Remember, first, that the sciatic nerve lies posterior to the GT at this level. It is considered advisable to identify it at this stage of the approach, and to make a mental note of its position to avoid damage.
- Identify the piriformis tendon (the only linear tendinous structure leading straight into the piriformis fossa of the femur). Cut it transversely as far up into the piriformis fossa as possible and retract it.
- This exposes the dome of the posterior hip capsule as it stretches across the posterior

aspect of the femoral head. Incise directly down to bone through the capsule in a horizontal curvilinear fashion. Extend the incision distally along the posterolateral aspect of the femur through the tendinous origins of the other external rotators en masse.

♦ The hip joint is thus opened up sufficiently to easily dislocate it posteriorly.

♦ At this point if using the anterolateral approach to the hip, having incised into the hip capsule (usually in the shape of a 'T', with the two arms of the 'T' skirting along the anterior borders of the acetabulum), the hip is also easily dislocated (anteriorly this time).

♦ With the hip dislocated make the femoral neck osteotomy with a powered saw. Different brands of hip replacement specify different precise levels at which to make the osteotomy. In this case, make the osteotomy 1cm proximal to the lesser trochanter and extend it into the piriformis fossa.

♦ With the femoral head excised, it is no longer obscuring the view of the acetabulum.

♦ The acetabular labrum can now circumferentially be excised down to the bony acetabular rim.

♦ The acetabulum is now reamed using powered 'strawberry reamers' up to a diameter appropriate to the patient's bone stock, ready to accept the acetabular component at this point. There are fundamentally two types of acetabular components that can be inserted: cemented and uncemented. For the purpose of exams you need only learn about cemented cups as these are the most common in current practice.

♦ Drill key holes into the reamed acetabulum.

♦ Drop a ball of cement into the acetabulum and compress it with a proprietary compressor (or the old swab-in-a-glove technique).

♦ The acetabular component (polyethylene most commonly, but it is possible to use ceramic or metal less commonly) is inserted on its jig into the cement and oriented 45° to the vertical and approximately into 20° of anteversion. It is held in compression in the socket until the cement has set (approximately ten minutes).

♦ The femoral shaft is then rasped (again there are cemented and uncemented types of femoral prosthesis, but as cemented is the more common, this is covered here), after

lateralising the entry point with the box chisel, as for hemi-arthroplasty of the hip.

♦ Rasp the femoral canal up to a diameter appropriate to the patient's bone stock. The rasp can then be left *in situ* with a trial (plastic) femoral head on its trunion, and a trial reduction performed to assess length and stability. Slight repositioning, or a longer femoral head can be performed at this stage, and this configuration remembered for the definitive insertion of a prosthesis later.

♦ Place an appropriately sized cement restrictor 1-2cm further down the femoral shaft than the length of the femoral prosthesis.

♦ Use a pulsed lavage washout of the femoral canal.

♦ Pack the canal with a swab.

♦ Place the cement into the canal retrograde with the cement gun, i.e. from distal to proximal to avoid cavitation.

♦ Pressurise the cement with the obturator tightly applied to the neck osteotomy on the cement gun.

♦ Insert the femoral prosthesis into the shaft to the depth determined by earlier trialling. Maintain pressure on the prosthesis and cement while the cement sets, for a good cement mantle.

♦ When set, reduce the hip with a trial (plastic head). If the stability is good, then apply the definitive head, impact it on the trunion, and finally reduce the hip.

♦ Close in layers with 1 vicryl.

♦ Suture the capsular incision.

♦ Suture the piriformis and the rest of the external rotators back to the femur.

♦ Suture the fascia lata.

♦ Use 2.0 vicryl to fat.

♦ Clips to skin.

Complications

Early
♦ Wound infection.
♦ Deep infection, effectively septic arthritis.
♦ Dislocation.
♦ Sciatic nerve palsy.
♦ Bleeding.

◆ Haematoma.
◆ Leg length discrepancy (long or short).

Late

◆ Dislocation (has a bimodal distribution, i.e. early or late) which may require revision surgery.
◆ Deep infection, causing septic loosening of the implant (requiring revision surgery and antibiotics).
◆ Aseptic loosening (requiring revision surgery).

Total knee replacement

This is the replacement of both (or all three if resurfacing the patella as well) articulating surfaces of the knee, usually in the form of a cemented tibial plateau, cemented femoral component and a polyethylene spacer between them.

Indications

◆ The most common indication is symptomatic osteoarthritis of the knee (resistant to analgesia, activity modulation, use of a stick and physiotherapy).

Other possible indications are:

◆ Post-traumatic arthritis.
◆ Rheumatoid arthritis.

Surgical technique

There are different approaches to the knee, but overwhelmingly the most common is the medial parapatellar approach.

◆ The patient is placed supine on the operating table and a tourniquet is inflated on the thigh (velband underneath to protect the skin) to 250-300mm of mercury.
◆ The knee is flexed up to 90° and held there with a sandbag under the foot, and a bolster to the lateral side of the thigh.

◆ A vertical incision is made using the patella as the central landmark and the tibial tuberosity as a distal landmark. The incision is extended proximally until the fibres of vastus medialis are visible at their musculotendinous junction.
◆ Incise through fat and delicately through the filmy fascia underlying the fat (as its vascular arcades are derived from this fascial layer).
◆ Peel the fat/fascia layers medially and laterally exposing the quadriceps tendon, patella and patellar tendon.
◆ The medial parapatellar incision can now be made. This extends from the musculotendinous junction of the vastus medialis with the quadriceps tendon (leaving a cuff of tendon proximally to suture back together at the end), skirts medially round the patella (again leaving a generous cuff of tendon), and extends along the medial border of the patellar tendon (on its border with the medial patellar retinaculum) distally as far as the tibial tuberosity's medial border.
◆ The knee is straightened, the patella everted, and the knee flexed up again. With the patella now out of the way, the knee joint is completely visible.
◆ There are many different types of knee replacement, but the most common type is the cemented knee replacement. (There are, of course, other subtleties of prosthesis type and surgical technique, which are not covered here.)
◆ The periosteum on the medial aspect of the proximal tibia is dissected from the bone; this allows the soft tissues to reflect away, giving a better exposure of the knee.
◆ The retropatellar fat pad is dissected away from the posterior patellar tendon; this affords better visibility of the knee joint, at the expense of compromise to patellar blood supply, which is through the fat pad.
◆ A drill hole is made in the intercondylar groove (the trochlea) of the distal femur. This allows placement of the intramedullary guide up the femoral shaft.
◆ It is from this guide that the distal femoral cut can be measured with a jig; it is a cut in 5° of valgus.
◆ From the flat surface of the distal femoral cut, another jig (appropriately sized to the patient's

bone stock) can be applied, enabling the anterior and posterior femoral condylar cuts as well as the two oblique chamfer cuts to be performed. These cuts give the distal femur the shape of half an octagon when looked at from either side. This is the shape of the inner surface of the femoral prosthesis which will be applied later.

♦ The tibial cut can be made using either an intramedullary guide (as for the femur) or extramedullary guide (which wraps around the ankle distally). Controversy still exists on the relative merits of the two systems.

♦ Using whichever guide is preferred, a horizontal cut is made across the tibial plateau, perpendicular to the axis of the tibial shaft.

♦ A trial femoral prosthesis is applied to the cut femur. A trial tibial prosthesis (metal) is then applied to the plateau, and a spacer (polyethylene) applied to the tibial trial.

♦ The knee is put through a range of movement, ensuring it is not too tight or too loose in either 90° of flexion or full extension. The thickness of the poly spacer can be varied, or ligamentous releases can be performed as required to achieve the correct soft tissue balancing of the knee.

♦ The position of the tibial prosthesis is marked on the tibia with diathermy.

♦ The femoral and poly spacer prostheses are removed, leaving behind the tibial tray. Through this a drill hole is made and keel cuts are made in the bone to accommodate the real tibial prosthesis.

♦ The tibial tray is also now removed.

♦ The cut bone ends are washed thoroughly with pulsed lavage and covered with a clean swab.

♦ The definitive femoral and tibial prostheses are cemented *in situ* with pressurisation until the cement is set and an appropriately sized polyethylene insert is applied at this stage.

♦ A drain, preferably of the re-transfusion variety (blood collected can be transfused back to the patient), is placed into the joint, exiting laterally.

♦ The medial parapatellar cut is closed with 1 vicryl interrupted.

♦ 2.0 vicryl to fat.

♦ Clips to skin.

Note

– The issue whether or not to resurface the patella has not been addressed here, but it is not relevant at this exam level. Nationally, the split lies between always resurfacing, never resurfacing, and those who selectively resurface based on the appearance of the patella articular surface at the time of surgery.

Complications

♦ Wound infection.
♦ Deep infection, effectively septic arthritis.
♦ Bleeding.
♦ Haematoma.
♦ Stiffness.
♦ Persistent pain.

Knee arthroscopy

This is keyhole surgery of the knee, 'arthros' meaning joint and 'scopy' meaning to look. This is not simply diagnostic, i.e. you are not simply looking, it is a therapeutic modality as well. The most commonly performed procedure arthroscopically is trimming of meniscal tears.

Indications

♦ MRI proven or clinically likely meniscal lesions of the knee.
♦ ACL tear.
♦ MRI proven or clinically likely osteochondral lesions of the femoral condyles (rare on the tibial condyles).
♦ Septic arthritis of the knee, for arthroscopic washout.
♦ Assessment of anterior knee pain. It is no longer indicated for osteoarthritic knees in the elderly. The assessment of degree of arthritis can be done radiologically, and studies have shown there is no benefit in terms of symptom relief in an arthroscopic washout of the knee in osteoarthritis.

Surgical technique

♦ Perform an examination under anaesthetic (EUA) of the knee at this stage, looking for range of movement, varus-valgus stability, anterior drawer, Lachman's test, and pivot shift test.

♦ Lie the patient supine on the table. Inflate a tourniquet on the thigh (velband underneath) to 250-300mm Hg.

♦ Place a bolster on the lateral thigh, to allow you to place a valgus force across the knee whilst performing the arthroscopy.

♦ Flex the knee up to 90°. Palpate the 'soft spot' on the lateral side of the knee (a triangle bounded medially by the patellar tendon, inferiorly by the tibial plateau, and laterally by the edge of the lateral femoral condyle).

♦ In the soft spot, stab the scalpel into the joint in the direction of the centre of the joint.

♦ Place the trocar into the joint in the same line as the initial incision and remove the trocar portion leaving behind the arthroscopic portal.

♦ Note whether any effusion fluid escapes through the portal at this stage.

♦ Place the camera into the portal and fill the knee with water (turn on the tap on the portal).

♦ Make a second incision on the medial 'soft spot' under direct vision of the camera in the joint.

♦ The hooked probe can be inserted through the medial portal.

♦ A system for looking round the knee should be in place to ensure that nothing is missed.

One such system is to:

• start in the suprapatellar pouch and inspect the retropatellar surface;

• move to the medial parapatellar gutter looking for loose bodies;

• move to the medial joint and lever the knee into valgus against the bolster; this opens up the joint for a better view. Assess the femoral condyle and tibial plateau for osteoarthritis grade and the presence of osteochondral defects. Assess the meniscus for tears and trim or repair as appropriate;

• move to the ACL and assess it for a visible tear. Look for the classical empty medial wall of the lateral femoral condyle (the site of its normal origin; it appears empty if torn off). Use a probe to test its strength;

• move across to the lateral joint and place the foot across onto the other leg with the knee flexed, i.e. a 'figure of four'. This opens up the lateral joint by placing a varus force across it. Assess the femoral condyle and tibial plateau for osteoarthritis grade and the presence of osteochondral defects. Assess the meniscus for tears and trim or repair as appropriate;

• look in the lateral parapatellar gutter (for loose bodies).

♦ It is sensible practice to photograph the relevant operative findings and record these in an operative note.

♦ Squeeze the fluid out from the joint while a portal is still *in situ*.

♦ Either close the incisions with a single suture, e.g. 3.0 Prolene, or simply place steristrips across them.

♦ Pad the incisions with blue gauze and wrap the knee in velband and crepe.

♦ The patient can fully weight bear and go home on the day of surgery. The knee will be sore for a week or so.

Complications

Arthroscopy is a low-risk procedure. Complications are:

♦ Wound infection.
♦ Septic arthritis (very rare).
♦ Persistent pain at the portal sites (very rare).

Carpal tunnel decompression

This is surgical release of the transverse carpal ligament in the wrist to relieve pressure on the median nerve.

Indications

♦   Carpal tunnel syndrome.

There is little agreement on the definitive indications for surgery. Common indications include:

♦   Night symptoms (paraesthesiae in the radial three and a half digits of the hand) that intrude on sleep.
♦   Persistent symptoms despite steroid injection(s).
♦   Progressive motor weakness.

Surgical technique

♦   The incision commences at the distal flexor crease just medial to the thenar eminence, continuing distally approximately 3cm (beware the superficial branch of the median nerve and the recurrent motor branch to the thenar muscles).
♦   Once through skin and subcutaneous fat, incise through the flexor retinaculum gently, enough to be able to pass a McDonald under the retinaculum to protect the underlying median nerve from the scalpel as the incision is completed distally and proximally.
♦   Direct the incision a little towards the ulnar side at the distal end of the incision, in an attempt to avoid the recurrent motor branch of the nerve.
♦   Divide all fibres of the retinaculum.
♦   Close the skin, only, with interrupted sutures.

Complications

♦   Wound infection.
♦   Wound haematoma.
♦   Persistence of symptoms.
♦   Pillar pain (pain on pressure on the region of the palm at the site of the incision lasting longer than can be explained by surgery alone).
♦   Reflex sympathetic dystrophy (RSD).

Zadek's operation

This is excision of a toenail (most commonly from the great toe) and ablation of the germinal matrix to prevent regrowth of the nail in patients with persistent ingrowing toenails.

Indications

♦   It is indicated for chronic ingrowing toenails, especially if wedge excision of the side of the toenail has been attempted and failed. It is contraindicated in the acutely infected toenail and patients with peripheral vascular disease.

Surgical technique

♦   A tourniquet can be used, i.e. rubber ring placed at the base of the toe (it is advisable to place a clip on the band as a reminder to remove it at the end of the procedure, otherwise it is easily forgotten, left on and can result in iatrogenic digital necrosis).
♦   Separate the nail from the nailbed with the McDonald instrument.
♦   Remove the whole toenail from the nailbed.
♦   Make two oblique incisions approximately 0.5-1cm from the two corners of the nailbed extending towards the sides of the toe.
♦   Retract the skin of the germinal matrix and excise the matrix for the whole width down, as deep as the periosteum of the underlying distal phalanx.
♦   The use of phenol is optional at this stage, as it is cytotoxic and kills the cells of the germinal matrix. One must beware not to spill the phenol on other tissues, and to wash it off the operation site with sterile saline after 30-60 seconds application. (In vivas if you mention phenol in your answer, be prepared to answer questions on the subject).
♦   Suture the two skin incisions and dress.

Complications

♦   Recurrent ingrowth of spikes of nail left from the residual germinal matrix.

VASCULAR PROCEDURES

Amputation

This is removal of part (or all) of a limb.

Indications

♦ 80-90% of amputations are performed for ischaemic limb disease (most frequently in the lower limb).

Common causes of ischaemic limb disease include diabetes, Buerger's disease, atherosclerotic disease and embolic disease.

Ideally, amputation is performed with the fitting of a prosthesis to the limb stump for early mobilisation. Exceptions to the above rule are people with severe OA, paralysis and fixed flexion deformity, where prosthetic fitting would serve little functional purpose and would be merely cosmetic.

A PAM aid is a post-amputation mobility aid. It is a pneumatic, does not require fitting and can be applied while still an inpatient post-amputation.

Types of amputation (Figure 4.3)

You are not expected to know every last detail of surgical technique for amputations at this level. You are, however, expected to be aware of the following different types of amputations and some of the basic facts about each:

♦ Guillotine. This is done in the emergency setting and is performed at the level of ischaemia. It is done with a view to the patient returning three to five weeks later to close the wound and fashion an appropriate stump.
♦ Toe, e.g. diabetic toe gangrene.
♦ Foot:
  • transmetatarsal, i.e. at the level of the metatarsal necks. The only prosthesis required is a shoe filler. This type of amputation is good for forefoot ischaemia;
  • a ray amputation is removal of an individual toe as well as its metatarsal. It is ideal for diabetic toe gangrene with ascending infection up the foot.

♦ Heel. Syme's amputation. Rarely performed as it is difficult to fit a prosthesis. It is preferable to have a below-knee amputation. In the heel, the foot is removed at the level of the ankle joint; the malleoli are sawn off.
♦ Below-knee amputation (aka BKA). This is the operation of choice in below-knee ischaemia, because it is a successful operation in terms of complications and quality of prostheses.

Note

— BKA is also the amputation type that most frequently comes up as a question topic in exams, followed by the ray amputation for diabetic gangrene.

Two types of BKA are performed:
• long posterior flap (Burgess);
• skew flap (Kingsley-Robinson).

Note

— The reasoning behind these two types of skin flaps for closure of the wound after amputation is to provide skin cover for the stump, while keeping the suture line away from the axis of the leg where it would be subject to the weight of the patient passing through it as they tried to mobilise on any prosthesis. This would result in pain and wound complications. The Burgess has a long posterior flap and hence the suture line is anterior to the axis of the leg and in the Kingsley-Robinson, the long flap is skewed from medial skin and hence sutured to lateral skin away from the axis of the leg.

♦ Through-knee amputation. Infrequently performed.
♦ Supracondylar. 'Gritti-Stokes' patella applied to the distal end of the femoral shaft. Infrequently performed.
♦ Above-knee amputation. Performed for ischaemia which extends above the level of the knee. It is also seen in the trauma setting.
♦ Others - disarticulation of the hip, hind quarter, upper limb. Seen in bone tumour surgery and

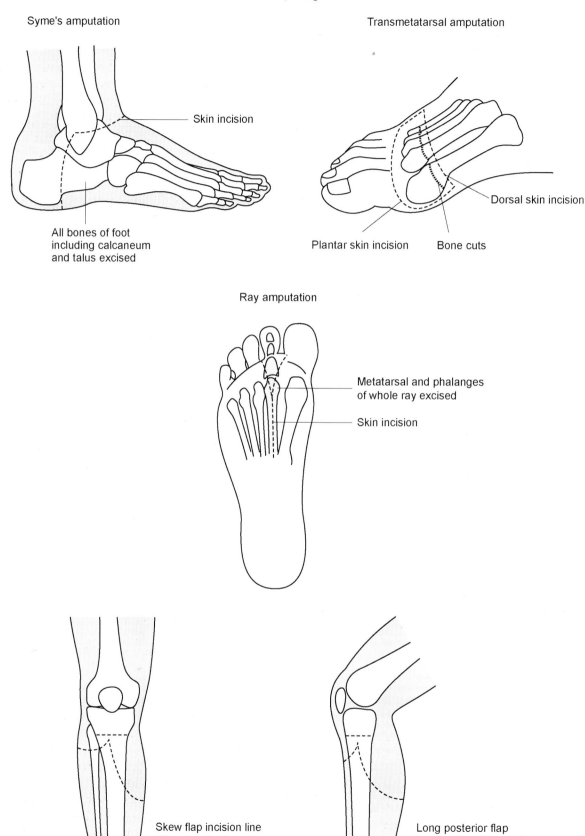

Syme's amputation

Skin incision

All bones of foot
including calcaneum
and talus excised

Transmetatarsal amputation

Dorsal skin incision

Plantar skin incision   Bone cuts

Ray amputation

Metatarsal and phalanges
of whole ray excised

Skin incision

Skew flap incision line
(Kingsley-Robinson)

Long posterior flap
incision line (Burgess)

Figure 4.3. Types of amputation.

other rarer indications, e.g. osteomyelitis, arteriovenous malformations, etc.

Alternatives to amputation

In ischaemic limb disease, alternatives to amputation are arterial bypass surgery, embolectomy or thrombolysis. Amputation, for obvious reasons, is very much end-of-the-line surgery, only to be performed when all other alternatives have been considered. This having been said, excellent results can be achieved with an appropriately crafted amputation and prosthesis.

Complications of amputation

This is a common question in exams and the following list should be remembered:

- Infection.
- Haematoma.
- Wound breakdown.
- Pressure ulcer.
- Osteomyelitis.
- Spurs.
- Osteophyte formation
- Stump neuroma.
- Phantom limb.

Varicose vein stripping and high tie

This is the physical removal (stripping) of varicose veins and tying off the greater saphenous vein at the level of its junction with the femoral vein in the groin (high tie).

Indications

- Presence of venous ulceration.
- Symptomatic varicose veins (dull ache on prolonged standing).
- Cosmetic appearance can be an indication so long as the patient is made aware of the risks of surgery. (Although all patients should be informed of the risks as a matter of course, it is in those operations done for cosmetic reasons alone that the associated risks are even more relevant.)

Surgical technique

- Prior to surgery the varicosities should be marked on the patient's leg (with them standing, as this accentuates the varicosities) with an indelible marker pen.
- The surgery treats the saphenofemoral incompetence present in the majority of severe varicose veins, as well as stripping the great saphenous vein from the thigh above the knee, and ligating those perforating varicosities in the leg (below the level of the knee).
- The intial incision is made parallel to the groin crease, inferior to it, and the landmark on its medial edge is pulsation of the femoral artery at this level.
- Dissect down through fat to the veins; these are tributaries of the great saphenous vein, and hence following these will lead you to it.
- Then follow the great saphenous vein down to the cribriform fascia, which it pierces before joining the femoral vein at the saphenofemoral junction.
- Ligate the tributary veins to the great saphenous vein.
- Ligate (twice!) the great saphenous vein flush with the femoral vein, to avoid a leak into the groin wound, risking haematoma, wound dehiscence and infection.
- Divide the great saphenous vein near to the ligation point.
- You may now pass the stripper wire through the vein opening down as far as the level of the knee.
- Incise at this level to expose the great saphenous vein.
- Ligate it distally.
- Divide the vein proximal to the ligation point, and pass the wire out through this cut end.
- Place an olive tip on the end of the wire (at its distal end); it is of greater diameter than that of the vein, thus gentle continuous traction from the proximal end strips the vein retrogradely.
- Apply manual pressure along the course of the stripped vein for 3-4 minutes (or as long as is necessary) to prevent subcutaneous bleeding from the torn branches. Some surgeons wrap the leg in a tight sterile bandage for a few minutes at this time for the same effect.
- This completes the saphenous tie and stripping component of the procedure. The perforators

that had been marked with a pen prior to surgery can then be excised and tied off.

- This is done by incising at the marked levels, exposing the tortuous perforating vein, grabbing it with an artery clip, ligating its base, then excising it.
- The groin wound is closed with a buried absorbable continuous suture (e.g. 2.0 vicryl or 3.0 monocryl). The stab wounds are closed with interrupted non-absorbable sutures (e.g. 3.0 Prolene), which are removed some 10 days later.
- The leg is bandaged tightly with velband and crepe.
- The patient may mobilise with this on.

Complications

- Wound bleeding.
- Persistent wound serous ooze.
- Wound haematoma.
- Wound dehiscence.
- Wound infection.
- Painful scars.
- Recurrence of varicosities.
- Damage to saphenous or sural nerves (closely associated with the veins).

Carotid endarterectomy

This is the coring out of the carotid artery to increase the narrow luminal diameter due to the presence of atherosclerosis.

Indications

- Transient ischaemic attack (TIA).
- Amaurosis fugax.

Randomised controlled trials dictate that patients with >70% carotid stenosis who are symptomatic should be offered carotid endarterectomy and patients for whom symptoms remain uncontrolled on antiplatelet medication also warrant operation.

The benefit is a six-fold reduction in stroke, compared with best medical management. The mortality rate is 1-2%.

Surgical technique

- The tissue layers comprise the skin, superficial fascia, platysma, deep cervical fascia, sternocleidomastoid (SCM) and carotid sheath.
- The incision is over the anterior border of SCM; the internal jugular vein is mobilised posteriorly. Care should be taken to preserve the vagus and hypoglossal nerves.
- The carotid sinus nerve is blocked with local anaesthetic to prevent excessive variations in BP during dissection. (These would be sensed as apparent changes on pressure by the carotid sinus, which would repeatedly fire off signals to the heart and peripheral vasculature, resulting in random pressure fluctuations).
- Systemic heparin is given when the vessel is ready for clamping.
- Make the arteriotomy from beneath the plaque to above it.
- Many surgeons use a shunt (Javid or Pruitt type) to allow blood flow while operating.

Note

- Remove the full extent of the plaque. Do not raise an intimal tear and do not leave behind any disease; otherwise, it becomes a thrombogenic projection. Close the arteriotomy, with or without a vein patch to prevent late restenosis.
- One can differentiate Internal from external carotid arteries by virtue of the internal carotid having NO branches, and the external carotid having MANY branches.

Complications

- Stroke (intra-operative risk 1-2%).
- Myocardial infarction.
- Infection.
- Recurrent laryngeal nerve palsy and facial nerve palsy.
- Recurrence of occlusion.
- Death (remember these patients are severe cardiopaths to begin with).

Abdominal aortic aneurysm (AAA) repair

This is the surgical insertion of an artificial lumen within the aneurysmal section of the aorta (there is also an endovascular, i.e. percutaneous and non-surgical, alternative to open surgery for aneurysmal repair).

Indications

- Emergency. Ruptured AAA.
- Urgent. Very large or rapidly expanding AAA.
- Elective. Any aneurysm >5.5cm should be repaired unless the patient has significant comorbidity.

Two recent publications by the Aneurysm Detection and Management Veteran Affairs Cooperative Study Investigators have clearly defined the rupture rate of AAA at various diameters:

- <5.5cm = 1% per year rupture rate.
- 5.5 to 5.9cm = 9.4% per year rupture rate.
- 6.0 to 6.9cm = 10.2% per year rupture rate.
- >7cm = 32.5% per year rupture rate.
- >8cm = 6-month rupture rate of 25.7%.

The surgical mortality rate for elective AAA repair ranges between 3.5% and 7.5%. According to the UK Small Aneurysm Trial (1998), there is no improvement in overall mortality among patients with aneurysms measuring 4-4.5cm who are offered early surgery. It is therefore recommended that patients with aneurysms <5.5cm should remain under close observation.

Surgical technique

- The procedure is performed under general anaesthetic with the patient positioned supine.
- Prep and drape the entire abdomen and both groins, in case access to the femoral arteries is required.
- The aorta may be accessed via a long midline incision from the xiphisternum to pubis, or via a long transverse incision midway between the xiphisternum and umbilicus. The latter gives excellent exposure and tends to heal more favourably, being orientated along the skin creases.
- Displace the omentum and large bowel superiorly and place the small bowel with its mesentery in a bowel bag to the right.
- Carefully displace the duodenum before dissecting the peritoneum off the aorta. Expose the inferior mesenteric artery and ligate it close to the sac of the aneurysm.
- Identify the upper and lower limits of the aneurysm, in particular the relation of the neck to the renal arteries. The majority (95%) of AAAs are infrarenal. Dissect enough room either side of the proximal aorta and common iliac arteries to place clamps from the front.
- In elective cases, give IV heparin three minutes prior to closing the clamps and always forewarn the anaesthetist.
- Open the aneurysm sac longitudinally and scoop out the thrombus and atheromatous material. A specimen should be sent to microbiology for culture.
- Identify back-bleeding from the lumbar arteries and close them at their origin with 3.0 Prolene.
- Construct an end-to-end anastomosis between the proximal aorta and a suitable prosthetic graft. This may be straight or Y-shaped, depending on the involvement of the common iliac arteries. The needle is passed from outside the graft to in, then inside the aorta to out. This creates an everted suture line. Test the proximal anastomosis by applying a soft clamp to the distal end of the graft and releasing the proximal clamp. Carefully repair any leaks.
- Construct the distal anastomosis in a similar fashion. Just prior to closing the distal anastomosis, flush the graft with heparinised saline. Perform a 'backwash' by manually compressing the femoral arteries at the groin with the distal clamps opened in sequence. This evacuates any clots which may have formed during the procedure. You should also check for adequate bleed-back from the iliac arteries. It may be necessary to pass an embolectomy catheter to retrieve distal blood clots.
- Once you are entirely happy with your repair, warn the anaesthetist and release the clamps

one at a time (first the proximal, then each common iliac clamp in turn). This minimises the risk of declamping shock. Ensure haemostasis. Oozing between anastomotic sutures can be stopped by applying Surgicell.

◆ The redundant aneurysm sac can now be closed over the graft with a continuous Prolene suture. This prevents direct contact between bowel and graft, thereby reducing the risk of an aorto-enteric fistula forming.

◆ Close the peritoneum over the sac and return the bowel to the abdomen. Close the abdominal wall using the mass closure technique.

◆ The patient must be carefully monitored in ITU in the immediate postoperative period.

Complications

◆ Bleeding.
◆ Limb ischaemia.
◆ Graft thrombosis.
◆ Intra-operative emboli.
◆ MI.
◆ Respiratory failure.
◆ Stroke.
◆ Prolonged ileus.
◆ Colonic ischaemia.
◆ Aorto-enteric fistula.
◆ Dialysis dependence.
◆ Graft infection.
◆ Wound infection.

Femoropopliteal bypass

This is surgical bypass of stenosed or occluded portions of the femoral artery(s) using autograft or prosthetic material grafts.

Indications

◆ Critical limb ischaemia.
◆ Claudication.

Surgical technique

◆ This should be performed in the supine patient under general anaesthesia.

◆ The whole leg should be prepped and draped from groin to ankle.

◆ Two incisions are required at the groin: the first is a 10-12cm longitudinal incision overlying the common femoral artery, i.e. midinguinal point aiming towards the adductor tubercle; the second is again longitudinal over the great saphenous vein from the saphenous opening to just below the knee. This forms a skin bridge between the two incisions.

◆ Dissect out the common femoral artery placing arterial slings over the branches.

◆ Dissect out the great saphenous vein, ligating and dividing its tributaries. Tie off the proximal end of the great saphenous vein as it joins the superficial femoral vein; then divide it 1-2cm distal to the termination (allowing you to regain control should your knot slip).

◆ At the distal end of the saphenous incision, you can continue to dissect medially to the popliteal fossa, identifying the neurovascular bundle as it passes between the two heads of gastrocnemius. Isolate the artery and place an arterial sling around it.

◆ Divide the distal end of the great saphenous vein, test it using hep-saline for leaks and turn it so that the distal end is now proximal.

The alternative to a saphenous vein graft is a polytetrafluoroethylene (PTFE) synthetic graft. Obviously if this is being used, then the steps involving saphenous vein harvest become unnecessary.

◆ Heparinize the patient and wait a few minutes.
◆ Clamp and control the femoral and popliteal arteries and all their branches.
◆ Perform the proximal arteriotomy and anastomose the distal end of the saphenous graft using 5.0 Prolene end-to-side.
◆ Pass the vein subcutaneously and perform the distal arteriotomy and anastomosis, leaving a small blow hole. Release the proximal clamp to test the anastomosis allowing any thrombus to be flushed out of the blowhole.
◆ Replace the clamp, suture the blowhole and any leaks; then release both clamps. Place drains in both the groin and the popliteal fossa.
◆ Close the fascia and skin separately in layers.

Complications

These are high risk patients, in the main because they are, by definition, cardiopaths.

- Death.
- Graft occlusion.
- Amputation.
- Re-do surgery involving extension of the graft to the below-knee position.
- Graft infection (more likely in PTFE than saphenous grafts).

ENT PROCEDURES

Tonsillectomy

This is surgical excision of tonsillar tissue generally for problems of recurrent tonsillitis.

Indications

Relative indications
- Repeated attacks of tonsillitis.
- Peritonsillar abscess (Quinsy).

Absolute indications
- Sleep apnoea syndrome, if due to tonsillar size.
- For histology if suspicious of malignancy.

Surgical technique

Dissection (generally with bipolar diathermy)
The patient is intubated using an orotracheal tube. The surgeon identifies the tonsillar tissue and excises it from the posterior pharynx by the method of his choice. Haemostasis is then achieved.

Note

— Tonsillectomy is performed under general anaesthetic, not local.

Complications

- Referred ear pain, which is very common, and is frequently misdiagnosed as infection (remember the glossopharyngeal nerve supplies both the posterior pharynx and ear).
- Formation of a membrane over the tonsillar bed, frequently misdiagnosed as infection.
- Primary haemorrhage, within 24 hours postoperatively by definition, but commonly occurs within the first 12 hours. This is due to inadequate or incomplete haemostasis at the time of surgery.
- Secondary haemorrhage. Greater than 24 hours postoperatively by definition, but is usually 5-10 days postoperatively.

Note

— Both primary and secondary haemorrhages are serious and are potentially life-threatening events. Both need haemostasis by direct pressure with pads (hydrogen peroxide or adrenaline soaked), or by ligation under GA (if left too long, haemorrhage can be fatal).

- Sepsis.

Tracheostomy

This is surgical opening up of an airway by incising the trachea.

Indications

- Upper respiratory obstruction.
- Aspiration of secretions, e.g. acute exacerbation of chronic obstructive airways disease (COAD), with an inability to clear secretions.
- Protection of the airway, e.g. aspiration risk when gag is lost secondary to neurological conditions.
- Comatose states.
- Mouth or pharyngeal wounds.
- Respiratory muscle paralysis.
- Reduction of dead space to help ventilation.

Surgical technique

This is a relatively uncommon question in clinical and viva exams, but it does crop up occasionally.

- Split the skin, subcutanous fat and platysma.
- Push apart the sternohyoid and sternothyroid.
- Incise through the deep cervical layer, then the pretracheal fascial layers.
- Split the isthmus of the thyroid.
- Penetrate the trachea.
- Look out for the tracheobronchial lymph nodes, cardiac plexus, inferior thyroid vein and thyroidea ima artery.
- Insert the tracheostomy tube itself (this can be the definitive article or a temporary [uncuffed] version for 72 hours or so).

Complications

- Pneumothorax.
- Haematoma.
- Tracheostomy obstruction or displacement.
- Wound infection.
- Late tracheal stenosis.

BREAST PROCEDURES

Mastectomy

This is the surgical excision of breast tissue in toto.

Indications

- A large or centrally located carcinoma (bearing in mind the size of the breast).
- Multifocal carcinoma.
- Multifocal or extensive ductal carcinoma *in situ*.
- Prophylactic mastectomy in BRCA1/2 mutation carriers and women at risk of hereditary breast cancer.
- Paget's disease of the breast.
- Other malignancies, such as squamous cell carcinoma and sarcoma.

Simple mastectomy is the excision of the entire breast, including the overlying skin and nipple/areolar complex. A more radical operation may be performed, depending on the level of tumour invasion and lymph node involvement:

- Modified radical (Patey) mastectomy is a simple mastectomy combined with axillary clearance.
- Halsted radical mastectomy is removal of all breast tissue, axillary lymph nodes and the pectoralis major muscle. It is rarely used in modern practice.

In patients with early stage invasive breast cancer, breast-conserving therapy (lumpectomy with levels I and II axillary node dissection, plus radiotherapy) provides comparable overall and disease-free survival to modified radical mastectomy.

Surgical technique (modified radical mastectomy)

All patients undergoing mastectomy should be provided with adequate pre-operative counselling. They should be aware that breast reconstruction is available to them and should be offered this option, either as an immediate or delayed procedure.

- The operation is performed under general anaesthetic with the patient supine and the ipsilateral arm abducted on an arm board.
- Prepare the skin of the breast, shoulder, arm and axilla. Place the drapes to allow access to the breast and the axilla.
- Start by marking the position of the lump and draw on the skin an ellipse for your incision. This should be transverse or oblique and encompass the nipple/areolar complex with about 5cm of skin around the lesion. Ensure that you will be able to approximate the wound edges.
- Make your incision. Use a scalpel or scissors to elevate the skin and subcutaneous tissue as flaps. Your plane of dissection should correspond to Scarpa's fascia between the subcutaneous fat and mammary fat. Ask an assistant to elevate the skin flaps as you

dissect. Take care not to traumatise the skin edges or make the skin flaps too thin, as this can cause skin necrosis or buttonholing. Raise the upper flap to the upper limit of the breast. This corresponds to within 2cm of the clavicle or the second intercostal space. Raise the lower flap to the lower limits of the breast, below the inframammary fold.

- Identify the fascia of the pectoralis major muscle at the upper limit of the breast. Mobilise the breast by using a plane of cleavage between the breast and pectoralis major. Work from superior to inferior, dissecting the breast tissue away with the pectoralis fascia.
- Control bleeding from perforating blood vessels with diathermy or ligatures.
- Elevate the breast laterally until it is only attached at the axilla.
- Place dry packs under each skin flap.
- Now proceed with axillary clearance. The borders of the axillary dissection are the lateral border of pectoralis major anteriorly, anterior border of latissimus dorsi posteriorly, axillary vein superiorly, and serratus anterior medially. Clear the axillary contents from along the lateral border of pectoralis major.
- Identify the underlying pectoralis minor muscle. Pass a finger under the insertion of pectoralis minor to free it from the underlying structures. Ask your assistant to retract the muscle forward and medially in order to expose the axillary contents of level II. To access level III nodes, pectoralis minor can be divided at its insertion into the coracoid process. The subpectoral area is best exposed by flexing and abducting the shoulder and flexing the elbow, so that the forearm lies across the patient's face. Gently stroke the axillary contents away from the underlying nerves and vessels using a swab. Identify and preserve the long thoracic nerve and thoracodorsal nerve which lie close to the chest wall. The intercostobrachial nerve crosses the mid-axillary region and should also be preserved.
- Remove the breast and axillary contents, mark them for orientation (e.g. a silk suture in the 12 o'clock position) and send for histological examination.
- Once you are satisfied that you have achieved adequate haemostasis, two suction drains should be placed. Position one in the axilla and the other along the inferior skin flap. The drains should pierce the skin below the incision in the axilla.
- Close the subcutaneous fat with absorbable sutures (e.g. Vicryl) and the skin with an absorbable subcutaneous suture (e.g. Monocryl).

Complications

- Haematoma.
- Wound infection.
- Seroma.
- Lymphoedema.
- Necrosis of skin flap.
- Chronic pain.
- Numbness of the upper arm (intercostobrachial nerve damage).
- Injury to the thoracodorsal nerve, long thoracic nerve, axillary vein or brachial plexus.
- Postoperative frozen shoulder.
- Phantom breast syndrome.

UROLOGY PROCEDURES

Transurethral resection of the prostate (TURP)

This is removal of the prostate using endoscopic means via the tract of the urethra.

Indications

- Urinary retention secondary to benign prostatic hypertrophy (if renal function is not impaired, then a trial without a catheter can be attempted).
- Obstructive uropathy.
- Recurrent UTIs with prostatic bladder outflow obstruction (BOO).
- Bladder calculus secondary to BOO.
- Significant recurrent haematuria from the prostate gland.

Relative indications

- Moderate to severe symptoms of bladder outflow obstruction (hesitancy, nocturia, poor stream, incomplete sensation of voiding).
- Poor response to (failure of) medical treatment.

It is worth noting that the prostate specific antigen (PSA) level can be used as a relative indicator of the progression of the disease and risk of acute urinary retention. This can be of use in deciding when to operate.

Surgical technique

- Perform a pre-operative PR exam to assess the size of the gland.
- An IV prophylactic antibiotic injection is intended to reduce the postoperative UTI/sepsis risk.
- Place the patient in the lithotomy position.
- A resectoscope is passed per urethra, after dilatation with incrementally increasing diameter sounds. This enables visualisation, as well as controlled cutting, coagulation and vaporisation of prostatic tissue.
- Before proceeding to resection the relevant anatomical landmarks must be identified, specifically the verumontanum, the neck of the bladder and both ureteric orifices.
- As with all endoscopic techniques, a fluid medium is required for irrigation. There are two basic choices: glycine, which has the advantage of conducting electricity enabling unipolar diathermy, and is non-haemolytic; or, saline, which has the advantage of not being associated with TUR syndrome. It does, however, necessitate the use of a bipolar diathermy resectoscope.
- The resection must take place in a systematic manner. The exact system used is less important, but the fact that a system is used will avoid incomplete resection. A classic system is the Nesbit technique. This involves, in the first instance, resection at the level of the bladder neck, followed by resection of the prostate adenoma in quadrants (right, followed by left), starting at the 12 o'clock position and working down. This has the advantage of allowing the lateral lobes to fall in. And finally, the tissue located at the apex is resected.
- After resection look in the bladder to ensure no resection tissue is present. Inspect the margins of resection.
- Pass a large diameter three-way catheter and secure to the thigh with tape.
- Consider irrigation (saline) overnight if there are problems of passage of clot.
- Plan the catheter removal at 24-48 hours.

Complications

Early

- Bleeding.
- Clot retention.
- Infection (can progress to severe septicaemia).
- TUR syndrome (more likely with glycine than saline irrigation during the procedure). This is a syndrome of fluid intoxication secondary to the irrigation fluid getting into the circulation resulting in metabolic consequences such as confusion, and potentially affecting consciousness.
- Epididymo-orchitis.

Late/delayed

- Retrograde ejaculation.
- Secondary/delayed haemorrhage.
- Erectile dysfunction.
- Urinary incontinence.
- Urethral stricture.

Section 2

Clinical surgery

Chapter 5

General surgery

Oesophageal motility disorders (dysphagia)

Presentation

Dysphagia simply means difficulty in swallowing. There are different types of dysphagia, which can be subdivided by asking the following questions:

- Is it difficult to swallow fluids and solids from the start of the swallowing process? Yes suggests a motility disorder; no suggests a stricture.
- Is it difficult to make the swallowing movement? Yes suggests a bulbar palsy (neurological in origin).
- Is it painful on swallowing? Yes suggests either a malignant stricture or oesophagitis (the most common cause of oesophagitis is acid reflux).
- Is the dysphagia intermittent, constant or worsening? If intermittent, this may be suggestive of an oesophageal spasm; if constant and worsening, this suggests a malignant stricture.
- Is there a neck bulge or gurgle when drinking? If yes, consider a pharyngeal pouch.

Causes of dysphagia (Figure 5.1)

Malignant stricture
- Oesophageal carcinoma.
- Gastric carcinoma.
- Pharyngeal carcinoma.

Benign stricture with extrinsic pressure
- Lung carcinoma.
- Thyroid goitre.
- Mediastinal carcinoma.

Motility disorder
- Diffuse oesophageal spasm.
- Achalasia.
- Systemic sclerosis.
- Bulbar palsy.

Other
- Oesophagitis (which can be caused by either infection or reflux).

Investigations

- Barium swallow.
- Endoscopy and biopsy.
- CT scan (to assess anatomy and resectability of tumour).
- Oesophageal manometry.
- FBC, ESR.

Treatment

Obviously treatment varies according to the primary diagnosis, which more commonly takes the form of either a malignancy or oesophagitis resulting from oesophageal reflux.

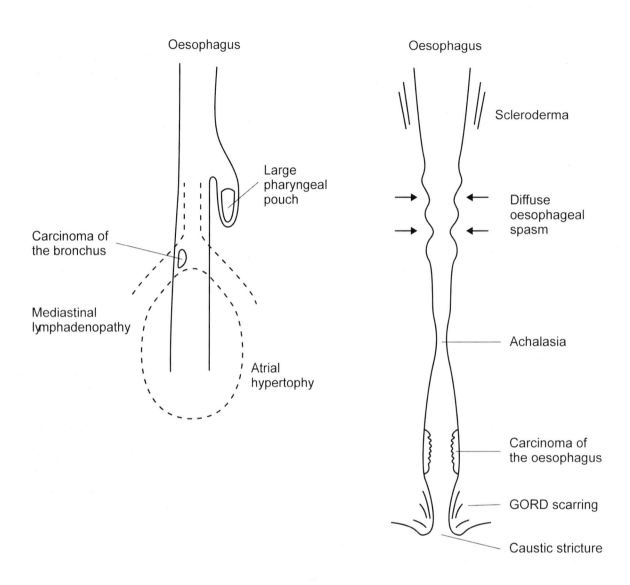

Figure 5.1. Oesophageal motility disorders.

The decision to proceed to oesophagectomy surgery is a complicated one involving an experienced surgeon's assessment of resectability, nutritional status of the patient, as well as the patient's ability to withstand a major surgical insult (see p209 for more detail on the Ivor Lewis oesophagectomy). Some series suggest that 50-60% of patients present with an unresectable tumour, necessitating palliative treatment. The major symptom to palliate is the dysphagia (that can otherwise result in rapid weight loss and aspiration of saliva with consequent pneumonia); this can be treated with an oesophageal stent, dramatically improving quality of life.

Currently, the treatment of oesophagitis is for the most part medical, in the form of proton pump inhibitors (PPIs).

Greater detail on treatment of the individual causes of dysphagia mentioned above can be found in their respective specialised sections.

Complications of oesophagectomy surgery

◆ Anastomotic leakage.
◆ Failure of re-inflation of the right lung on a postoperative radiograph check.
◆ Basal atelectasis, pneumonia, respiratory failure.
◆ Delayed gastric emptying.
◆ Recurrence of disease. Unfortunately, oesophageal carcinoma carries a high recurrence rate, despite attempts at curative surgery in well selected patients.

Diffuse oesophageal spasm
This is intermittent dysphagia with solids and liquids and chest pain. A barium swallow shows abnormal contractions.

Achalasia
This is a failure of oesophageal peristalsis and relaxation of the lower oesophageal sphincter due to loss of ganglia from Auerbach's plexus.

Presentation
◆ Dysphagia of both liquids and solids, chest pain and regurgitation.
◆ Barium swallow shows a grossly expanded oesophagus tapering to a tight oesophageal sphincter.
◆ Chest X-ray shows an 'air-fluid-level' behind the heart.
◆ A double right heart border can also be seen (representing an expanded oesophagus).

Treatment of achalasia
Achalasia is treated (medically) with hydralazine or nitrates; this is a short-term solution, however. Cardiomyotomy (surgical incision and resulting dilatation of the cardia [lower end] of the oesophageal sphincter) or balloon dilatation are more permanently effective treatments.

Benign oesophageal strictures
Benign oesophageal strictures, caused by oesophageal reflux, corrosives or trauma, are treated with endoscopic dilatation.

Webs

Plummer-Vinson syndrome
This is a fine web usually found immediately above the cricopharyngeal sphincter. Associated features include glossitis, dysphagia and iron deficiency anaemia. The web is often diagnosed by barium swallow and can be ruptured endoscopically.

Gastro-oesophageal reflux disease

Presentation

Relaxation of the lower oesophageal sphincter results in acid reflux from the stomach (which has mucosal defenses against acid) to the oesophagus (which does not).

Symptoms are as follows:

◆ Heartburn. This is a lay term, referring to the sensation of a burning retrosternal pain, felt from the throat extending down to the epigastrium. It is classically worse with stooping or lying down, and with drinking hot drinks.
◆ Waterbrash. The mouth fills with a bitter tasting (acidic) saliva and stomach acid combination.
◆ Nocturnal cough and wheeze. A reactive bronchospasm from exposure to refluxed stomach acid.

Aetiology

◆ Smoking, alcohol and obesity (these are associatiations, rather than proven causes).
◆ Hiatus hernia. The herniation of the stomach through its diaphragmatic opening results in disruption to the cardiac sphincter and, hence, causes reflux.

There are two basic types of hiatus hernia:

● sliding. The gastro-oesophageal junction slides through the hiatus and lies above the diaphragm;
● rolling. The sphincter remains below the diaphragm but part of the stomach rolls up through the hiatus alongside the oesophagus.

Note

– Hiatus hernia alone does not cause symptoms. It is when it is associated with reflux that it becomes symptomatic.

◆ Drugs (tricyclic antidepressants, anticholinergics, nitrates).

Investigations

◆ Barium swallow (shows a hiatus hernia).
◆ 24-hour pH monitoring.
◆ Oesophageal manometry (shows the pressure at the cardia, and hence its ability to prevent reflux, or not).

Differential diagnosis

◆ Peptic ulcer disease (gastric or duodenal).
◆ Swallowed corrosives (usually apparent from the history).
◆ Infection.

Treatment

◆ Alginates, e.g. Gaviscon, acting as a barrier between the stomach or oesophageal wall and the acid.
◆ Malox (magnesium hydroxide and aluminium hydroxide). Again, a form of barrier antacid.
◆ Proton pump inhibitors, e.g. omeprazole, directly inhibit the parietal cells of the stomach from secreting acid. The proton pump is so termed because H$^+$ is a proton, and is the cation of HCl, i.e. acid.
◆ Fundoplication creates an artificial sphincter by folding the gastric fundus around the distal oesophagus.

Lifestyle changes

◆ Decrease intra-abdominal pressure (lose weight and avoid tight belts/trousers).
◆ Raise bed head (improves nocturnal posture, providing a slope up which acid must travel before it is able to reflux).
◆ Small, low-fat meals (because fat delays gastric emptying, thus avoiding it promotes faster gastric emptying).
◆ No eating for three hours before bed.

Complications

◆ Peptic ulcer or erosions.
◆ Anaemia (from chronic bleeding, either from an ulcer or from oesophageal erosions).
◆ Benign stricture.
◆ Barrett's oesophagus (glandular metaplasia of the oesophageal mucosa secondary to chronic exposure to stomach acid). This is a premalignant condition that can lead to oesophageal cancer.

Tumours of the oesophagus

Benign oesophageal tumours

Leiomyomas - these are extremely rare.

Malignant oesophageal tumours

Malignant oesophageal tumours are more common than their benign counterparts, either as adenocarcinomas or squamous cell carcinomas. The male:female ratio is 3:1. They usually result from Barrett's metaplasia. Metaplasia means abnormal growth, resulting from chronic exposure of the oesophageal mucosa to acid from reflux from the stomach. The most common cause of such reflux is hiatus herniation.

Risk factors

◆ Barrett's oesophagus (squamous metaplasia on a background of chronic gastric acid reflux).
◆ Alcohol consumption.
◆ Smoking.
◆ Genetic predisposition (rare).
◆ As yet unproven, but suspected high dietary nitrosamines, low vitamin A or C.

Also, there is an increased risk seen in patients with oesophageal webs, achalasia and alkaline strictures (all these have oesophageal stagnation as a common vector).

Presentation

Presents insidiously and progressively with the following:

◆ Dysphagia (difficulty swallowing).
◆ Retrosternal discomfort.
◆ Pneumonia (aspiration).
◆ Persistent cough (tracheobronchial fistula).
◆ Anaemia.
◆ Haematemesis.
◆ Malnutrition.
◆ Disseminated cancer.

Investigations

◆ Oesophago-gastroduodenoscopy (OGD) and barium swallow (for anatomy and tissue diagnosis).
◆ Liver scan and/or laparoscopy (staging, looking for presence of metastases).
◆ CT and/or endoluminal ultrasound (USS probe in the lumen of the oesophagus, looking for the possibility of resectability of the affected segment).
◆ Respiratory function tests (most Western patients with oesophageal cancer are heavy smokers, i.e. a risk factor).

Treatment

Surgical

The decision to proceed to resection surgery for an oesophageal tumour is a complex one, and is best made by an experienced surgeon. It is based on imaging (CT and endoscopy), tissue diagnosis (endoscopic biopsy), absence of distal metastases (abdominal, hepatic), medical comorbidity, degree of malnutrition, and the patient's ability to withstand a major surgical insult.

For oesophageal tumours of the middle and distal thirds, the operation is an Ivor Lewis oesophagectomy. This is an operation encompassing two parts: the first is a laparotomy to look for peritoneal metastases (that are often otherwise missed), and to mobilise the stomach on vascular pedicles, such that it can be raised for the oesophagogastric anastomosis; the second is a right thoracotomy (in the 4th interspace) to expose the oesophagus, dissect off its anatomical relations, and resect the segment containing the tumour, leaving a cut end of oesophagus for anastomosis. It should be mentioned that this second part of the procedure requires single lung ventilation (deflation of the right lung, ventilation of the left).

The stomach is raised through the diaphragmatic hiatus in its entirety, the lesser curvature resected and the cut end of the oesophagus and stomach are anastomosed either by hand or with a staple gun. A nasogastric tube is placed across the anastomosis at the time of surgery, and is not removed until a gastrograffin swallow has been performed confirming its integrity, usually on day six postoperatively. Total parenteral nutrition is given in the intervening time.

It can safely be said that the (many) finer points of this complex surgery are beyond the remit of this book, but it is important to realise that there is significant morbidity and mortality associated with the procedure, and that it requires a specialist surgical (and anaesthetic) unit. HDU or ITU surveillance is required postoperatively.

Medical
◆ Radiotherapy treatment has a poor outcome for adenocarcinoma, but a good outcome for squamous cell carcinoma.
◆ Stenting.
◆ Endoscopic laser.

Complications of surgery

◆ Anastomotic leakage.
◆ Failure of re-inflation of the right lung on postoperative radiograph check.
◆ Basal atelectasis, pneumonia, respiratory failure.
◆ Delayed gastric emptying.

◆ Recurrence of disease. Unfortunately, oesophageal carcinoma carries a high recurrence rate, despite attempts at curative surgery in well selected patients.

Note

— Overall, the results for medical compared with surgical treatment for oesophageal cancer are said to be equal.

Oesophageal varices

Presentation

Oesophageal varices characteristically present with an upper gastro-intestinal (GI) bleed. They are caused by portosystemic hypertension, commonly secondary to hepatic cirrhosis.

Note

— Portosystemic hypertension is a backup of blood in the portal circulation as a result of liver disease. There are points of anastomosis between the portal and systemic blood circulations, mainly oesophageal in this context, at which the rise in pressure results in venous dilation, and hence bleeding risk (see p103 for more detail on portosystemic anastomoses and venous drainage).

Oesophageal varices result in death of one third of cirrhotics by haemorrhage. Non-surgical treatment is best, as this group of patients do not tolerate surgery well.

Investigations

Diagnosis is best made by OGD. However, because upper GI bleeds can be severe and life-threatening, investigation takes place along the lines of acute resuscitation, i.e. send off for an emergency FBC (to know the starting Hb), U+Es (to know the renal function

and potassium level), LFTs (to see how deranged they are), and a clotting screen (CS) (often there is deranged coagulation, needing urgent correction to help stop the bleed). An appropriate number of units should be grouped and cross-matched urgently.

The gastroenterologists on call should be called upon for OGD in severe bleeds, as this represents both investigation (confirms the diagnosis of variceal bleed or, peptic ulcer bleed as the main differential diagnosis) and treatment, i.e. band ligation or sclerotherapy can be performed via this route.

Treatment

As mentioned above the treatment is divided into stopping the bleeding, as well as supporting the patient's cardiovascular (and coagulation) system (acute), and addressing the portal hypertension that has caused the varices in the first place (long term). This means that rapid fluid resuscitation with placement of two large-bore cannulae needs to be started. The fluid of choice is, of course, blood, when available, but while waiting for the cross-match, Hartmann's solution is appropriate. If the FBC shows a very low platelet count, then two units of platelets should be given. If the clotting screen shows grossly disturbed coagulation, then two units of fresh frozen plasma (FFP) should be given.

Emergency treatment options
◆ Sclerotherapy, e.g. adrenaline, ethanolamine.
◆ Rubber band ligation.
◆ Sengstaken-Blakemore tube (complications of aspiration and pressure necrosis of oesophagus).
◆ Transjugular intrahepatic portosytemic shunt (TIPS). This causes a shunt by passage of a catheter from the jugular vein into one of the intrahepatic branches of the portal vein.
◆ Octreotide infusion.

Elective treatment options
In patients in whom oesophageal varices have been identified, the risk of them going on to bleed is 30%, if they have never had a bleed before. Where patients have already had one or more bleeds, the risk of a re-bleed is more like 70%.

Pharmacological

Propranolol reduces the first bleeding risk by 40%; it also reduces the frequency of re-bleeding, but does not affect survival.

Note

— Glypressin has a similar prophylactic function.

Surgical

◆ Liver transplantation is the definitive treatment, but the patient population is at a high surgical risk, being very medically unfit.
◆ Total shunt (however, the encephalopathy rate is high).
◆ Partial shunts (the encephalopathy rate is lower and it is difficult surgery).
◆ Devascularisation procedures.

Note

— Surgery does not show any increase in survival time, compared with medical treatment.

Complications

The different treatment modalities have their own specific complications as follows.

Liver transplantation

These can be divided into mechanical and non-mechanical groups.

Mechanical complications relate to the structures that were anastomosed in the transplant:

◆ Hepatic artery thrombosis, stenosis or pseudo-aneurysm.
◆ Biliary leak or stricture.
◆ Portal vein thrombosis or stenosis.
◆ Inferior vena cava thrombosis or stenosis (less common).

Non-mechanical complications include:

◆ Ascites.
◆ Postoperative pyogenic abscess.

◆ Non-function of the grafted liver.
◆ Graft rejection.
◆ Viral re-infection of the graft by the host.
◆ Recurrent hepatic malignancy.
◆ Post-transplantation lymphoproliferative disease.

Partial shunt (TIPS being the most commonly performed)

◆ Thrombosis, stenosis, or occlusion of the shunt.
◆ Puncture of the hepatic capsule.
◆ Intraperitoneal bleed.
◆ Stent migration.
◆ Sepsis.
◆ Recurrent encephalopathy.
◆ Haemolysis.

Gastritis and peptic ulcer disease

Presentation

Patients complain of epigastric pain (dyspepsia), which may radiate round to the back (suggesting posterior ulceration).

It is possible for food to relieve the pain in some cases.

Patients can present with the complications rather than the symptoms of peptic ulceration, e.g. the sequlae of chronic haemorrhage (iron deficiency anaemia), or an acute upper GI bleed (haematemesis or melaena), or with peritonitis secondary to perforation of a peptic ulcer, or with gastric outflow obstruction symptoms secondary to a chronic duodenal ulcer causing narrowing of the pylorus (post-prandial vomiting, sometimes projectile).

Finally, it should be mentioned that some gastric malignancies present as ulcers. One should look out for constant epigastric pain associated with weight loss in the history.

The differential diagnosis of epigastric pain is unsurprisingly broad (considering the number of anatomical structures in and around the area): myocardial ischaemia or infarction, PE, cholecystitis, pancreatitis, gastro-oesophageal reflux disease, gastric cancer and irritable bowel syndrome.

Aetiology

Peptic ulcer disease is common, but since the advent of successful medical treatment, first with H_2 receptor antagonists (e.g. ranitidine), but more commonly now with proton pump inhibitors (PPIs, e.g. omeprazole), symptomatic disease rates are considerably decreased. Certainly the need for surgery has fallen dramatically.

Pathogenesis

It is important to know the background information on mucosal defence mechanisms against the effects of gastric acid. Fundamentally this falls into three categories:

- Extramucosal factors. A lining of mucus on the stomach lumen and bicarbonate secreted as a form of buffer.
- Mucosal factors. Resistance to acid of the stomach lining cells, the presence of tight junctions between cells, and a reaction involving migration of adjacent mucosal cells to the site of damage.
- Vascular factors. The presence of an alkaline tide neutralising acid. It is at this stage of the defence systems that prostaglandins, as well as neuropeptides and nitric oxide, have roles in regulating the defence.

Failure of one of the above systems can result in ulceration or gastritis, or erosions.

Commonly, one sees patients on anti-inflammatory drugs, which interfere with the prostaglandin vascular defence mechanism presenting with peptic ulcer disease.

Investigations

Obviously, a full history and examination should be taken, looking for the aforementioned presenting complaints and physical findings.

Routine blood tests should be performed, looking for anaemia, raised inflammatory markers, amylase, deranged LFTs and renal function (to aid the differential diagnosis and assessment of fitness for surgery if necessary).

In the case of upper GI bleeds, peritonitis or other acute presentations, a group and save (G+S), if not urgent cross-match, may be indicated.

The investigation that will make the diagnosis, though, is endoscopic assessment (OGD). This gives direct visualisation of the ulcer (or erosions or tumour), and enables biopsies to be taken for a tissue diagnosis.

Breath testing for *Helicobacter pylori* is also a useful adjunct. *H. pylori* hydrolyses urea to CO_2, which if radioactively labelled can be measured, and the presence of *H. pylori* can be inferred indirectly.

In the case of suspected perforation, an erect CXR may show free air under the diaphragm.

Note

- The presence of multiple ulcers, especially ulceration distal to the second part of the duodenum, are highly suggestive of the rare Zollinger-Ellison syndrome (a gastrin-secreting tumour, stimulating the stomach to oversecrete acid).

Treatment

For the most part the management of peptic ulceration, when fully investigated, is medical. Use of PPIs is extremely successful. OGD can be used to treat acutely bleeding ulcers with injection of sclerosants (e.g. adrenaline), laser or, a thermocautery probe. However, in cases refractory to medical treatment it may be necessary to proceed to surgical treatment. Gastric ulcers can be treated with the Bilroth type I partial gastrectomy. Duodenal ulcers can be treated by placing an under-running suture at the base of the ulcer by open surgery.

In the emergency situation of a perforated duodenal ulcer, an open duodenal oversew of omentum, as well as a thorough peritoneal lavage, should be performed. Gastric perforation can be treated with the Bilroth type I partial gastrectomy.

Pyloric stenosis can be treated by pyloroplasty or a bypass procedure such as a gastrojejunostomy.

Complications

♦ Wound infection.
♦ Dumping, early or late (covered in the 'Gastric cancer' section below).
♦ Diarrhoea.
♦ Prolonged ileus.
♦ Reflux.

The emergency presentations (peritonitis, perforation, acute life-threatening GI bleeds) carry a significant mortality.

Gastric cancer

Presentation

Gastric cancer may present in the following ways:

♦ Indigestion.
♦ Nausea +/- vomiting.
♦ Anorexia.
♦ Epigastric pain.
♦ Weight loss.

Clinical findings include:

♦ Abdominal mass (typically epigastric).
♦ Virchow's node (supraclavicular, also known as Troisier's sign).
♦ Hepatomegaly.
♦ Cachexia.
♦ Jaundice.
♦ Haematemesis.
♦ Melaena.

Pathology

Normally presents as an adenocarcinoma, i.e. a cancer originating from glandular tissue.

Macroscopically, it can take on the appearance of:

♦ An ulcerating lesion.
♦ A convex growth (cauliflower appearance).
♦ Linitis plastica ('leather bottle' stomach). This is a diffuse infiltration of the submucous tissue of the stomach by the tumour.

The majority of tumours arise at the pre-pyloric region (64%).

Spread

Gastric cancer is a tumour capable of spread via the following routes:

♦ Direct invasion (through the stomach wall into adjacent structures).
♦ Lymphatic.
♦ Haematogenous (via the blood stream).
♦ Transcoelomic (via the peritoneum).

Note

— Gastric secondaries in the ovaries are termed 'Krukenberg tumours' with a characteristic 'signet-ring' cell appearance.

Epidemiology

Gastric cancer is more common in men than women, the incidence being greatest between the ages of 40 and 60 years. It appears more commonly in people of blood group A.

Investigations

♦ Barium meal (shows the outline of the ulcer or mass).
♦ OGD enables direct visualisation and an opportunity for tissue diagnosis with a biopsy.
♦ FBC (looking for anaemia).
♦ U&Es (looking for renal failure secondary to dehydration).
♦ LFTs (looking for hepatic infiltration).
♦ Liver ultrasound (also looking for hepatic invasion, the presence of which renders the tumour inoperable as it signifies metastatic spread).

BILROTH II GASTRECTOMY + ROUX-EN-Y

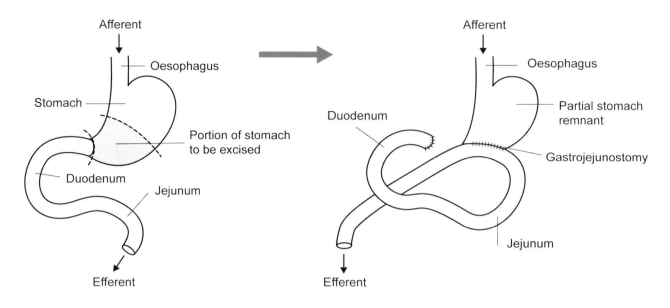

TOTAL GASTRECTOMY + ROUX-EN-Y

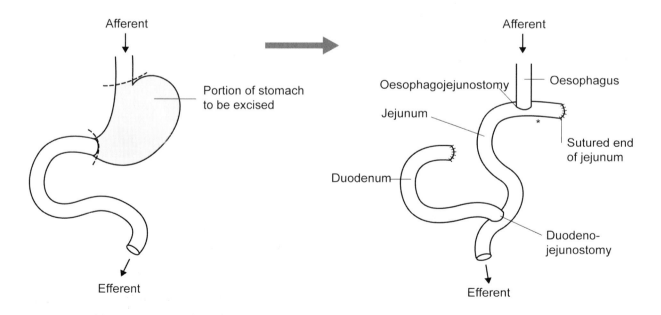

* Note small end of jejunum left free to act as a reservoir of sorts. There are numerous variations of reservoir types involving sutured-together loops of bowel

Figure 5.2. Gastric cancer treatment.

Treatment (Figure 5.2)

The only curative treatment is surgery, which takes the form of a total or a subtotal gastrectomy. The local lymph nodes must also be excised. If the aim of surgery is palliation rather than cure, i.e. there is evidence of distant metastasis, then surgery is indicated only for relief of obstruction.

Note

— Before surgery it is important to place the patient on a clear fluid diet, if there is any evidence of gastric outlet obstruction. This is to empty the stomach of food residue which would otherwise be a contaminant at the time of surgery.

Partial gastrectomy

This is suitable for cancers arising in the distal stomach, i.e. pre-pyloric region in the majority of tumours.

The pylorus, antrum and lesser curvature of the stomach are excised, and the lesser curvature is sewn up. The remaining open portion of the distal stomach is anastomosed to a loop of jejunum as an end-to-side anastomosis (end of stomach to side of jejunum). The duodenal stump is closed. This is a Bilroth II (Polya partial) gastrectomy and reconstruction.

Note

— The 'Roux-en-Y' is a variation on the enterostomy loop mentioned. It is a procedure designed to avoid the complication of bilious vomiting. It differs from the above only in the addition of the division of the proximal jejunum, anastomosing proximal loop to a more distal loop of jejunum, and having the gastrojejunal anastomosis as an end-to-end anastomosis (instead of the end-to-side). This results in a much greater distance that the bile would have to travel retrogradely to produce bilious vomiting and, hence, considerably reduces its incidence.

Total gastrectomy

Total gastrectomy is indicated if the tumour is more proximal, i.e. lesser curve or the body of the stomach. The entire stomach is excised, leaving a duodenal and oesophageal stump. The oesophageal stump is anastomosed to a mobilised loop of jejunum. The duodenal stump is closed.

Oesophageal anastomoses are temperamental to put it mildly; they are at risk of leak and anastomotic breakdown. It is common practice to pass an NG tube beyond the anastomosis into the jejunum in an attempt to protect it.

Note

— It is sometimes necessary to perform the operation through a thoraco-abdominal approach, particularly in total gastrectomy, if the exposure is insufficient in the abdominal approach.

Complications

General complications
- Wound infection.
- Dehiscence.
- Bleeding.
- Haematoma.
- Chest infection.
- Basal atelectasis.
- DVT.
- PE.
- Incisional hernia.

Specific complications
- Bilious vomiting.
- Anastomotic dehiscence.
- Early dumping.
- Late dumping.
- Diarrhoea.

Bilious vomiting occurs characteristically 15-30 minutes post-meal, and is more common soon after surgery but tends to resolve. The problem can be solved, if it persists, by the aforementioned Roux-en-Y anastomosis (it can also be prevented by performing it as part of the original procedure).

Dumping can be early or late. Early dumping is due to rapid emptying of the stomach. A high osmotic load thus enters the small intestine, increasing splanchnic blood flow and hence a fluid shift from the systemic circulation to the intestinal circulation. Symptoms are sweating, flushing, tachycardia, palpitations, nausea, vomiting and diarrhoea.

Late dumping is a reactive hypoglycaemia in response to the large insulin secretion following the earlier hyperglycaemia secondary to the sudden load of gastric contents into the small intestine. The symptoms are similar to those of early dumping, but delayed.

Early dumping occurs immediately post-meal, and late dumping occurs within 1-2 hours post-meal.

Inflammatory bowel disorders

Characteristically thought of as meaning ulcerative colitis and Crohn's disease only. However, amoebic dysentery (*Entamoeba histolytica*), bacillary dysentry (shigellosis), schistosomiasis, Campylobacter, Yersinia and *Clostridium difficile* can all cause dysentery, i.e. diarrhoea with passage of blood PR, hence causing inflammation of the bowel, specifically the colon.

Ulcerative colitis (UC)

- Unknown aetiology.
- Damage is to the mucosa only (unlike Crohn's, which is transmural).
- Involves the rectum and then spreads proximally (unlike Crohn's which affects any part of the bowel and has skip lesions).
- Can relapse and remit (as can Crohn's).
- When severe, can cause toxic megacolon (unlike Crohn's, typically, although it is accepted that toxic megacolon can occur in proven Crohn's).
- Over time, this results in dysplasia, which puts the patient at a severe risk of malignant change. It has, in fact, been demonstrated that eight years of total colitis results in a definite increase of malignant change (Crohn's can predispose to malignant change, but the incidence is less). A colectomy should be considered if severe dysplasia is found on routine biopsy.

Presentation

Ulcerative colitis clinically presents as bloody diarrhoea, cramping and abdominal pain which, if severe, can result in malnutrition, dehydration and electrolyte loss.

Extra-intestinal symptoms include:

- Skin (pyoderma gangrenosum, erythema nodosum).
- Mucous membranes (apthous ulceration of mouth and vagina).
- Eyes (iritis).
- Joints (ankylosing spondylitis, arthritis, sacro-iliitis).
- Liver (chronic active hepatitis, sclerosing cholangitis, cirrhosis, cholangiocarcinoma).
- Renal (amyloidosis).
- Fingernail (clubbing).

Investigations

- PR.
- AXR.
- Sigmoidoscopy.
- Colonoscopy combined with biopsy.
- FBC.
- U&Es.
- LFTs.
- ESR.
- CRP.
- Albumin (Alb).

Treatment

Medical or surgical (the best management is said to be with an aggressive gastroenterologist and a conservative surgeon).

Medical treatment

Steroids and salicylic acid derivatives (e.g. Asacol), which can prolong remission and codeine phosphate to prevent diarrhoea. Additionally, azathioprine and cyclosporin are used as second-line medical treatments.

Surgical treatment

Indications for surgery can be acute (severe episode failing to respond to medical measures), or chronic (again failing to respond to medical measures). The preferred operation is a subtotal colectomy with a mucous fistula, i.e. leaving the rectum behind, certainly in the acute phase, as the morbidity of excising it in such a sick patient is considerable.

Complications of surgery

◆ Pelvic sepsis.
◆ Anastomotic dehiscence.
◆ Incontinence.
◆ Stricture formation (usually responds to simple dilatation).

Crohn's disease

Presentation

◆ Can involve any part of the GI tract from the mouth to the anus.

Note

— UC does not involve the anus; this is almost diagnostic of Crohn's disease.
— Never say never - it is possible for UC to cause peri-anal and perineal enterocutaneous fistulae; however, it is very uncommon.

◆ The most common part of the bowel involved is the terminal ileum.
◆ Chronic granulomatous disease in 60% (unlike UC which has no granulomas).
◆ Transmural disease (unlike UC which only involves the mucosa).
◆ Causes fissures and ulceration.
◆ Causes marked thickening of the bowel wall with a characteristic 'cobblestoning' appearance (unlike UC).
◆ Mucosal thickening can result in stricture formation, and hence obstructive symptoms usually requiring surgery if they do not settle (unlike UC).
◆ Crohn's can cause perforation, fistulation and abscess formation (unlike UC).

Investigations

◆ Sigmoidoscopy or colonoscopy combined with a biopsy/barium enema to demonstrate possible skip or string lesions.
◆ FBC.
◆ U&Es.
◆ ESR.
◆ CRP.

A string sign is characteristic of Crohn's disease and refers to the appearance on a contrast study of a narrow stretch of lumen resulting from the mucosal thickening of Crohn's.

Treatment

Note

— This is an incurable condition, therefore, management should be as conservative (i.e. medical) as possible, because the patient will eventually run out of bowel when too much has been resected, the so-called short bowel syndrome.

Medical

Flare-ups in disease activity are treated by steroids with or without azathioprine.

Surgical

If an acute flare up of Crohn's presents with complete obstruction which does not resolve with non-operative management ('drip and suck', i.e. nil by mouth [NBM] and nasogastric [NG] tube), then a laparotomy to identify the obstructed segment, with local excision and primary anastomosis, is indicated.

Formation of an abdominal abscess presents with abdominal pain, ileus, pyrexia and an acute abdomen. This is successfully treated by laparotomy and peritoneal lavage, and will likely require excision of the affected segment of bowel.

For symptomatic strictures, an endoscopic stricturoplasty (balloon dilatation) can be performed. The advantage is that this is 'bowel conserving', i.e. does not involve excision of yet more bowel from the patient.

Complications

As per other procedures involving laparotomy in the acute setting and bowel anastomosis, the complications can be local or general.

Local

◆ Wound infection.
◆ Anastomotic failure.
◆ Persistent ileus.

- ◆ Incisional hernia formation.
- ◆ Stricture formation at the anastomosis site.

General

- ◆ Pneumonia due to splinting of the diaphragm.
- ◆ Cough inhibition secondary to pain from the abdominal incision.
- ◆ CVA.
- ◆ MI.
- ◆ DVT.
- ◆ PE.
- ◆ Acute renal failure.

Stricturoplasty carries with it a risk of bowel perforation, failure to expand the lumen successfully and recurrence of the stricture.

Diverticular disease (Figure 5.3)

Presentation

A diverticulum is an 'A by-road' (from the Latin derivation). They are mucosal extrusions at weak points in the bowel wall. Diverticular disease most commonly affects the sigmoid colon (NEVER the rectum).

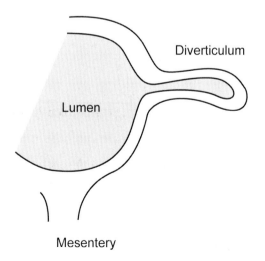

Figure 5.3. Diverticular disease: section through a loop of sigmoid colon.

It is thought to occur due to low fibre, high constipation and high intraluminal pressure. This is the reason why it is more common in the West than in, say, African countries. The above factors result in extrusion at weak points (i.e. anti-mesenteric border), where the vessels perforate the wall. The incidence is over 30% of people >60 years old in the Western world.

It is important at this stage to emphasise the correct use of terms involving the word diverticulum. Diverticular disease refers to the finding of diverticulae on colonoscopy or contrast enema; this is a potentially symptom-free condition. Diverticulosis refers to symptomatic diverticular disease, specifically generalised cramping abdominal pains in the abscence of pyrexia. However, the two terms are used relatively interchangeably in common parlance.

Diverticulitis refers to the inflammation of diverticulae, i.e. pyrexial patient, left iliac fossa pain with or without a diverticular bleed. A diverticular bleed is self-explanatory.

A diverticular mass is the formation of an inflammatory mass or abscess adjacent to an inflamed diverticulum. A diverticular perforation is self-explanatory.

Pathology

Diverticular disease can cause:

- ◆ No symptoms.
- ◆ Intermittent discomfort.
- ◆ Inflammation, hence 'diverticulitis', due to inspissated faecal matter resulting in mucosal ulceration.
- ◆ A PR bleed as a result of the inflammation.
- ◆ A pericolic abscess.
- ◆ A fistula as a result of rupture of the abscess. These can be vesicocolic, enterocolic, colocutaneous and colovaginal.
- ◆ Generalised peritonitis as a result of rupture of the abscess into the peritoneal cavity.

Investigations

As for an upper GI bleed, the investigations relate to resuscitation during an acute bleed, but in the non-acute setting, the investigations relate more to imaging/visualising the source of the bleed.

An emergency FBC (to know the starting Hb), U+Es (to know the renal function and potassium level), LFTs (to see how deranged they are), and a clotting screen (often there is deranged coagulation, needing urgent correction to help stop the bleed) should be requested. An appropriate number of units should be grouped and cross-matched urgently.

The patient should be regularly reviewed during an acute bleed for evidence of dehydration, pyrexia, and developing an acute abdomen (suggesting perforation or a diverticular mass).

In general terms, sigmoidoscopy picks up the majority of diverticulae, as this is the most common site for them to be found, but to exclude a diverticular source of bleeding, in the presence of a negative sigmoidoscopy, a full colonoscopy must be performed, as there may be other sources of lower GI bleeds to be found.

Angiography can localise the source of bleeding and has the potential to treat it by embolisation. It depends on local facilities and expertise as to its availablity.

Contrast studies, such as barium enemas, are not generally used for identifying sources of lower GI bleeds.

Treatment

80% of lower GI bleeds resolve spontaneously with conservative management. The risk of a re-bleed is 30% if this is the patient's first; otherwise it rises to 50%.

Conservative management is by fluid rehydration, keeping an eye on the Hb and renal function (U&Es, and catheter urine output), and replacing blood when necessary during the bleed.

Note

— The risk of a re-bleed, if the pathology is angiodysplasia, is higher than the above mentioned figures.

The majority of the time the acute bleed resolves with these conservative measures alone. Endoscopic or angiographic means can be used to stop the bleeding if conservative measures fail. If all fails, then surgical resection of the bleeding segment can be all that is left in terms of therapeutic options.

Complications

Endoscopic cautery of a diverticular bleed carries a small risk of bowel perforation.

Angiographic embolisation of a diverticular bleed carries a risk of necrosis of the affected section of bowel, as well as the vascular cannulation site risks of haematoma, infection and pseudo-aneurysm formation.

Laparotomy and excision of the bleeding section of bowel carries with it, as previously mentioned, the general risks of laparotomy.

Local
- Wound infection.
- Anastomotic failure.
- Persistent ileus.
- Incisional hernia formation.
- Stricture formation at the anastomosis site.

General
- Pneumonia due to splinting of the diaphragm.
- Cough inhibition secondary to pain from the abdominal incision.
- CVA.
- MI.
- DVT.
- PE.
- Acute renal failure.

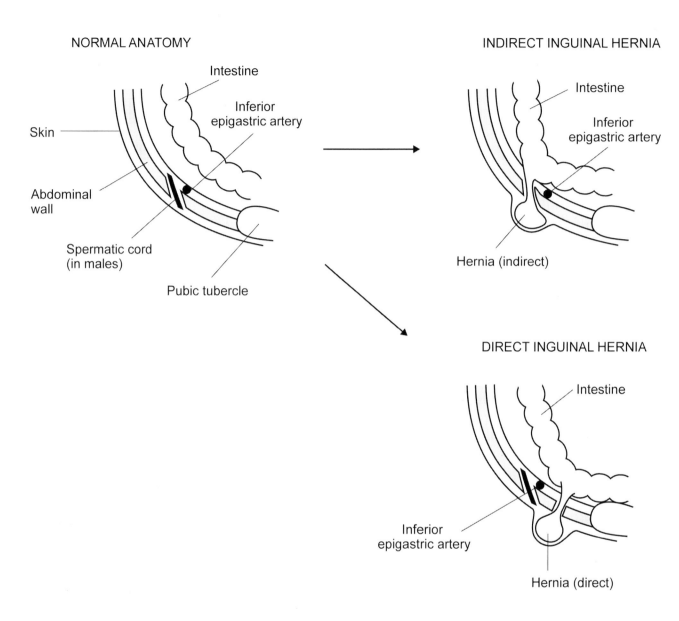

Figure 5.4. Inguinal hernias.

Hernias

The definition of a hernia is the protrusion of all or part of a viscus through a wall that normally contains it.

Presentation

Groin hernias present with groin pain, especially when straining, e.g. at work, or when passing water or a bowel motion (especially in prostatism or constipation), or when lifting weights. They also present with the sensation of a mass.

They can present in the emergency setting with a painful irreducible mass, with or without intestinal obstruction (colicky abdominal pain, absolute constipation, abdominal distension, nausea and vomiting). They can also present with an acute abdomen in the rare case of intestinal perforation.

Inguinal hernias (Figure 5.4)

Presentation

An important concept to be clear on is the difference between direct and indirect hernias. Direct inguinal hernias pass 'directly' through the abdominal wall medial to the internal inguinal ring. Indirect inguinal hernias take an 'indirect' route through the abdominal wall, i.e. they enter the abdominal wall at the internal inguinal ring, travel along the inside of the inguinal ligament, and exit at the external inguinal ring.

If the hernia is indirect, this is due to a congenital defect in a male, a patent processus vaginalis resulting from descent of the testicle.

Inguinal hernias are more common on the right (the right to left ratio is 5:4) and indirect hernias occur less frequently in females.

Note

– A female child with an indirect hernia should be checked for testicular feminisation (perform a chromosome check).

Children can present with incarcerated herniae. Two schools of thought exist as to the correct treatment (in children). Many books advocate conservative treatment, i.e. placing them in the Solomon's position (Gallow's traction), the thinking behind this being that incarceration rarely leads to strangulation in inguinal hernias in children. However, general surgeons will advocate close observation of the child, repeatedly on the ward, with a relatively low threshold for proceeding to surgery.

In adults, 65% of inguinal hernias are indirect, 35% are direct, and 5% are a combination of the two.

Direct hernias are more common in elderly men, indirect hernias are more common in young men. Women rarely develop direct hernias.

Predeterminates for indirect inguinal hernias

◆   Prematurity.
◆   Low birth weight.
◆   Twin birth.
◆   African race (this is postulated to be due to the greater forward tilt of the pelvis, which results in the insertion of external oblique being less effective at preventing herniation).

Indirect hernias can occur as a complication of intraperitoneal fluid accumulation (e.g. CCF, cirrhosis, malignant ascites); this opens up the processus vaginalis.

Femoral hernias (Figure 5.5)

Presentation

Femoral hernias herniate into the femoral canal, below and lateral to the pubic tubercle.

The femoral canal is a space within the femoral sheath (an opening from the peritoneal cavity to the lower limb, containing the femoral nerve, artery and vein) which peritoneum or bowel can herniate through. The femoral canal is that space medial to the femoral vein shown in the diagram.

Femoral hernias become incarcerated in the inextensible neck of the femoral sheath (it is a point of semantic argument that it is not the sheath that is the cause of obstruction; it is in fact the neck which provides the constriction). However, it is possible for it to emerge through the fossa ovalis and then bend upwards and over the inguinal ligament, known as a bubonocoele.

Femoral hernias are 2.5 times more common in females.

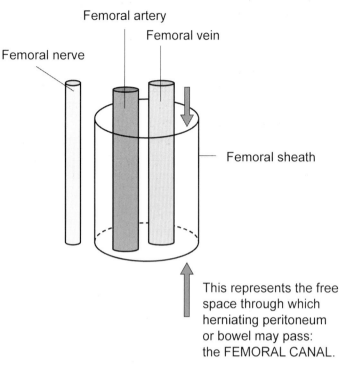

Figure 5.5. Femoral hernias.

This represents the free space through which herniating peritoneum or bowel may pass: the FEMORAL CANAL.

Differential diagnosis of groin hernias

- Hydrocoele.
- Ectopic testicle.
- Lipoma of spermatic cord.
- Inguinal lymphadenopathy.
- Femoral canal lipoma.
- Saphena varix.
- Psoas abscess.
- Ileofemoral aneurysm.

Note

— This is a vital list to commit to memory for clinical exams; it is frequently asked when asked to examine the groin of a patient (hernias are common; therefore, they are likely to come up in the exam).

Umbilical hernias

Presentation

These are congenital hernias, which tend to disappear after the child's first 3-4 years of life.

In adults, umbilical hernias are due to raised intra-abdominal pressure, e.g. ascites, multiple pregnancies, obesity.

There is equal incidence in males and females.

Umbilical hernias have a tendency towards strangulation, therefore an elective operation is advisable. The Mayo 'vest over pants' repair is a double layer of sutured, folded linea alba over the internal defect and was the preferred type of repair before the advent of mesh.

Investigations

Hernias themselves usually do not require investigation, being a clinical diagnosis. In cases of clinical doubt, herniography can be performed. This is injection of a radiopaque dye into the peritoneal cavity under local anaesthetic. X-rays are taken while the patient performs a Valsalva manoeuvre, thus raising their intra-abdominal pressure, which pushes the dye into the hernia sac, showing up on the X-ray.

If surgery is contemplated, then routine pre-operative bloods are indicated, as well as a chest X-ray and ECG if appropriate.

Treatment

The indications for inguinal and femoral hernia repair have been alluded to in Chapter 4 'Operative surgery'. To recap, symptomatic hernias in the elective setting may warrant surgical repair, but the associated risks of surgery (wound infection, wound dehiscence, hernia recurrence, and anaesthetic risks) must be discussed with the patient beforehand. The reason for surgery is the potential for the hernia to strangulate in the future, and to relieve the patient of their symptoms. These are relative indications only. Remember, if the risks of surgery outweigh the benefits, then non-operative management is best.

Hernias can be repaired via open or laparoscopic means. In either case, this is usually day-case surgery. For the most part, the repair involves the use of a mesh to cover the defect. For more detail, refer to the 'Operative surgery' chapter.

Complications

Whether open or laparoscopic there is a risk of wound infection. Wound dehiscence is less likely in laparoscopic surgery. The risk of recurrence appears similar for both approaches. The anaesthetic risks are pneumonia, CVA and MI.

Note

— Inspect other sites of concurrent hernias, e.g. femoral. ALWAYS mention this in exam situations.

Gallstones

Presentation

This is the pathological crystallistion of bile salts or cholesterol in the gallbladder to form stones. There are three types of stone: bile stones, cholesterol stones and mixed stones. Their presence can cause pain, flatulent dyspepsia (stomach ache and burping), a predisposition to cholecystitis, and occasionally obstructive symptoms.

Investigations

As you will have noted the presenting symptoms are somewhat vague, and a diagnosis of gallstones must be made prior to considering treatment. The investigation of choice is abdominal ultrasound. This picks up the presence of gallstones, but also provides a measure of bile duct dilatation, indicative of biliary obstruction.

Routine pre-operative investigations are warranted in the presence of gallstones: bloods, G+S, chest X-ray, ECG. LFTs must be performed to look for any derangement indicative of biliary obstruction.

In the much less common case of suspected cholecystitis (infected gallstones and gallbladder contents), in a patient who is pyrexial, systemically unwell, with right upper quadrant pain, the following should be looked for: a raised white cell count, raised ESR and CRP, as well as deranged LFTs. This warrants antibiotics and an urgent cholecystectomy.

Treatment

While it is possible to treat some stones pharmacologically or by lithotripsy, the relapse (reformation of stones) rate approaches 100%. Currently, the only permanently effective treatment for symptomatic gallstone disease is excision of the gallbladder (cholecystectomy). This is performed laparoscopically for the most part; it may be occasionally necessary to convert to open cholecystectomy due to the presence of adhesions which, when severe, make laparoscopic dissection impossible. Adhesions are a recognised sequela of cholecystitis or previous local surgery.

Complications

The complications of laparoscopy itself can relate to induction of the pneumoperitoneum, instrumentation within the abdominal cavity, the gas used in the pneumoperitoneum, and the use of diathermy or thermal instruments.

Induction of the pneumoperitoneum can result in damage to bowel (perforation), other solid organs (liver, spleen, bladder, uterus) and abdominal blood vessels, pneumothorax (perforation of the diaphragm or pleura), or damage to the omentum.

Abdominal instrumentation can result in damage to abdominal organs (bowel, liver, spleen, bladder, uterus, blood vessels).

Pneumoperitoneum gas is generally carbon dioxide (CO_2), as it is relatively inert and non-combustible. However, CO_2 is converted to carbonic acid in the peritoneum which is painful; the pain tends to be referred to the shoulder tip postoperatively. There exists the possibility of gas embolus and cardiac arrhythmia (from absorbed CO_2 into the circulation).

Diathermy instruments, as well as being able to damage the abdominal contents already mentioned, can also result in skin burns at the site of laparoscopic port insertion (from capacitance induction or direct conduction; see the section on 'Diathermy' in Chapter 2).

Laparoscopic cholecystectomy carries with it additional specific complications as follows:

- Common bile duct damage (bile leak).
- Cystic artery bleed.
- Gallbladder fossa bleeding.

Acute pancreatitis

Presentation

Patients present with acute severe abdominal pain, which is diffusely located. There is no guarding, no rebound and normal bowel sounds. The pain can also radiate round the back.

More importantly, acute pancreatitis, as well as the pain, can present with multi-organ failure (MOF). As one might expect, the greater the number of organ systems in failure, the greater the mortality. Acute pancreatitis is a severe and potentially life-threatening condition (see Ranson's criteria below, as this is effectively based on the number of failing organ systems using various markers to represent each system and hence can be correlated to mortality).

Inflammation of the pancreas is associated with acinar cell injury. It causes an acute onset of pain due to enzymatic necrosis and inflammation of the pancreas.

Pathology

- Proteolysis.
- Vascular necrosis (acute haemorrhagic pancreatitis).
- Lipolysis (fat necrosis, which results in precipitation of insoluble calcium salts in the abdominal cavity; seen on abdominal X-ray (AXR). This, however, is only seen in chronic pancreatitis.
- Associated acute inflammatory reaction.

Aetiology

Gallstones, ethanol/trauma (surgical or ERCP), steroids, mumps, autoimmune disease, scorpion sting, hyperlipidaemia, hypercalcaemia, hypothermia, and diuretics (thiazide). A mnemonic for remembering the above in order is: GETSMASH'D.

Note

- Everyone remembers the part of this medical school mnemonic of the 'Scorpion bites'. Of course, the bite of the scorpion is as inoffensive as a human bite (less, in fact, due to the polymicrobial load of human saliva). It is the sting of the scorpion that has been linked to pancreatitis.

The most common causes of acute pancreatitis are gallstones and ethanol in fairly equal proportion. However, in a significant number of patients presenting with acute pancreatitis, no cause is found, despite investigation, i.e. idiopathic.

Severity scores (Imrie or Ranson)

Imrie
- Age >55.
- WCC >15 x 10^9/L.
- Glucose (Glu) >10mmol/L.
- Alb <32g/L.
- Urea >16mmol/L.
- pO_2 <8kPa (on air).
- LDH >600UL.

- Aspartate transaminase (AST) >200UL.
- Calcium <2mmol/L.

The presence of three or more of the above in the first 48 hours indicates a severe attack, increasing the predicted mortality.

Ranson's criteria

On admission:

- Age >55yrs.
- WCC >15 x 10^9/L.
- Glu >10mmol/L.
- LDH >350UL.
- AST >250UL.

Within 48 hours:

- Decrease in Hct >10 points.
- Increase in urea >5mmol/L.
- Ca^{2+} <2mmol/L.
- pO_2 <60mmHg.
- Base deficit >4.
- Fluid deficit >6L.

Ranson's criteria, like Imrie's, give prognostic information for the likely severity and, hence, mortality associated with the bout of pancreatitis.

A useful way of trying to remember the various criteria listed above is to think of the organ systems that they represent, i.e. the number of organ failures (haematological, hepatic, respiratory, renal).

Investigations

The appropriate tests need to be performed to document Ranson's criteria, i.e. FBC, U+Es, CS, LFTs, G+S, arterial blood gases (ABGs). Urine output and IV fluid input should be monitored.

In the emergency investigation of acute pancreatitis, do not forget to look for a treatable cause of the attack. Most commonly this will take the form of gallstones, which should be investigated by abdominal ultrasound. MRI shows the pancreas to be inflamed, confirming the diagnosis, but not generally

contributing to the diagnosis of the actual cause of the attack. The other common cause, ethanol abuse, can be inferred from the history and, if the patient is a severe alcoholic, the gamma GT and mean cellular volume (MCV) will be elevated.

Treatment

Treatment of an acute attack of pancreatitis is for the most part supportive, i.e. support of the failing systems that are identified by the tests. Powerful analgesics are given as required (opiates or anti-inflammatories, unless contra-indicated). An oxygen mask is applied and IV fluids are administered while keeping the patient NBM. This rests the pancreas (remember its exocrine function is to secrete pancreatic enzymes into the second part of the duodenum for proteolytic purposes in response to the presence of food in the stomach). A urinary catheter is inserted to monitor the fluid balance and renal function.

If the patient goes into MOF, they require intensive care admission for a greater degree of system support than can be provided on the ward.

If the patient continues to deteriorate, with pyrexia and large system failure, the only surgical option left open is pancreatic necrosectomy. This is a last ditch attempt to remove some of the necrotic tissue in the pancreas that is perpetuating the cycle of inflammatory multi-system failure. It is effectively a laparotomy, approaching the pancreas in its retroperitoneal position and scooping out the obviously necrotic tissue. Needless to say this is a procedure associated with a high mortality, because the patient is in a life-threatening condition before surgery.

The most common natural history of an acute pancreatitis attack is a period of hospitalisation for 4-5 days, NBM, gradually increasing to sips, and then diet. These patients require large analgesic doses. If ethanol abuse is identified, then chlordiazepoxide, folate and vitamin B12 should also be given. If gallstones are identified, then a date should be set (soon) for laparoscopic cholecystectomy, when the patient has fully recovered.

Complications

◆ Pseudocyst.
◆ Multi-organ failure.
◆ Pancreatic abscess or necrosis.
◆ Colonic infarction.
◆ Pancreatic fistula.
◆ Chronic pancreatitis.

Pancreatic carcinoma

Presentation

Classically, pancreatic carcinoma is a late presenting condition. This is one of the major reasons for the very poor prognosis. It presents with epigastric pain and obstructive jaundice.

Note

— Courvoisier's sign is a palpable distended gallbladder in the RUQ with associated obstructive jaundice, which is highly suggestive of pancreatic carcinoma (as opposed to other causes of jaundice).

Other clinical features are weight loss, pruritis (associated with the jaundice), and hepatomegaly (with metastatic spread). Rarely, one sees steatorrhoea.

Pathology

Most commonly it appears as an adenocarcinoma, although squamous, cystic, mucinous and ciliated varieties exist, rarely. The most common site of the tumour is in the pancreatic head. It is capable of local spread, invading the duodenum, pancreatic duct, pancreatic body and tail, and local lymph nodes. Distal spread is characteristically to the liver. A less common site for the tumour to originate is the ampulla of Vater; this is of relevence, as the results of resection in this subgroup are markedly improved.

Aetiology

The incidence increases with age and it is more common in smokers, diabetics, and sufferers of chronic pancreatitis.

Investigations

◆ Ultrasound is highly sensitive in picking up pancreatic masses, cholestasis and the presence of liver metastases.
◆ Contrast-enhanced CT is excellent at identifying the operability of the tumour, invasion into local structures, and metastatic spread.
◆ Endoscopy is also useful in identifing ampullary lesions, and looking for the site of obstruction causing jaundice.
◆ Pancreatic biopsy can be performed percutaneously, ultrasound-guided for a tissue diagnosis.
◆ Routine bloods should include G+S, FBC, U&Es, LFTs, ESR and CRP. There are no reliable tumour markers in common usage.

Treatment

There is only really one curative option: surgery. Chemotherapy and radiotherapy have poor results.

The operative option is the Whipple procedure. This is a radical pancreatoduodenectomy involving excision of the head of the pancreas, the gallbladder, part of the common bile duct, the duodenum, and sometimes a portion of the stomach, with gastrojejunostomy, choledochojejunostomy, and pancreatojejunostomy. At the beginning of the procedure it is important to do a full exploratory laparotomy looking for spread and, if positive, it is inadvisable to proceed with a full resection; instead, palliate where necessary and perform a choledocho-duodenostomy for biliary decompression or a gastrojejunostomy for duodenal obstruction.

This is a very major and technically challenging procedure, the details of which are beyond the remit of this book.

There is a very significant mortality associated with this surgery (up to 25%), and unfortunately a low cure rate. It follows, therefore, that patient selection, and thorough investigation form the mainstay of ensuring the best possible result.

Do not forget that ampullary carcinomas stand a much improved chance of cure with resection.

Complications

General complications

- Chest infection.
- Basal atelectasis.
- DVT.
- PE.
- Wound infection or dehiscence.
- High mortality rate (as previously mentioned, as high as 25%).

Specific complications

- Pancreatic fistula breakdown (leak, abscess, fistula formation, haemorrhage).
- Biliary leak.
- Ascending cholangitis.

Hepato- and splenomegaly

If you are asked to examine an abdomen in the clinical section of exams, and you find either an enlarged spleen or liver, you must have a list of possible causes, as this is an obvious follow-up question.

Causes of hepatomegaly

- Cirrhosis (do not forget that the liver can also be shrunken in late cirrhosis).
- Tumours:
  - primary - hepatoma;
  - secondary - lung, colon, etc.
- Congestive cardiac failure.
- Hepatitis.
- Leukaemia/lymphoma.

Causes of splenomegaly

- Infective: leishmaniasis, CMV, HIV, malaria, etc.
- Haematological: hereditary spherocytosis, ITP, myelofibrosis, myelodysplasia.
- Malignant: lymphoma/leukaemia.
- Portal hypertension.
- Rheumatoid arthritis (very rare).

Benign colonic tumours

The definition of a polyp is an abnormal elevation of an epithelial surface. This is a common question leading on to the classification of different types of polyps seen below; an easy question if you are prepared.

Polyps are divided into neoplastic and non-neoplastic types.

The following focuses on colonic polyps, although there are other types to be found. It is simply that colonic polyps are more common in clinical practice and in exams, and they have the classic adenoma-carcinoma progression.

Non-neoplastic colonic polyps

Metaplastic
These are flat and do not progress to malignant change; they are symptomless.

Hyperplastic
As for metaplastic.

Hamartomatous
The juvenile polyp or the Peutz-Jeghers' polyp are good examples. They represent a polyp made up of normal tissue, but, from another part of the body.

Inflammatory
Associated with Crohn's disease or ulcerative colitis.

Note

- Important exceptions to the above classification lie within the syndrome of juvenile polyposis, and Peutz-Jehgers' polyps, which have been shown to be premalignant.

Neoplastic colonic polyps (Figure 5.6)

- Adenomatous (tubular, villous, tubulovillous).
- Lymphoma.
- Lipoma.

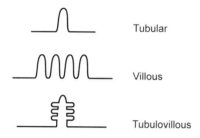

Figure 5.6. Neoplastic colonic polyps (adenomatous polyps).

- Leiomyoma.
- Haemangioma.

You will be expected to know the above two lists in relation to types of polyps as well as further detail mostly on adenomatous polyps.

There is another type of adenomatous polyp called the serrated adenoma, which is an adenomatous polyp found within an erythroplastic polyp.

The most important and common of the above neoplastic polyps are, of course, the adenomatous polyps, as they are involved in the adenoma-carcinoma sequence.

A colonic adenoma is a benign tumour of the colonic glandular epithelium, i.e. the lining of the wall of the bowel.

As stated above, adenomatous polyps can be tubular, villous, or a combination of the two, tubulovillous. Tubular means shaped like a tube (and smooth in contour) and villous means that it has fronds (like villi) on its surface.

Tubular adenomas can be pedunculated (hanging by a thread) or sessile (smooth-contoured polyp with a similar diameter base as its tip). Villous adenomas have villous fronds around them. Tubulovillous adenomas are intermediate in shape and surface contour.

The risk of malignant change of a polyp has been shown to increase significantly as its diameter grows beyond 1cm. Villous adenomas have a 30% overall risk of malignant change.

Histology of polyps

Neoplastic adenomatous polyps show dysplasia (variations in the norm in size, shape and orientation of cells). The gradual change of severity of dysplasia to malignancy is the adenoma-carcinoma sequence. As long as dysplastic glands remain above the muscularis mucosae they are termed dysplastic. The dysplasia may be to a mild, moderate or severe degree. As there are no lymphatics in the lamina propria, it is questionable as to whether the term carcinoma *in situ* should be used. Once there is invasion through the muscularis mucosa this is termed focal carcinoma. If invasion of the stalk (of a polyp) has occurred this is termed focal carcinoma with stalk invasion.

These stages have implications regarding treatment. The deeper the invasion, the worse the differentiation of the tumour, and the more likely there is a lymphocytic invasion, then a more radical operation is required.

Note

- The important message from the above is that these tumours are only considered malignant if they have invaded through the muscularis mucosa; until then they are termed carcinoma *in situ*.
- It is proven that adenoma can progress to carcinoma; however, it is NOT proven that ALL carcinomas have their origin in adenomas.

The adenoma-carcinoma sequence is important to understand because adenomas are localised and can easily be completely excised using an endoscope. This provides a complete cure and potentially prevents the progression to carcinoma and the consequent need for major surgery.

Whilst screening of populations that are at high risk of polyp formation (i.e. familial adenomatous polypi, or first degree relatives of colonic cancer patients, or patients who have already had polyps or colonic cancer themselves) is in place, it is a key fact that adenomas are easy to treat and are known to have pre-malignant potential.

Familial adenomatous polyposis (FAP)

This is an inherited condition of massive numbers of colonic adenomatous polyps. These polyps form in such numbers that these patients (untreated) invariably progress to colonic cancer between the ages of 20 and 40 years.

Definitive treatment of this population is a prophylactic colectomy and ileorectal anastomosis (followed then by rectal surveillance), preventing malignant progression before it can happen. This is surgery with considerable associated morbidity (and a finite mortality), but it is considered worthwhile because of the invariable progression to malignancy without it. The alternative to the above operation is a restorative proctocolectomy.

FAP may represent a cluster of syndromes that end in polyposis; its aetiology has been identified as a specific genetic mutation, which is inherited in some cases (autosomal dominant mutation of chromosome 5), and spontaneous in others.

Clinical presentation of polyps

- No symptoms.
- PR bleed.
- Mucus.
- Tenesmus (a painful sensation of rectal distension, but the passage of stool does not relieve it).

- Intussusception (an invagination of one part of the bowel into another, which results in bowel obstruction).
- Metabolic disturbance from severe fluid and electrolyte loss (uncommon - occurs as a result of hypersecretion of albumin and potassium from the polyp associated with diarrhoea).

Investigations

The mainstay of investigation is endoscopic sigmoidoscopy or colonoscopy. This enables direct visualisation, photography, biopsy and, hence, histological diagnosis. This is performed as a day-care procedure with minor sedation.

Treatment

Sigmoidoscopy/colonoscopy are used to identify and remove appropriately sized polyps for histological grading. Thereafter, the decision can be made regarding the removal of the affected portion of the colon and surrounding lymph nodes.

Note

— Regular follow-up is required with sigmoidoscopy and/or colonoscopy after polypectomy/colectomy.

The treatment algorithm for polyps is covered in the 'Malignant colonic tumours' section below.

Complications

- Bleeding from polypectomy site (usually mild and self-limiting, but occasionally severe).
- Bowel perforation, either by the tip of the colonoscope or by the diathermy instrument.
- Problems relating to sedation medication (allergic reaction, respiratory depression, death).

Malignant colonic tumours

Colorectal cancer

The risk is increased by a high fat, low fibre diet (?changes in gut flora), UC and FAP. Epidemiologically, there is a high incidence in the West, a low incidence in Africa. It usually presents between the ages of 50-70 years old. Fifty percent of colorectal tumours are rectal, the remaining 50% are 25% sigmoid and 25% caecal. The vast majority are adenocarcinomas and they are present as polyps which undergo malignant change, i.e. easily curable if found in polypoid form.

Presentation

- Altered bowel habit.
- PR bleeding.
- Palpable mass.
- PR mucus.
- Weight loss.
- Anorexia.
- Abdominal pain.
- Anaemia.
- Tenesmus (sensation of incomplete emptying of the rectum).

Spread

- There is direct invasion, usually lateral, and not longitudinal. This is especially relevant when considering resection margins in colectomies, exemplified in Bill Heald's paper 'A Close Shave', referring to the fact that you can have smaller resection margins, longitudinally, than was previously accepted, as there is a predisposition for these tumours not to spread in this fashion.
- Lymphatic spread is upwards along the superior rectal and inferior mesenteric vessels.
- Blood-borne - to liver, lungs, bone, adrenals and kidneys.
- Transperitoneal. If spread reaches the ovaries by this route, it results in Krukenberg tumours.

Investigations

- A FBC is necessary to look for anaemia, as these tumours tend to bleed (chronically, but can be acute).
- U+Es demonstrate renal function.
- LFTs may show deranged function due to secondaries (but >60% of the liver is thought to need to have been affected before this is noted on blood testing).
- Clotting screen.
- Group and cross-match four units for any planned surgery.
- Chest X-ray may show pulmonary secondaries.
- Abdominal ultrasound may show hepatic secondaries, or hepatosplenomegaly.

All the above are necessary. But the diagnosis is generally made by colonoscopy, as it visualizes and enables tissue diagnosis by biopsy.

Dukes' staging

Initially described by Sir Cuthbert Dukes for rectal cancer only, the UK now uses a modified Dukes' system for colonic cancer:

- A. Restricted to bowel wall.
- B. Extends through bowel wall without lymph node (LN) spread.
- C. LN involvement (C2 = highest LN, C1 = other LNs).
- D. Distant metastatic involvement.

The five-year survival rate for Dukes' A = 90%, B = 65%, C = 23%, D = 5%.

Treatment

Adjuvant therapies are radiotherapy and chemotherapy (5FU [fluorouracil] and folinic acid). 5FU is used because of its relatively low toxicity, as all agents used so far have poor proven benefit, i.e. 5FU is as effective but less dangerous than its competitors.

Depending on the location of the tumour, a left or a right hemicolectomy is performed for descending or ascending colonic tumours, respectively, a sigmoid colectomy for sigmoid tumours and an AP (anteroposterior) resection for rectal tumours.

Prior to any colectomy operation, the abdominal cavity is thoroughly examined for hepatic secondaries, peritoneal spread, spread from the colon to other local structures and for a 'second primary' in the bowel.

Depending on operative conditions, a primary anastomosis should be attempted, rather than a colostomy or ileostomy. These are performed either as palliation for an inoperable tumour (defunctioning of the bowel), or if there is faecal contamination at the time of surgery of the abdominal cavity. The anastomosis is monitored by means of a drain for five days. If it suddenly starts to drain significant amounts, and the patient seems to develop an acute abdomen, an anastomotic leak should be suspected.

Complications

- ◆ Obstruction (usually left-sided annular lesions, results in colicky pain, distension and absolute constipation).
- ◆ Perforation.
- ◆ Fistula formation, e.g. vesicocolic, colo-cutaneous, etc.
- ◆ Complications of the surgery itself include an anastomotic leak, bleeding, ileus and wound infection.

Postoperative follow-up

Postoperatively, patients should be followed up with colonoscopy at three months, six months, one year, and then yearly, for a minimum of five years.

Volvulus

Volvulus is a rotation of greater than 360° of a section of bowel about its mesenteric attachment (most common in the sigmoid colon, then the caecal colon), resulting in closed loop obstruction, and potentially leading to ischaemic necrosis of the affected bowel.

Strangely, the rotation always seems to be anti-clockwise (this is of relevance to the operating surgeon, as he knows to 'de-rotate' it clockwise).

Sigmoid volvulus

This is more common by far than caecal volvulus; however, it is much less common a cause of intestinal obstruction than colonic carcinoma, which accounts for 65% of all causes of colonic obstruction, other causes being pseudo-obstruction and diverticulitis. Sigmoid volvulus probably accounts for 4% of causes of colonic obstruction.

Pathology

The redundant loop of sigmoid rotates anti-clockwise on its sigmoid mesentery and obstructs.

The longer the obstruction persists, the greater the chance of ischaemic necrosis and, hence, perforation and peritonitis.

Aetiology

This seems to occur in people who have had long-standing problems with constipation and laxative use. The theory is one of a redundant loop of distended sigmoid colon that is more likely to twist than in a normal individual.

Presentation

- ◆ Colicky abdominal pain.
- ◆ Abdominal distension.
- ◆ Nausea and vomiting.
- ◆ Absolute constipation.

The abdominal examination findings are of a distended (tympanic) abdomen and a generalised tenderness, with absent (or tinkling) bowel sounds. Rebound, guarding, tachycardia and hypotension may be found in cases of peritonitis.

Investigations

A plain abdominal X-ray is the main source of information needed. It shows a grossly distended loop of large bowel with its base in the left iliac fossa, and its convexity directed towards the right upper quadrant.

Occasionally, where diagnostic difficulty exists, and the patient is not peritonitic, a barium enema can be performed to investigate futher. However, this is not normally required.

If the patient is showing signs of peritonism or cardiovascular compromise, this becomes a surgical emergency and they should be prepared for emergency theatre. FBC, U&Es, G+S, ECG, CXR and any other relevant investigations should be determined by history and examination.

Treatment

In the absence of signs of peritonism, it is safe to make an attempt at passing a flatus tube past the rectum into the sigmoid colon. The pressure of the released flatus (and liquid stool) is the stuff of legend! The word to the wise is to stand back (or preferably off to one side). This effectively decompresses (as well as untwists) the volvulus.

Depending on the practice in your department, the patient may then be admitted for observation or sent home, if they are well. Occasionally, there is a need to leave the flatus tube *in situ* for 24 hours or so. However, if the patient shows signs of peritonism, or if the passage of the flatus tube proves impossible, they may need to be taken to theatre. At laparotomy, the volvulus can be untwisted (clockwise), and the viability of the bowel assessed. In the case of ischaemic bowel, a sigmoid colectomy is indicated. In the case of gross faecal contamination, the surgeon may elect to perform a defunctioning colostomy and come back at a later date to anastomose the bowel.

Complications

Passage of a flatus tube is a relatively benign intervention and so the complications are more likely to be due to the condition than the passage of the tube, i.e. perforation, recurrence of the volvulus,

inability to deflate the volvulus by this means alone (necessitating laparotomy).

Laparotomy in the acute setting carries the risks mentioned previously.

Local
- Wound infection.
- Anastomotic failure (if performed for perforation or ischaemic section of bowel in this condition).
- Persistent ileus.
- Incisional hernia formation.
- Stricture formation at the anastomosis site.

General
- Pneumonia due to splinting of the diaphragm.
- Cough inhibition secondary to pain from the abdominal incision.
- CVA.
- MI.
- DVT.
- PE.
- Acute renal failure.

Caecal volvulus

This is less common than sigmoid volvulus and does not have the same aetiology at all. There seems to be an anatomical predisposition to caecal volvulus formation with a caecum and right colon that are less adherent to the posterior abdominal wall than the norm.

The presentation is similar (colicky pain, abdominal distension, nausea and vomiting), with a similar predisposition to proceed to ischaemic necrosis, perforation and peritonitis.

The abdominal X-ray shows a grossly distended loop of large bowel with its origin in the right iliac fossa, and its convexity extending towards the left upper quadrant. It looks like a large 'coffee bean'.

The simple passage of a flatus tube in this case is not an option; instead the surgeon should expeditiously proceed to laparotomy to untwist the volvulus (clockwise).

Controversy still exists as to whether to leave it at that and close up, or to perform a caecostomy, or caecopexy (repair) or even a right hemicolectomy.

Obviously the management of peritonitic findings will be as above for sigmoid volvulus as it applies to the caecum.

Anal conditions

Fissure-in-ano

- Longitudinal tear in the anoderm, almost always in the midline.
- In males 90% are posterior, 10% are anterior.
- In females 80% are posterior, 20% are anterior.
- There is an equal sex ratio, common in young adults.
- The aetiology is uncertain. Constipation has a 'chicken and egg' relationship, i.e. is it a cause of the problem or result of the problem?

Presentation
Pain on defaecation (and for 1-2 hours later), PR bleed (on paper), pruritis, watery discharge and constipation.

Investigations
Diagnosis is made by parting the anal margin and inspecting the area affected.

Treatment

Conservative
Soften stool with laxatives, topical GTN, or topical 0.2% diltiazem.

Surgical
Lateral sphincterotomy or anal dilatation (which is now only very rarely performed).

Note

- There is a risk of incontinence which is increased when performing an anal dilatation, if the patient has already had obstetric sphincter damage.

Complications

A lateral sphincterotomy can result in:

- Pain.
- Pruritis.
- Discharge.
- Wound abscess.
- Bleeding.
- Constipation.
- Faecal incontinence.

Anorectal sepsis

Presentation
The aetiology is development of an abscess in the anal glands, which normally drain mucus into the anus through the crypts of Morgagni.

This can result in the following:

- Simple peri-anal abscess (the treatment is to incise and drain it).
- Intersphincteric abscess (needs laying open when internal opening is found by a probe).
- Trans-sphincteric abscess (complicated surgery involving the use of a seton [Latin for bristle], as these cannot be laid open without causing faecal incontinence [the incision would have to cross the anal sphincter muscle]).

Ischio-anal (ischiorectal) or suprasphincteric abscesses have similar surgical management problems to trans-sphincteric abscesses.

Goodsall's rule

Posterior fistulae always drain into the midline and anterior fistulae drain radially to the corresponding region of the anteror anus.

Pruritis ani

Presentation
- Is a symptom, NOT a disease.
- Can be part of a general dermatosis.

- Can have a local anal cause.
- Can be an allergic reaction to creams and ointments.
- Unfortunately, whatever the precipitating factor, it can become a vicious cycle (faecal soiling/moisture causes more pruritis even in the absence of the precipitant).

The list of causes of pruritis ani is long, but it is broken down into:

- Primary. Part of generalised dermatosis, peri-anal disease (fissure, carcinoma, Crohn's disease, infection, allergy).
- Secondary. Skin damage due to moisture and irritants, i.e. poor anal hygeine, haemorrhoids, rectal prolapse, fistula-in-ano, diarrhoea, incontinence, others).

Treatment
The management of pruritis ani is to avoid the allergen, do not use abrasive paper, wash without soap after defaecation, and avoid creams and LA preparations.

This is a common case to be seen in the general surgical outpatient. While it would be unlikely to have a case of pruritis ani in a clinical exam, the subject comes up sufficiently regularly that you should have the above list of advice ready to give people who present with it, and you should also be aware of the classification of primary and secondary causes.

Pilonidal sinus

Presentation
- The word pilonidal means 'nest of hairs'.
- Refers to anywhere in the body where the growing end of a hair has become a subcutaneous tissue, i.e. a nidus for infection. Examples where this can happen are in the natal cleft, the finger webs of barbers or, in the axilla.
- Affects young adults, the male to female ratio being 4:1.

Aetiology
In the case of a classic pilonidal sinus, i.e. in the natal cleft between the buttocks, the aetiology is undecided between congenital (natal cleft and hence hair ingrowth) and acquired (hair ingrowth despite the possible absence of the natal cleft; it can even be the result of a scalp hair falling between the buttocks). It presents as an abscess or a chronic discharging sinus.

Treatment
Treatment is by drainage of the abscess in the acute phase. The patient should return for excision of the sinus tract electively.

Complications
Incision and drainage of the abscess can be complicated by recurrence of the abscess, pain, bleeding, and formation of a persistent sinus.

Excision of the sinus tract actually has exactly the same potential complications.

Haemorrhoids

Presentation
Haemorrhoids are classified into three different types. First degree haemorrhoids are effectively 'internal' piles, i.e. a saccular distension of the anal veins that does not prolapse beyond the anal margin. These can bleed and cause pain or pruritis. Second degree haemorrhoids are piles that intermittently prolapse, and can be replaced intra-anally by the patient. These can have the same symptoms as first degree haemorroids, as well as the sensation of prolapse. Third degree haemorrhoids are permanently prolapsed piles that cannot be reduced by the patient.

Treatment
- Nothing.
- Dietary advice.
- Laxatives.
- Injection sclerotherapy.
- Banding.
- Surgical haemorrhoidectomy.
- Anal stretch.

The above list is in order of increasing intervention, i.e. each treatment modality is increasingly interventional.

First degree haemorrhoids generally do not require treatment other than to address any problems of constipation with dietary advice or laxatives.

Second degree haemorrhoids, if symptomatic, despite non-operative treatments, warrant banding or injection sclerotherapy. Some perform a Lord's stretch if anal stenosis is considered to be at the root of the problem (a forced dilatation of the anus under general anaesthetic).

Third degree haemorrhoids, if symptomatic, despite non-operative treatments, warrant haemorrhoidectomy surgery.

It may be expected of you to describe how you would perform a haemorrhoid banding. This is done in the outpatient department requiring the use of a suction device over the end of which an elastic band has been stretched. The sucker draws the haemorrhoid into its tip, at which point the release trigger of the device is depressed releasing the elastic band around the neck of the haemorrhoid. The patient is warned that he/she may be sore for a couple of days, may have a little bleeding, and will notice the husk of the haemorrhoid drop off within a week or so.

One should never band haemorrhoids whose origins are distal to the dentate line of the anus, as these have a somatic nerve supply, resulting in severe pain as a result of the procedure.

Complications

Banding of haemorrhoids can be complicated by:

- Pain (although a lower incidence than for surgical haemorrhoidectomy).
- Failure of treatment (i.e. band falls off or haemorrhoid fails to resolve).
- Bleeding.

Surgical haemorrhoidectomy can be complicated by:

- Pain.
- Failure of treatment (although a lower incidence than for banding).
- Bleeding.

Note

- There is a separate clinical entity known as the thrombosed external pile, for which the two management options are ice and analgesia with delayed haemorrhoidectomy, or immediate haemorrhoidectomy.

Stomas

Types of stomas and the indications for their use in surgery are a very common case to be presented with in clinical examinations. Part of the reason for this is that there are large numbers of patients out there with longstanding stomas, they are quite stable, and easily accessible for the surgeon trying to find cases for his/her part in the organisation of the exam.

The first thing to say about a stoma is that it means 'mouth' or 'opening'. The word stoma is incorporated into the terms colostomy and ileostomy meaning a new opening made into the colon and ileum, respectively. Specifically in the surgical sense, the opening is from the abdominal cavity to the outside.

It is a common question in exams to speculate on the origin of a patient's stoma, i.e. whether it represents an ileostomy or colostomy. Subsequently, you may be asked what original pathology may have been the indication for the patient's stoma.

Two generalities will help you at this point:

- Stomas located in the right iliac fossa tend to be ileostomies (if asked to justify this statement, one can fall back on basic anatomy: the ileum ends at the ileocaecal valve and the caecum is reliably to be found in the right iliac fossa [RIF]).
- Stomas found on the left (or right) side of the *upper* abdomen tend to be colostomies. Usually the transverse colon is used (upper abdomen) as it is freely mobile on its mesentery, and the ascending and descending colons are retroperitoneal.

LOOP COLOSTOMY

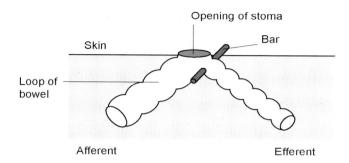

HARTMANN'S

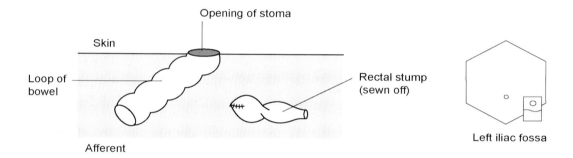

Left iliac fossa

ILEOSTOMY

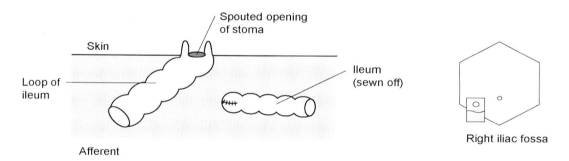

Right iliac fossa

MUCOUS FISTULA

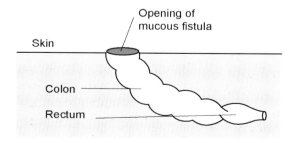

Figure 5.7. Types of stoma.

The two major reasons for formation of a stoma are visceral perforation (and hence peritoneal soiling) and tumour. Obviously the two can be related, i.e. tumour obstruction can result in perforation.

Diverticulitis can result in colonic perforation. At laparotomy, the peritoneal cavity is faecally soiled, and attempting to re-anastomose the bowel runs the risk of anastomotic dehiscence. Thus, the surgeon performs peritoneal lavage, bringing out the stoma proximal to the point of perforation. This is left for a period of time (eight weeks is adequate) and the patient returns for a reversal of the colostomy and a bowel anastomosis.

The above reasoning can be applied to colonic perforation secondary to obstructing tumour, obstructing hernia and Crohn's perforation. If a tumour is unresectable, the bowel proximal to it must be brought out as a stoma, which is permanent in this case.

Inflammatory bowel disease is another important indication, under certain circumstances for formation of a stoma, e.g. the toxic megacolon of ulcerative colitis despite maximal medical therapy (steroids and 5-ASA drugs). This requires pan-proctocolectomy and formation of a permanent ileostomy.

Occasionally you will see stomas brought out to defunction the bowel in an attempt to protect an area of sepsis from faecal soiling, for example, a severe peri-anal tear or sepsis.

Complications

- Parastomal hernia is a specific complication of stoma formation. It is, as the term suggests, a weakness in the abdominal wall at the site of the stoma resulting in protrusion of peritoneum and bowel.
- Stomal stenosis: a tightening of the stoma at its exit.
- Skin excoriation: a result of the proteolytic enzymes, more commonly in ileostomies, acting on the skin surrounding the stoma.
- Bleeding from the stoma or the surrounding skin.

- Prolapse: extrusion of bowel beyond the abdominal wall.
- Retraction: invagination of the stoma into the abdominal cavity.
- Fistulation: seen more frequently in Crohn's disease, a fistula from bowel to abdominal wall, a type of enterocutaneous fistula.

After reversal of a stoma, it is possible for an incisional hernia to occur.

Types of stoma (Figure 5.7)

Loop colostomy
A loop of bowel is brought out to the abdominal wall surface and a bar is placed under the loop to stop it falling back in. This defunctions the bowel distal to the stoma. It has the advantage of being easily reversible, i.e. one can form the anastomosis of the two bowel ends without having to open the abdomen again and allow the anastomosed ends to fall back into the abdominal cavity, closing the defect behind it.

Hartmann's
This is a left iliac fossa colostomy. The proximal portion of colon is brought out as the stoma and, specifically, in this eponymous operation, the rectal stump is sewn off (closed). This is performed as a defunctioning colostomy, for example, for an unresectable rectal tumour.

Ileostomy
A useful tip for clinical exams where you are frequently asked to identify the type of stoma on the patient in front of you, is that the ileostomy is characteristically to be found in the right iliac fossa (remember the terminal ileum finishes at the ileocaecal valve which is to be found in the RIF). Conversely, colostomies are much more commonly found in the left iliac fossa. Other useful identifying features of the ileostomy are the liquid nature of its contents (colostomies have more formed stools) and the occasional presence of a spout, to help avoid the constant presence of the stool which, from the ileum, has a high content of proteolytic enzymes, resulting in

the high incidence of excoriations of the surrounding skin. Ileostomies are performed to defunction the colon, for example, in fulminant colitis (ulcerative colitis or Crohn's colitis), or in proximal colonic obstruction, e.g. tumour.

Mucous fistula

The proximal end of the distal bowel segment is brought out as a stoma to allow it to decompress. It is easily found when the stoma is later reversed, e.g. for subtotal colectomy or colitis.

Hodgkin's lymphoma

Hodgkin's lymphoma is a tumour of white cells, usually found within lymph node clusters, although it has extranodal potential.

It is characterised by the Reed-Sternberg cell on microscopy (looks like an owl's face, with two large eyes - nuclei).

Subtypes

- Lymphocyte predominant.
- Lymphocyte depleted.
- Mixed cellularity.
- Nodular sclerosing.

Presentation

- Painless discrete lymphadenopathy, e.g. neck, axilla.
- Incidental mass on CXR.
- 'B symptoms' (fever, night sweats, weight loss).

Classification (Ann Arbor)

- I. Single lymph node (LN) cluster (or single extranodular site).
- II. Two or more LN clusters on the same side of the diaphragm (or LN cluster and extranodal site on the same side of the diaphragm).
- III. LN clusters on either side of the diaphragm (with or without spleen involvement or localised extranodal site).
- IV. Diffuse/disseminated involvement of one or more extranodal organs, e.g. liver, lung, bone, skin.

Investigations

- FBC.
- ESR.
- U&Es.
- LFTs.
- CXR.
- CT chest, abdomen and pelvis.
- Anaemia (usually 'late', anaemia implies the bone marrow is involved).
- Neutrophilia.
- Lymphopaenia (poor prognosis).
- Raised ESR (association with B symptoms).
- Renal failure (rare).
- Hypercalcaemia (rare).

Note

- CT is very useful at identifying enlarged LN groups for staging.

Treatment

- Stages I-II - radiotherapy.
- Stages III-IV - chemotherapy.

Note

- The exception is the presence of B symptoms, which is an indication for chemotherapy.
- A relapse after radiotherapy requires the use of chemotherapy.

Complications

Chemotherapy can be complicated by the following:

- Acute toxicity:
  - bone marrow suppression;
  - gastrointestinal bleed or long-term fibrosis;
  - alopecia.
- Long-term toxicity:
  - carcinogenesis;
  - gonadal damage.
- Bladder:
  - fibrosis;
  - haematuria.

Radiotherapy can be complicated by the following:

- Skin:
  - inflammation and desquamation.
- Gastrointestinal:
  - nausea and vomiting;
  - bleeding;
  - oesophagitis;
  - abdominal pain;
  - fibrosis, causing stricture.
- Bone marrow:
  - bone marrow suppression.
- Gonadal:
  - infertility.
- Lymph tissue:
  - lymphoedema.

Lung cancer

Presentation

From primary
Cough, haemoptysis, pleuritic chest pain and dyspnoea.

From secondaries
Bone pain, weight loss and paraneoplastic symptoms.

Types of lung cancer

- Small cell. This is highly malignant which has usually metastasised by the time of onset of symptoms. Treatment is rarely surgical, but more often is with chemotherapy. The mean survival time, even with treatment, is nine months.
- Adenocarcinoma.
- Squamous.
- Large cell.

Note

- Adenocarcinoma, squamous and large cell lung cancer are termed non-small cell carcinoma as a group, of which 10-15% are amenable to surgery.

- Pancoast's tumour. An apical lung tumour, causing local pain because of invasion of the first rib. It can affect the brachial plexus and also the sympathetic trunk, resulting in Horner's syndrome (this is unilateral: ptosis [drooping eyelid], enophthalmos [sunken eye], anhydrosis [absence of sweat], miosis [constriction of the pupil]). It can also invade the subclavian artery or vein.

Treatment

Pneumonectomy or segmentectomy are the operations of choice in surgically amenable lesions. The decision as to the suitability for surgery is taken, based on the tissue diagnosis (from a biopsy), absence of metastases and, a high definition CT scan, which looks for the degree of invasion of the tumour into local structures.

Complications

- Pneumonia.
- Empyema.
- Cardiac arrhythmias.
- Persistent air leak.
- Wound infection.
- Bronchopleural fistula (rare).

Pearce's Surgical Companion *Essential notes for postgraduate exams*

Chapter 6

Trauma and orthopaedic surgery

Fractures and their general complications

These are a common theme throughout exam questions relating to trauma, particularly in clinical exams. You should have a list of potential complications of fractures on the tip of your tongue, classified as follows.

Early

- Infection in open fractures.
- Compartment syndrome. An emergency which must be treated by urgent fasciotomies.
- Fracture blisters.
- Vascular injury: vasospasm, intimal tear, vascular laceration, vascular transection.
- Nerve injury: neurapraxia, axonotmesis, neurotmesis.
- Haemarthrosis.
- Ligamentous injury or tendon injury (can be trapped in the fracture, preventing reduction) and rupture.

Late

- Delayed union.
- Non-union. Hypertrophic or atrophic.
- Malunion. Out of alignment, i.e. rotated, angulated, displaced.
- Stiffness.

- Chronic regional pain syndrome (CRPS), previously known as reflex sympathetic dystrophy (RSD), or algodystrophy. A syndrome of pain and stiffness is present after healing has occurred.
- Nerve compression/entrapment.
- Volkmann's ischaemic contracture, a sequela of compartment syndrome, due to myonecrosis of the affected compartment.
- Avascular necrosis (AVN) in specific fractures, e.g. scaphoid waist, femoral neck, proximal humeral fractures. The blood supply beyond the fracture can be compromised resulting in AVN of the affected segment of bone.

This list and classification applies to whichever fracture you are being examined on.

Note

- When fractures are described as dorsally/volarly angulated (or displaced), it refers to the fragment of bone distal to the site of the fracture's position.

Non-union

Before giving the definition for non-union, it is perhaps advisable to give that of delayed union: a fracture that has failed to unite as expected, but continues to show some biological activity. There is no reference made to time since fracture and in this case, biological activity refers to the taking of serial radiographs which continue to show some progression to union.

Non-union is defined as a fracture without clinical or radiographic evidence of healing 6-9 months after injury.

There are fundamentally three different types of non-union:

- ◆ I. Atrophic non-union. The bone ends at the fracture site are atrophied to points, and are avascular. This represents a failure of biology to cause healing. Thus, the biology needs to be jump-started. In this case this is done with surgical freshening of the bone ends, bone grafting and fracture stabilisation, e.g. plate, X-fix or IM nail.
- ◆ II. Hypertrophic non-union. The bone ends are hypertrophied and look like two opposed elephant's feet. This represents a biological ability to heal, but it is mechanical stability that is lacking. It is sufficient, therefore, to plate the fracture; bone grafting is not required.
- ◆ III. Infected non-union. The presence of infection at the fracture site inhibits bony union. The treatment modalities are highly individual to each case. The treatment should include stabilisation of the fracture and eradication of the infection with a combination of surgical debridement and prolonged antibiotic treatment.

UPPER LIMB TRAUMA

Clavicular fractures

This is a common fracture of childhood and young adults. These fractures always look terrible on X-ray (grossly displaced), but do remarkably well with conservative treatment (broad arm sling).

The clavicle is divided into thirds: medial, middle and lateral. Fractures are named after the position, most commonly the middle third, and are usually between the costoclavicular and coracoclavicular ligaments (as they are stronger than the bone).

Middle third fractures left alone heal with invariable malunion leaving a lump which usually disappears with time. It is advisable not to operate on middle third fractures as they have been shown to do worse.

Lateral third fractures, when displaced, signify coracoclavicular ligament disruption, and carry a greater risk of non-union than medial third fractures. Some argue for surgical fixation on this basis.

Note

- − Associated brachial plexus and vascular injuries are rare.
- − Malunion after a clavicular fracture is invariable (always present). This is due to the weight (downwards) of the arm on the lateral clavicle, and pull (upwards) of the SCM muscle on the medial clavicle. However, the rate of union is upwards of 95% when treated non-operatively in a sling.

Shoulder dislocation

The glenohumeral (shoulder) joint is unstable by nature. It is a ball and socket type joint, although the socket is very shallow.

Stabilisers of the joint are static and dynamic.

Static stabilisers:

- ◆ Concavity of the glenoid.
- ◆ Labrum around the glenoid (deepens the concavity).
- ◆ Joint capsule and ligaments.

Dynamic stabilisers:

- ◆ Pull of the rotator cuff muscles.
- ◆ Negative pressure (suction) of the capsule and its synovial fluid.

Traumatic shoulder dislocation can result from an axial load (landing heavily on an outstretched arm) or a direct blow (classically, rugby on a Sunday afternoon). Dislocation is 95% anterior in nature. Posterior dislocations only tend to be seen in electrical shock cases or are associated with epileptic seizures.

The treatment is relocation, generally with sedation in the emergency department, with appropriate monitoring, by one of the following manoeuvres:

- Stimson. This is less traumatic than the Hippocrates or Kocher's methods. It involves either the patient lying prone with a weight suspended from the wrist or, lying on their back with the doctor applying gentle upwards traction on the arm, with or without small rotatory movements if traction alone is insufficient.
- Kocher's. A sequence of manoeuvres of forced external rotation, adduction, internal rotation, and abduction.
- Hippocrates. Counter traction (classically with the doctor's foot in the axilla) with a rolled towel looped under the axilla, and traction in line with the arm.

Always check for axillary nerve involvement with each of these methods by testing the sensation of the deltoid patch and documenting it prior to relocation.

Relocation is followed by a period of time protected in a sling (2-3 weeks) and physiotherapy to the shoulder.

The re-dislocation rate is higher the younger the patient at the time of their first traumatic dislocation. This generally reflects the higher energy of the trauma.

There are associated injuries possible with anterior dislocations: a Bankart lesion, which is damage to the anterior labrum and capsule origin at this site, with or without an associated 'bony' Bankart, i.e. a fracture fragment to the anterior glenoid margin; a Hill-Sachs lesion, an osteochondral fragment off the femoral head; and a greater tuberosity avulsion fracture from a traction injury from the supraspinatus insertion at this point.

Rarely is an open relocation required, unless for some reason the dislocation is chronic, i.e. has been 'out' for more than 48 hours.

Humeral shaft fractures

These occur as a result of a direct blow or a fall onto the outstretched arm. Occasionally, spiral shaft fractures are seen caused by the torsional stress of arm wrestling.

Generally speaking, so long as the arm is immobilised in good alignment using a collar and cuff alone, or in combination with a hanging cast, or a plastic humeral brace, then the ovewhelming majority of humeral shaft fractures proceed to union.

Indications for operative fixation are open fractures, or if the fracture occurs in the context of polytrauma, where the patient would benefit from the extra stability of the fixed fracture as part of their nursing, or attempted mobilisation.

Distal humeral and articular fractures of the elbow are not required knowledge for exams, except perhaps the supracondylar paediatric humeral fracture (see below). There is one eponymous fracture that is worth knowing: the Holstein-Lewis fracture. This is a fracture of the mid-distal third junction of the humerus which is associated with wrist drop, i.e. radial nerve entrapment. It is recommended that the nerve be explored in these fractures.

Supracondylar humeral fractures

A fall in a child onto the outstretched hand with the elbow flexed can transmit the load axially to the elbow, resulting in a supracondylar fracture.

These fractures are classified by Gartland's classification, I, II and III (Figure 6.1). Gartland's I and IIA can simply be treated with collar and cuff, with a satisfactory result anticipated, but Gartland's IIB and III (displaced) must be treated by manipulation and cross K-wiring to stabilise the fracture in a reduced position.

The specific potential complication of this type of fracture if malreduced (operatively or otherwise) is cubitus varus (cubitus in this context means elbow), or gunstock deformity of the elbow. This is due to the continued growth at the distal humeral epiphysis in the malreduced direction and can result in ulnar nerve symptoms as the deformity gradually progresses.

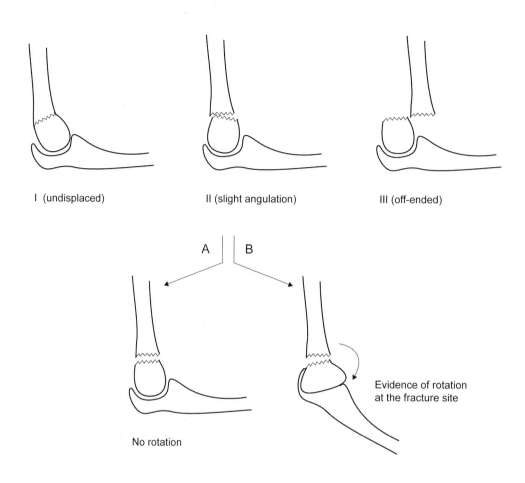

I (undisplaced)   II (slight angulation)   III (off-ended)

A   B

No rotation

Evidence of rotation
at the fracture site

Figure 6.1. Supracondylar humeral fractures: Gartland's classification (based on lateral elbow X-rays).

Olecranon fractures

The olecranon is that portion of the proximal ulna that articulates with the distal humerus (the trochlea). An olecranon fracture is therefore, generally, an intra-articular fracture. When displaced it requires operative fixation to ensure anatomical reduction. The displacement is caused by the cephalad pull of the triceps tendon on the proximal fragment of the olecranon.

The standard operative fixation technique is the tension band wire (Figure 6.2). The benefit of this technique is that it results in compression at the fracture site when triceps pulls on it, thus enabling early mobilisation.

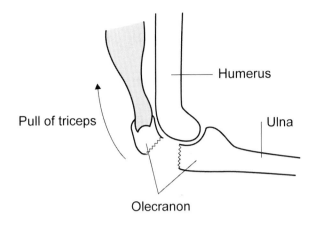

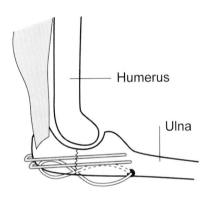

Consists of two parallel wires across the fracture and a loop of wire in a figure of eight, pulled tight across the fracture. The pull of triceps results in compression at the fracture site, hence, enabling early mobilisation.

Figure 6.2. Olecranon fractures.

Radius and ulna shaft fractures

These commonly occur in children falling from a height onto their outstretched hand. These fractures can be greenstick in nature, or off-ended.

They require manipulation under anaesthetic (MUA) if angulated, generally only in children, as their periosteal sleeve is thick enough to help maintain reduction. Adults require open reduction and internal fixation (ORIF) and immobilisation with an above-elbow cast. This prevents that element of pronation and supination that can be a deforming force if a below-elbow cast, alone, is used.

If, however, the fractured bones are off-ended (in adults or children), they require fixation, either by ORIF with plates (in adults or children) or, as advocated by a growing number of surgeons, with intramedullary wires passed across the fracture site (in children only) enabling percutaneous fixation. The wires do have to be removed at a later date.

The duration required in plaster is shorter for children, around 4-6 weeks, depending on the child's age and severity of the fracture, but adults require the full six weeks.

Distal radial fractures

Colles' fracture (Figure 6.3)

Described by Abraham Colles in Dublin in 1814 as a distal radial transverse fracture with dorsal displacement/angulation, caused by falling onto an outstretched hand.

If displaced and/or dorsally angulated, this fracture requires MUA as a minimum, but if it remains unstable, it then requires either supplementation with K-wires, or even ORIF using either a dorsal (low profile) plate or a volar (locked) plate.

Smith's fracture (Figure 6.3)

Described in 1834 (Smith was also from Dublin). As above, but with palmar displacement. It is caused by falling onto the dorsum of a flexed wrist.

Currently, there is very little place for non-operative treatment of displaced Smith's fractures. Their re-displacement rate, when treated in a cast (in extension), is unacceptably high. They must, therefore, be treated by volar buttress plating.

Colles' fracture

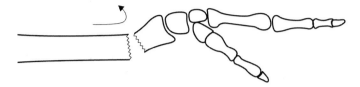

Fracture of distal radius with
dorsal angulation/displacement

Smith's fracture

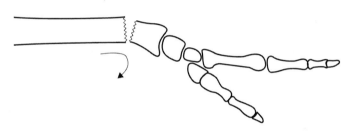

Fracture of distal radius with
palmar angulation/displacement

Figure 6.3. Colles' and Smith's fractures.

Open injuries of the hand

The structures that can be damaged are listed in the note below. These injuries normally require open exploration and debridement.

Note

- Fibrous flexor tendon sheaths, nerves, arteries, bones, tendons and ligaments.

Special cases are flexor tendons, which should not be repaired primarily in the presence of contaminants; these require delayed repair. Dead skin and muscle should be debrided.

Note

- Skin in the hand is a precious commodity, so split-skin grafts or advancement flaps should be considered where necessary.
- The Kessler technique of tendon repair refers to the clover leaf style of inserting sutures into the two severed ends of a tendon.
- It is essential to know if the patient is left or right-handed.
- It is important to know the patient's tetanus status.

Pulp space infection, paronychia, and flexor tendon sheath infections can occur, all of which require open treatment and cleaning out. Flexor tendon sheath infection requires urgent irrigation and antibiosis.

Note

— Human bites contain polymicrobial organisms. Both aerobes and anaerobes must be covered with antibiotic treatment. Do not primarily close bite wounds in the emergency setting; leave them open to heal by secondary intention. The only way to close these wounds, if needed, is by formal debridement and washout in an operating theatre.

LOWER LIMB TRAUMA

Proximal femoral fractures

Proximal femoral fractures, also known as hip fractures, are overwhelmingly more common in the elderly osteoporotic patient, classically in the female, although, given sufficient trauma, it is possible for these fractures to occur in the younger patient.

The key to understanding the different types of fracture in this region, is the blood supply to the femoral head, as it determines the treatment modalities used.

The femoral head receives its arterial supply from three main sources in the adult:

- Intramedullary vessels.
- Capsular vessels. These provide the predominant arterial supply to the femoral head. They are derived from a branch of the profunda femoris artery, becoming the lateral circumflex femoral artery which enters the capsule postero-superiorly, giving off numerous branches to the femoral head.
- Via a vessel in the ligamentum teres which is usually quite atrophic in the elderly, if present at all. It is derived from the obturator artery, becoming the foveal branch, also known as the medial epiphyseal artery.

As you might expect, fractures located within the region of the capsule (Figure 6.4) of the femoral neck (intracapsular), result in disruption to the arterial supply to the femoral head from both intramedullary vessels and capsular vessels. The disruption is greater when the fracture is displaced. This decreases union rates at the fracture and increases AVN of the femoral head, which results in painful osteoarthritis.

NORMAL

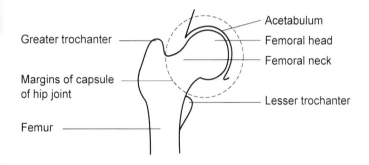

Figure 6.4. Proximal femoral fractures: normal anatomy.

The corollary to this is that extracapsular fractures have no effect on femoral head blood supply, and are more amenable to good results from fixation, rather than joint replacement.

Intracapsular fractures

These are classified by the Garden classification into I-IV classes. The exact details of this classification are less important than the realisation that I and II represent undisplaced fractures, which are more amenable to good results when fixed, and that III and IV represent displaced fractures, which have poorer results when fixed, and would be better treated by joint replacement (hemi-arthroplasty).

Fixation of undisplaced fractures is performed with three cannulated hip screws (Figure 6.5). This is a percutaneous procedure using the image intensifier for location. However, repeated studies have shown an approximate 40% complication rate (AVN of the

Undisplaced intracapsular fracture

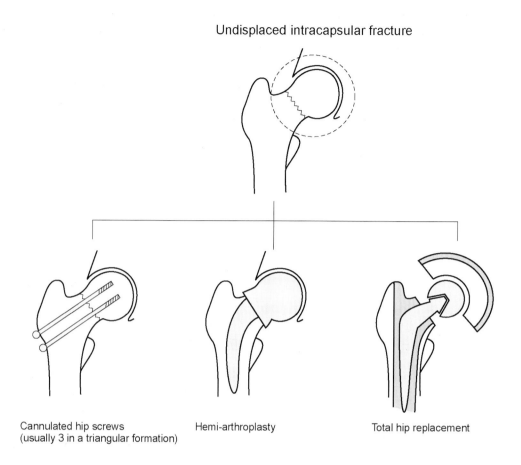

Cannulated hip screws
(usually 3 in a triangular formation)

Hemi-arthroplasty

Total hip replacement

Figure 6.5. Undisplaced intracapsular fractures.

femoral head or non-union) requiring conversion to total hip replacement within one year. The reasons to take these odds on board and still perform the operation is that the 60% who do well have retained their own hip joint, which is considered an advantage to a prosthetic joint and, that the operation itself is a minor one.

Another highly relevant point relating to cannulated screw fixation, is that it is necessary to partially weight bear the patient for a minimum of six weeks after the procedure to protect the fixation from the considerable forces through the hip during weight

bearing. This is particularly significant in the elderly, as they do not have the upper body strength, and sometimes co-ordination or cognitive function, to comply with partial weight bearing. In this case, they would be unsuitable for cannulated screw fixation.

The major alternative to fixation for intracapsular fractures is hemi-arthroplasty. This requires excision of the femoral head and replacement by a stemmed implant with a metal (stainless steel) head. These can be cemented (Thompson) or uncemented (Austen-Moore). Obviously, blood supply is no longer an issue in this case.

The hemi-arthroplasty operation takes longer, blood loss is greater, and wound infection rate is greater. The advantage, though, is the immediate ability to fully weight bear, and there is no AVN or non-union complications to require re-operation.

As a general rule, in the elderly, who are cognitively impaired, frail and have poor mobilisation, a hemi-arthroplasty should be performed. In the younger, mobile, compos mentis patient with an undisplaced fracture, cannulated screw fixation should be considered. For patients who fit between these two extremes, a surgeon's judgement call must be made.

Extracapsular fractures (intertrochanteric)

Intertrochanteric fractures can be in two, three or four parts (Figure 6.6) and either displaced or undisplaced.

The treatment modality is the same whatever the type of intertrochanteric fracture; it is only the technical difficulty of fixation that varies. The dynamic hip screw (DHS) is used in these cases.

The lag screw is passed up the femoral neck into the head. The barrel of the plate (usually four holes, with a neck shaft angle of 135°) is then passed over

the screw, immobilising the fracture fragments and allowing them to 'crunch down' on each other (to 'dynamise', hence the name).

The union rates are very good with a DHS. It does not share the same problems as cannulated hip screw fixation.

Extracapsular fractures (subtrochanteric)

These fractures are relatively unsuitable for fixation with the DHS. They are much less common than their intertrochanteric cousins, which is fortunate as they are technically more difficult to fix. The mainstay of fixation of subtrochanteric fractures is an intramedullary nail. It must be of a specific design termed cephalomedullary, an example of which is the gamma nail, although there are others (Figure 6.7). Like the DHS it has a lag screw up the femoral neck into the head, which passes through a hole in the proximal portion of the nail; thus, it has a fixed angle between the neck and the shaft. It allows postoperative weight bearing depending, to some extent, on the amount of comminution at the actual fracture site.

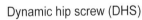

Dynamic hip screw (DHS)

Intramedullary fixation (e.g. gamma nail)

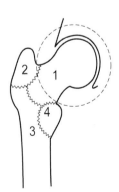
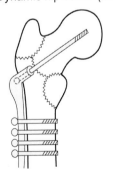
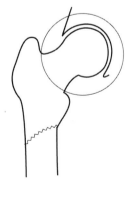
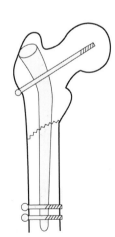

Figure 6.6. Intertrochanteric fractures (by definition this is extracapsular).

Figure 6.7. Subtrochanteric fractures (by definition this is extracapsular).

Femoral shaft fractures (Figure 6.8)

These are commonly seen in young men, e.g. motorcycle road traffic accident (RTA), or in children. They can be open or closed. Open fractures always require urgent debridement and washout.

In adults the mainstay of treatment is femoral nailing. It is percutaneous, involves very little disturbance of the soft tissues and has a very high union and low infection rate.

In children the physeal plates are still open, and hence the passage of a femoral nail can potentially damage the physes, resulting in a shorter leg. The mainstay of treatment of femoral shaft fractures in children is traction. The union rates are excellent. There is a tendency for the fracture ends to overlap, i.e. be up to 1cm short at the time of union. This, far

from being a disadvantage, is usually followed by bony overgrowth (common in young children post-fracture) bringing the leg back to an equal length with its uninjured partner.

An alternative to traction in paediatric femoral shaft fractures is the (still relatively uncommonly used) elastic nailing system. Two pre-bent wires are passed percutaneously from each femoral condyle proximally up past the fracture, after it has been reduced by indirect means. These wires cross each other twice on their way up to the proximal femur. The strength of the fixation is derived from the pre-bend on the wires giving them a tendency to want to spring apart, but being restricted from doing so by the femoral cortices. It does not seem to affect the physes, but they do have to be removed after union, though. The child can partially weight bear and does not have to spend time in traction.

Femoral supracondylar fractures

These are a difficult, but fortunately uncommon, type of fracture to treat. The subject is not required knowledge for exams.

The mainstay of treatment is either by using a dynamic condylar screw (DCS), which is a laterally placed plate with standard screws and a large fixed-angle condylar screw or, alternatively, a retrograde femoral nail can be placed, the entry point being through the knee joint between the femoral condyles and up the femoral shaft.

A more recent alternative is a locked plate placed percutaneously called the LISS (less invasive stabilisation system), which despite being a plate, has an advantage of less disturbance to the soft tissues than the DCS as it can be placed percutaneously.

Proximal tibial fractures

Tibial plateau fractures are caused by a varus or valgus force combined with axial loading, e.g. a fall from a height. It usually occurs in the 50-60 age range, but it can occur at any age. They often require CT to classify the fracture. Figure 6.9 shows the basic anatomy of the tibia.

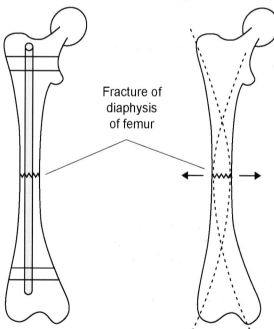

Femoral nail

Elastic/flexible nails
(formerly known as 'Noncy nails')

Fracture of diaphysis of femur

Figure 6.8. Femoral shaft fractures.

Anterior view, left tibia and fibula

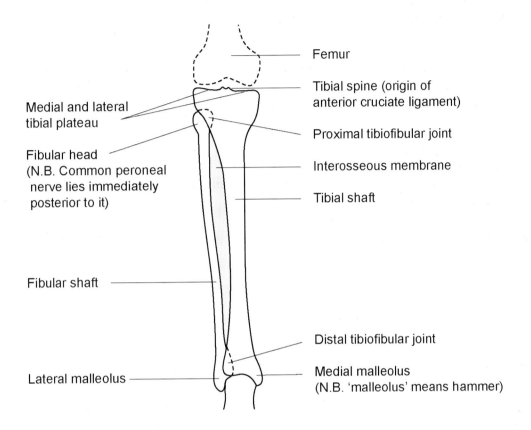

Femur

Tibial spine (origin of anterior cruciate ligament)

Medial and lateral tibial plateau

Proximal tibiofibular joint

Fibular head (N.B. Common peroneal nerve lies immediately posterior to it)

Interosseous membrane

Tibial shaft

Fibular shaft

Distal tibiofibular joint

Lateral malleolus

Medial malleolus (N.B. 'malleolus' means hammer)

Superior view, right tibial plateau

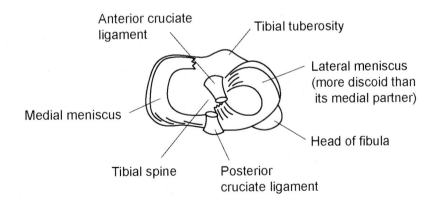

Anterior cruciate ligament

Tibial tuberosity

Lateral meniscus (more discoid than its medial partner)

Medial meniscus

Head of fibula

Tibial spine

Posterior cruciate ligament

Figure 6.9. The tibia.

Schatzker's classification of tibial plateau fractures (Figure 6.10)

- ◆ I. Lateral condyle only (sheared).
- ◆ II. Lateral condyle only (comminuted crush with depression).
- ◆ III. Lateral condyle only (sparing lip most laterally).
- ◆ IV. Medial condyle only (shear).
- ◆ V. Both condyles.
- ◆ VI. Combined condylar and subcondylar fracture.

Treatment

Modalities of treatment include:

- ◆ In the case of an undisplaced fracture, apply a hinged cast brace which prevents varus-valgus movements, but permits flexion and extension.

Encourage movement, but forbid weight bearing for 6-8 weeks.
- ◆ Surgical options include:
  - screw fixation;
  - buttress plate fixation;
  - bone graft areas of deficient bone, allowing the depressed articular surface to be 'pushed up' in a type III fracture.

Complications

Early
- ◆ Vascular injury.
- ◆ Compartment syndrome.

Late
- ◆ Joint stiffness.
- ◆ OA.
- ◆ Deformity.

Schatzker's classification of tibial plateau fractures

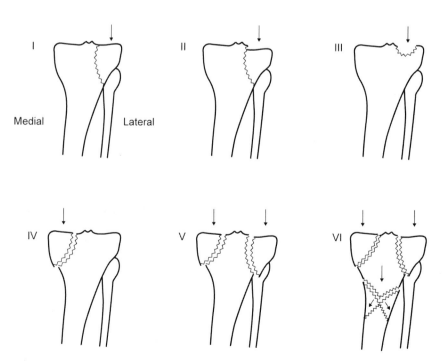

Figure 6.10. Tibial fractures.

Tibial shaft fractures

This is a common injury, as the bone is subcutaneous, and is often seen in motorcyclists. Fractures can be open or closed.

Gustillo Anderson classification of open fractures

This refers to fractures of any bone, not merely the tibia:

- I. Small puncture wound.
- II. Wound >1cm long (without extensive soft tissue damage).
- III. Severe laceration, soft tissue injury and comminuted (high energy) fracture pattern. Type III injuries are subdivided into three subgroups:
  - IIIA. Large soft tissue laceration that can nonetheless be directly closed without the need for skin grafting or muscle flaps (it is worth remembering that severely comminuted, or segmental, fractures are automatically classified into IIIA even if there is little external evidence of soft tissue damage);
  - IIIB. Extensive soft tissue loss and likely periosteal stripping. There is massive contamination and obvious bone exposed. Generally, muscle flaps and/or skin grafts are necessary for soft tissue cover;
  - IIIC. An arterial injury associated with the fracture that will require vascular repair.

Treatment of tibial fractures has some points of controversy. No one treatment is without its problems.

Tibial nails have the advantage of being percutaneous, disturbing the soft tissues very little, and being a relatively technically undemanding procedure. The down side is that there is a relatively high incidence of anterior knee pain at the site of the entry point in the knee.

Tibial plating allows anatomical reduction of the fracture, at the expense of exposing (and hence damaging) the soft tissues. The tibia is a subcutaneous bone and the blood supply to the overlying skin is poor. This results in a higher wound problem rate (infection or dehiscence), although, in the right case, it is a perfectly good treatment.

External fixation (X-fix) is relatively easy in the tibia, due to its subcutaneous location but, in common with all X-fixes, there is the problem of pin-site infection and loosening. Added to that is the social issue for the patient of having a frame on their leg for anything up to three months.

Ankle fractures

The ankle (Figure 6.11) is one of the most common anatomical sites fractured in adults. The mechanism is generally the combination of axial load with rotation, usually inversion of the ankle. The modality of treatment is dependent upon the classification of fracture.

There are two main classifications:

- Lauge-Hansen (1950). This is complex and little used in clinical practice.
- Weber (Figure 6.12). This is more commonly used. There are three types: A, B and C:
  - A. Fibular fracture distal to the syndesmosis, which is the name for the structure made up of both anterior and posterior tibiofibular ligaments together (see Figure 6.11). There can be an associated medial malleolar fracture and/or deltoid ligament rupture;
  - B. An oblique fibular fracture starting at the level of the joint line and extending proximally. The syndesmosis is intact, but the mortise joint is sometimes affected, resulting in 'talar shift'. Talar shift is seen on the mortise view X-ray as the talus sitting more laterally towards the fractured fibula and away from the tibial side. You will therefore see widening of the mortise joint on the tibial (medial) side. This is an indication for operative fixation;
  - C. Fibular fracture proximal to the syndesmosis, therefore, the syndesmosis and interosseous septum are necessarily ruptured, as the force of the injury has travelled up through, and hence disrupted, the structures from the talar dome to the exit point of the fracture. The mortise is thus disrupted.

Ankle, anterior view

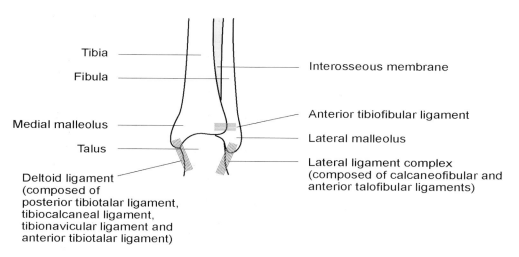

- Tibia
- Fibula
- Interosseous membrane
- Medial malleolus
- Anterior tibiofibular ligament
- Talus
- Lateral malleolus
- Deltoid ligament (composed of posterior tibiotalar ligament, tibiocalcaneal ligament, tibionavicular ligament and anterior tibiotalar ligament)
- Lateral ligament complex (composed of calcaneofibular and anterior talofibular ligaments)

Ankle, medial view

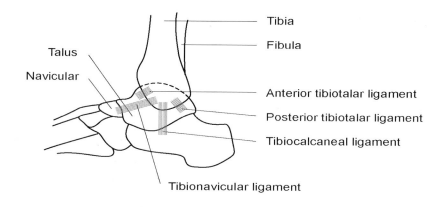

- Talus
- Navicular
- Tibia
- Fibula
- Anterior tibiotalar ligament
- Posterior tibiotalar ligament
- Tibiocalcaneal ligament
- Tibionavicular ligament

Ankle, lateral view

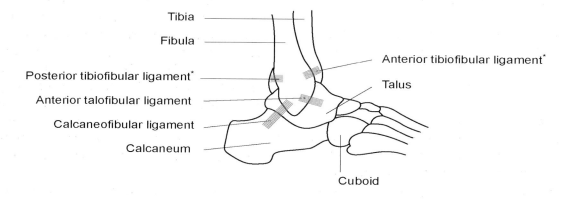

- Tibia
- Fibula
- Posterior tibiofibular ligament*
- Anterior talofibular ligament
- Calcaneofibular ligament
- Calcaneum
- Anterior tibiofibular ligament*
- Talus
- Cuboid

* Both together form the syndesmosis of the ankle

Figure 6.11. The ankle.

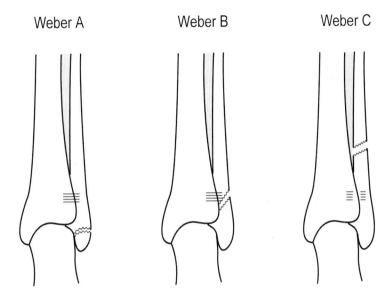

Figure 6.12. Ankle fractures (Weber classification).

Two X-rays are required, a lateral view and mortise view (not quite the same as an AP; it is in fact 15° internally rotated from an AP).

Treatment

Undisplaced Type A or B fractures can be treated with six weeks in plaster; Type B fractures with a talar shift and Type C fractures require ORIF.

In the case of Weber B fractures with a talar shift, a fibular plate is required. In the case of Weber C fractures, the fibula should be plated and a syndesmosis screw passed proximally to the syndesmosis from the fibula, across to the tibia, holding them together while the syndesmosis heals. This screw should be removed after ten weeks, as during the course of normal weight bearing the tibia and fibula do rotate through up to 5° with respect to each other, which could break the screw or the fibula.

Foot trauma

Foot trauma is a subject quite unlikely to come up in exams. It is included only briefly here for completeness.

The most commonly seen traumatic condition of the foot in orthopaedic practice is fracture of the base of the fifth metatarsal. It is a simple avulsion fracture from the point of insertion of the peroneus brevis tendon. It occurs as a result of an inversion of the ankle and a reflex contraction of the peroneus brevis in an attempt to resist the inversion. The bony insertion then suffers avulsion fracture. This is effectively a sprain and can be treated symptomatically. Those who can weight bear are safe to do so; those who need some immobilisation for pain relief can be put into a weight bearing plaster 'bootie' (a below-ankle, removable, light-weight material cast, which looks like a shoe).

Toes often fracture and need no management, unless they are open fractures or grossly deformed.

Metatarsal fractures are for the most part uncomplicated and require a short period of time in non-weight bearing below-knee casts.

A Lisfranc fracture dislocation is an indication for surgery. It is a fracture dislocation of the base of the index metatarsal, with lateral drift of the more lateral metatarsals with it. These must be wired or screwed back into their anatomical location for foot function to potentially return to normal.

Calcaneal fractures are a specialist subject and are fundamentally divisible into two groups: those that are undisplaced and do not involve the subtalar joint, which can be treated non-operatively with non-weight bearing below-knee casting; and, those that display loss of calcaneal height, an increase in calcaneal width, and involvement of the subtalar joint. These more complex fractures may require reconstruction.

Head injury

Layers of the SCALP

The layers of the SCALP (from superficial to deep) are: skin, connective tissue, aponeurosis, loose areolar tissue and the pericranium. (Remember the mnemonic of SCALP. All mnemonics have at least one contrived portion. In this case it is clearly the loose areolar tissue, but such a contrivance actually helps to remember the mnemonic.)

Meninges

Knowing which form of vascular structure is found within each meningeal layer forms the basis of understanding of the different types of intracranial bleed.

There are three meningeal layers:

- Dura mata - adherent to the periosteum.
- Arachnoid mata - lies between the dura mata (to which it is adherent) and the pia mata.
- Pia mata - the surface lining of the brain.

Important areas relating to intracranial bleeds are:

- Extradural - between the periosteum and the dura, containing the middle meningeal artery.
- Subdural - between the dura and arachnoid, containing bridging veins which drain to the venous sinuses.
- Subarachnoid - between the arachnoid and pia mata, containing CSF and arteries of the Circle of Willis, and cerebral arteries.

Types of intracranial bleed are:

- An extradural haematoma: an arterial bleed between the dura and the periosteum from the middle meningeal artery.
- A subdural haematoma: a venous bleed.
- A subarachnoid haemorrhage: an arterial bleed from the Circle of Willis or the cerebral arteries into the CSF.

Often the cause of bleeds can be a rupture of an arterial aneurysm, classically, the Berry aneurysms of the Circle of Willis.

Note

— Raised intracranial pressure (ICP) causes herniation of the uncus into the tentorium cerebelli pressing on the ipsilateral III cranial nerve (oculomotor), causing a dilated pupil on the ipsilateral side. This is very important, as it represents the mechanism behind the fixed dilated pupil in head injury patients that all junior doctors look for, but few understand its significance.
— Cushing's reflex is a vagal and sympathetic stimulation due to increased ICP, e.g. an intracranial bleed. It causes an increase in BP to maintain cerebral perfusion pressure and a decreased heart rate, quite different from shock where the drop in BP is accompanied by an increase in the HR.

Peripheral nerve injuries

A peripheral nerve is basically a bundle of neuronal processes (axons and dendrites, and their supporting structures) (Figure 6.13).

Axons are the functional unit of a neurone transmitting information away from the cell body. Dendrites are the functional unit of a neurone transmitting information towards the cell body (Figure 6.14).

Peripheral nerves conduct efferent (motor) information from the anterior horn cell to muscle fibres and afferent (sensory) information from peripheral receptors via the dorsal root ganglia to the anterior horn of the spinal cord (Figure 6.14). Peripheral nerves also conduct sudomotor (information to sweat glands) and vasomotor (information to vascular smooth muscle) fibres from the sympathetic chain.

Nerves are either motor, sensory or mixed. Myelin is a substance made by Schwann cells which lines motor axons and provides an insulated outer layer that prevents loss of signal from the axon as it transmits its information. The net result is that myelinated nerves are faster than their non-myelinated relatives. Outside the myelin layer is the endoneurium. Around the bundles of axons in the nerve is the perineurium (dividing up the bundles).

The nerve trunk itself is surrounded by epineurium. Nerves have a rich blood supply; these vessels (the vasa neuronum) run on the surface of the nerve trunk, which then form endoneurial capillaries. Damage to these results in nerve ischaemia.

Note

— The vessels supplying the nerve also have a sympathetic supply themselves. Damage to this is implicated in reflex sympathetic dystrophy (RSD) syndrome. There are ever-changing theories and nomenclature with regard to RSD. The term currently in use is chronic regional pain syndrome.

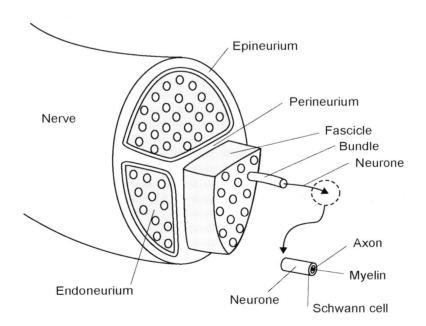

Figure 6.13. Anatomy of a peripheral nerve.

(a)

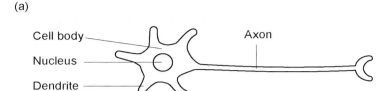

(b)

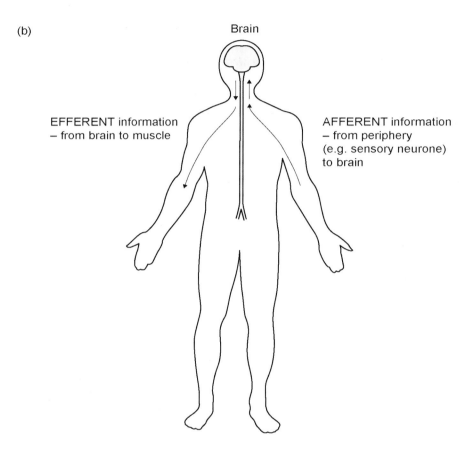

Figure 6.14. (a) A neurone; (b & c) examples of afferent and efferent neurones.

Types of peripheral nerve lesion

- Ischaemia caused by acute nerve compression. A sensation of tingling comes on after 15 minutes of compression, loss of pain sensibility after 30 minutes, muscle weakness after 45 minutes, and when compression is removed, this results in intense paraesthesiae (pins and needles) for 5 minutes, restoration of normal sensation after 30 seconds and full muscle power after 10 minutes. The damage is transient with no lasting sequelae.
- Neurapraxia, a term coined by Seddon in 1942, is defined as reversible physiological nerve conduction block followed by spontaneous recovery after a few days/weeks. The pathology is caused by mechanical pressure leading to segmental demyelination, e.g. in Crutch palsy/Saturday night palsy.
- Axonotmesis, which means literally axonal disruption. There is loss of conduction, but the nerve is in continuity (endoneurial tubes are intact). The pathology is termed Wallerian degeneration, which means that the neurones distal to the site of the lesion undergo phagocytosis of the axonal material along the remnant of their length.

Note

- Axonal regeneration begins within hours of damage at a maximum speed of 1-3mm per day.

- Neurotmesis, which means division of the nerve trunk, e.g. in an open wound. Wallerian degeneration is also present, but over a greater length of the nerve segment. There is no regeneration. A neuroma often forms at the ends of the severed nerve.

Clinical features

Clinical features of a peripheral nerve lesion are: pain, paraesthesiae, joint stiffness, deformity, wasting, anaesthetised skin which is smooth and shiny, possible trophic ulcers (especially the feet) and a palpable neuroma.

Prognostic factors

- Type of lesion. Neurapraxia always recovers fully; neurotmesis invariably recovers poorly/not at all.
- Level of lesion. The higher the lesion, the worse the prognosis.
- Type of nerve. Mixed nerves, that contain both sensory and motor information, do not recover as well as 'pure' nerves, i.e. that are either completely sensory or completely motor.
- Size of gap (between the two cut ends).
- Age. Children do better.
- Delay in surgical repair.
- Associated lesions and soft tissue damage, e.g. vessels, muscle, etc.

Treatment

- Nerve exploration.
- Primary repair.
- Delayed repair.
- Nerve grafting. A nerve graft will never do as well as a primary repair; however, it is indicated if there has been loss of nervous tissue.

Chapter 7

Cold (non-traumatic) orthopaedics

Conditions of the shoulder

Frozen shoulder

Presentation
This is a painful condition of the shoulder characterised by both pain and stiffness. It is a form of adhesive capsulitis. The most marked restriction of movement is in external rotation; there is characteristically none. It has been classified into three stages as it is a self-limiting condition, taking the best part of 18 months to resolve:

- I. Painful phase: a gradual onset of shoulder pain. No trauma.
- II. Stiff phase: a reduction in the range of movement.
- III. Thawing phase: a gradual resolution of both pain and stiffness.

Investigations
The pathogenesis is poorly understood. X-rays are normal but MRI shows thickening of the capsule. Arthrography can sometimes show loss of the axillary recess. Arthroscopy shows decreased joint space, a thickened capsule and the presence of intra-articular adhesions.

Treatment
Treatment is equally problematic. Early on in the phases, manipulation under anaesthetic (MUA) and steroid injection might help a little. Physiotherapy, especially during the painful phase, is counterproductive and can cause more pain. Surgical division of adhesions or capsular release surgery does not seem to help either. Waiting until the disease resolves forms the mainstay of treatment.

Complications
- Manipulation under anaesthetic risks causing more pain, potentially not improving the range of movement, fracturing the humerus and causing haemarthrosis.
- Physiotherapy does not risk a great deal apart from the potential to aggravate the painful symptoms.
- Surgery (open or arthroscopic) risks wound infection, septic arthritis, haemarthrosis, causing more pain, potentially not improving the range of movement, and reflex sympathetic dystrophy (RSD)/chronic regional pain syndrome (CRPS).

Impingement of the shoulder

Presentation
This is a condition that can come on in the absence of trauma, although a precipitating event does not preclude the diagnosis. It is the presence of pain as the shoulder is abducted close to 90° (sometimes less).

The coraco-acromial ligament and undersurface of the acromium are impinging on the superior rotator cuff (supraspinatus tendon) as it is pinched by the greater tuberosity of the humerus in abduction. This can be associated with a tear of the rotator cuff, or even degenerative changes to the cuff, but not necessarily so.

Investigations

The classical clinical test for impingement is Jobe's test involving abduction and internal rotation (point the patient's thumb downwards to the ground) of the shoulder. This causes a sudden sharp pain as the greater tuberosity rotates up to pinch the supraspinatus with the above structures. Neer's test involves the same movement, but noticing that the pain is abolished 20 minutes or so after injecting the joint with local anaesthetic and repeating the manoeuvre.

Standard X-rays of the shoulder tend to appear normal, even when the patient has impingement. However, one can sometimes see 'beaking' of the lateral inferior tip of the acromion. But the other use of the X-ray is its ability to identify osteoarthritis (OA), which is the major differential in shoulder impingement.

Ultrasound examination of the shoulder can show inflammation of the subacromial bursa and supraspinatus tendon. It can also show the presence of a rotator cuff tear or calcific tendonitis in the supraspinatus tendon. MRI can show the same information as ultrasound.

Treatment

Treatment modalities range from rest for a short period and resolution of mild cases or, injection of the subacromial bursa with local anaesthetic and steroid. In theory, this reduces the oedema of the supraspinatus tendon, hence giving more space in abduction and less impingement.

Finally, a subacromial decompression can be performed (either open or arthroscopic) by burring away the undersurface of the acromion and dividing the coraco-acromial ligament.

Complications

◆ Arthroscopic subacromial decompression risks persistence of symptoms, haemarthrosis, wound infection, septic arthritis, and RSD/CRPS.

Osteoarthritis of the shoulder

Presentation

This can be taken to mean either of two diagnoses: acromioclavicular joint (ACJ) or glenohumeral joint (GHJ) degenerative disease.

ACJ osteoarthritis (OA) presents as a gradual onset of high arc pain (pain on overhead activities) as the ACJ is under greatest strain in abduction greater than 90°.

It is possible to inject the ACJ (a small joint) with a small volume of steroid. This relieves the symptoms in a good proportion of cases. However, if surgery is indicated, an excision of the ACJ (either open or arthroscopic) can be performed which, when performed correctly, results in excellent pain relief with no loss of stability of the joint.

GHJ OA presents as an insidious onset of shoulder pain on all types of movement, as well as a gradual decrease in the range of movement. Swelling is often present, as it is common to have an associated joint effusion. Steroid injection may have a temporising effect, but is generally not very helpful in established OA.

Investigations

Standard X-rays are generally all that is required to make the diagnosis.

Treatment

In GHJ OA, joint arthroplasty is indicated when the symptoms have reached sufficient severity. This can take the form of a hemi-arthroplasty (humeral head only) or total joint arthroplasty (humeral head and glenoid replacement), depending on the surgeon's preference. There is a general trend towards hemi-arthroplasty because the results are as good as total joint arthroplasty, without the complication of the glenoid prosthetic loosening, which is still a problem with total joint implants.

Complications

◆ Haematoma or haemarthrosis.
◆ Wound infection.
◆ Deep infection. This can become chronic and severe, requiring excision of the implant for antibiotic treatment to work and a revision arthroplasty at a later date.
◆ Persistent shoulder pain despite successful arthroplasty.
◆ Stiffness and weakness of shoulder movements.
◆ Neurovascular damage.
◆ RSD.

Nerve disorders of the shoulder

You are expected to be able to recognise the clinical signs of these nerve lesions, but the finer points of management and investigation are beyond the remit of this book. General principles that are of use are as follows:

◆ The mainstay of investigation is nerve conduction studies.
◆ MRI can be used to look for nerve root avulsions.
◆ For severed or avulsed nerves there is the surgical option of nerve grafting, the results of which are mediocre.

Brachial plexus injury

This can be caused by traction injuries of the shoulder causing paraesthesiae in the distribution of the affected root and weakness in the relevant distribution. The injury can be a neurapraxia (demyelination of a portion of the sheath, but continuity of the axon with a 100% recovery), axonotmesis (axon and myelin sheath both disrupted with a poorer recovery), or neurotmesis (both epineurium and endoneurium disrupted, e.g. an avulsion of the nerve root, which has a very poor prognosis for recovery, even with surgical repair).

Long thoracic nerve (LTN) palsy

The LTN supplies motor innervation to the serratus anterior muscle, which is an anterior stabiliser of the scapula. Thus, a palsy to this nerve results in scapular winging. Depending on the cause, treatment can be expectant with good recovery, but occasionally it requires surgery, e.g. a pectoralis major transfer procedure.

Suprascapular nerve compression

The suprascapular nerve supplies motor innervation to the supraspinatus and infraspinatus muscles. The compression of the nerve results in a palsy and in wasting of these two muscles which is visible on inspection of the back, the acromium being more prominent. Weakness of initiation of abduction and of external rotation of the shoulder is present. Compressing masses such as ganglia or tumours can cause this. Surgical release is indicated if imaging suggests a mass compressing the nerve.

Carpal tunnel syndrome

Presentation

Carpal tunnel syndrome is a collection of symptoms relating to compression of the median nerve as it passes beneath the flexor retinaculum of the wrist, the carpal tunnel.

It can be primary or secondary, i.e. associated with another condition such as rheumatoid arthritis, pregnancy, peripheral oedema, hypothyroidism or local trauma, e.g. a fractured wrist.

The symptoms therefore reflect the function of the median nerve:

◆ Paraesthesiae in the thumb, index, middle and ulnar border of the ring fingers.
◆ When there is prolonged compression, there can be thenar eminence wasting and some weakness of grip.

Patients complain of an uncomfortable tingling in the hand, which is worse at night, occasionally causing them to drop objects. This can be exacerbated by activities involving prolonged gripping, e.g. driving. See the section on examination of the hand for greater details, but salient clinical findings are:

◆ Reduced sensation in the median nerve distribution.

♦ Thenar eminence wasting.
♦ Tinnel's sign is positive (see p401 in Chapter 13, Examination Techniques).
♦ Phalen's sign is postitive (see p401 in Chapter 13, Examination Techniques).

Investigations

Nerve conduction studies (NCS) can be used to confirm the diagnosis if clinical doubt exists. Distal sensory latencies of greater than 3.2 milliseconds or motor latencies of greater than 4.2 milliseconds (in electromyography [EMG], rather than NCS) are considered abnormal and contribute to the diagnosis.

Treatment

The treatment is to release the compression on the median nerve. This is done surgically by incising the flexor retinaculum. This is termed the carpal tunnel release operation.

The flexor retinaculum is a transverse fibrous band of tissue at the volar wrist crease, intended to prevent bow-stringing of the underlying flexor tendons. Thus, it may well be asked as to why there is no bow-stringing after the procedure. The answer seems to be that healing takes place at the flexor retinaculum and scar tissue bridges the gap in the two cut ends. Therefore, the continuity of the ligament is restored, but it remains more lax due to the presence of the bridging scar tissue.

Complications

♦ Wound infection.
♦ Haematoma.
♦ RSD/CRPS.
♦ Pillar pain. This is discomfort, which is permanent whenever the patient puts pressure on the palm, e.g. when leaning on a stick or gripping an object hard.
♦ Persistence of median nerve symptoms (incomplete release, i.e. technical error, wrong diagnosis in the first place, or unknown cause).
♦ Damage to the median nerve at the time of surgery.

The back

There are a number of separate causes of back pain that can be individually recognised by the following clusters of symptoms.

The point of this classification is that the modalities, and need, for treatment are entirely different.

The backache problem

Guide to differential diagnosis

♦ Transient backache following muscular activity represents a simple back strain, which needs rest followed by exercise.
♦ In sudden acute back pain and sciatica occurring in the <20-year-old age group, spondylolisthesis and infection need to be excluded (Figure 7.1). Both have characteristic X-ray changes. In the 20-40 year age group, it is more likely to be acute disc prolapse (Figure 7.2). There is a history of strain, definite sciatic tension and neurological signs. In the elderly population, it may be an osteoporotic compression fracture (Figure 7.3).
♦ With chronic low back pain with or without sciatica in the >40-year age group, with a previous history of disc prolapse and recurrent episodes of pain, the diagnosis is most likely facet joint dysfunction (Figure 7.4)/ osteoarthritis. The symptoms are aggravated by activity and are relieved by rest. Treatment is almost invariably conservative.
♦ Back pain and pseudoclaudication represents spinal stenosis (Figure 7.5). There is calf pain at irregular intervals during mild exercise, or exacerbation of symptoms by certain back postures. Surgical spinal decompression is required to relieve the condition.
♦ Severe and constant pain localised to a specific site represents local bone pathology, e.g. compression fracture, Paget's disease, a tumour, an infective focus.
♦ Chronic back pain syndrome is back pain that has (in addition to the pain) affective and psychosomatic symptoms (which are part of illness behaviour). This diagnosis can only be made if all organic causes of pain have been excluded.

(a)   (b)

(c)

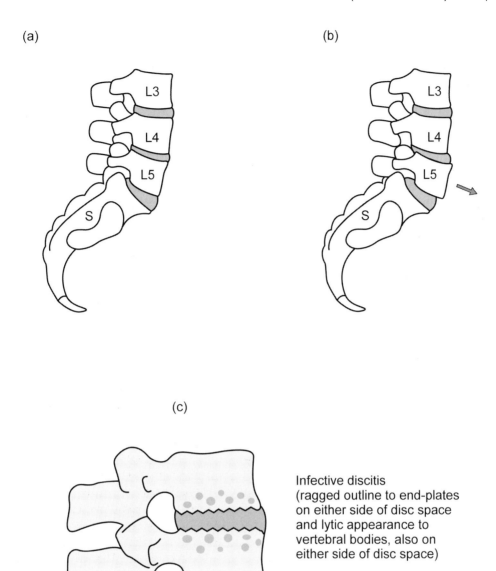

Infective discitis
(ragged outline to end-plates
on either side of disc space
and lytic appearance to
vertebral bodies, also on
either side of disc space)

Figure 7.1. The backache problem: (a) normal lateral view of lumbar spine; (b) spondylolisthesis of L5 on S1 (X-ray changes); (c) infection.

Acute lumbar disc rupture

Presentation

This can occur at any age, but it is most common in the 20-45 year age group, after stooping or an activity resulting in pain in the back, as well as the affected leg It is uncommon in the very young and very elderly. Both areas of pain are exacerbated by coughing and straining. Paraesthesia, numbness and muscle weakness may develop in one leg, but rarely, in both legs.

Note

- Cauda equina compression (rare) causes urinary retention and saddle anaesthesia.

Normal disc (basic anatomy)

Annulus fibrosus
(resilient cartilaginous
structure)

Nucleus pulposus
(liquid centre)

Disc showing prolapse

Prolapse of liquid from
nucleus pulposus
(v. gelatinous type
of viscocity)

Axial view of vertebral body (lumbar)

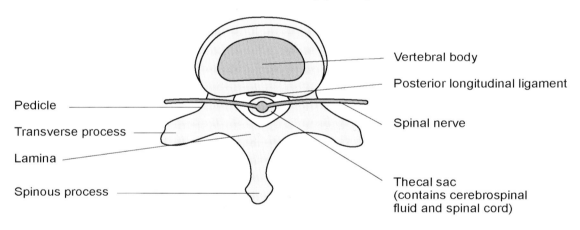

Vertebral body

Posterior longitudinal ligament

Pedicle

Transverse process

Lamina

Spinal nerve

Spinous process

Thecal sac
(contains cerebrospinal
fluid and spinal cord)

Axial view of vertebral body and overlying disc
with prolapse compressing nerve root

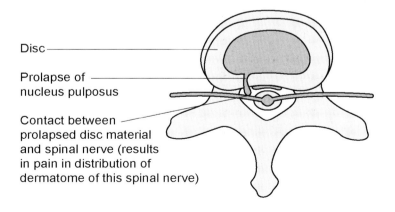

Disc

Prolapse of
nucleus pulposus

Contact between
prolapsed disc material
and spinal nerve (results
in pain in distribution of
dermatome of this spinal nerve)

Figure 7.2. The backache problem: acute disc prolapse.

Lateral view of spine

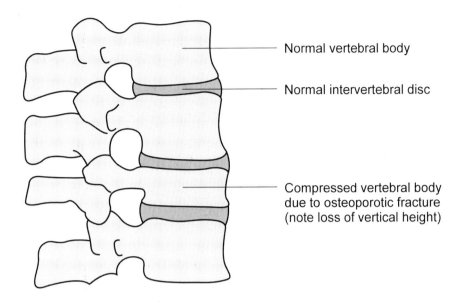

Normal vertebral body

Normal intervertebral disc

Compressed vertebral body due to osteoporotic fracture (note loss of vertical height)

Figure 7.3. The backache problem: osteoporotic compression fracture.

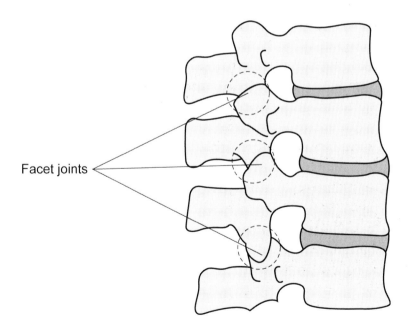

Facet joints

Figure 7.4. The backache problem: facet joint dysfunction.

Normal anatomy of vertebral canal

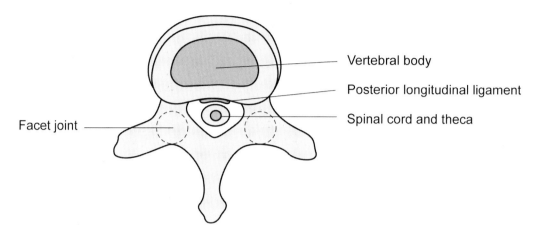

Vertebral body

Posterior longitudinal ligament

Spinal cord and theca

Facet joint

Anatomy of spinal stenosis

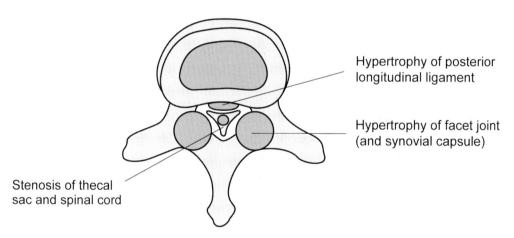

Hypertrophy of posterior longitudinal ligament

Hypertrophy of facet joint (and synovial capsule)

Stenosis of thecal sac and spinal cord

Figure 7.5. The backache problem: spinal stenosis.

A straight leg raise is the angle at which pain in the affected leg (ipsilateral) prevents further elevation. Pain in the back restricting further raising is not considered relevant. It is important that you are able to demonstrate this clinical sign. If the same pain is caused by a contralateral straight leg raise (the cross-over leg sign), the prolapse is large and central. Typically, the level of prolapse is at L4/5 or L5/S1.

On examination there is muscle weakness/wasting (late) and diminished reflexes/sensory loss. The patterns of neurology that you will most commonly see in the clinical setting are:

- L5 impairment. Weak big toe extension, weak knee flexion and a sensory loss to the outer side of the leg and dorsum of the foot.
- S1 impairment. Weak plantar flexion of the foot, weak eversion of the foot, depressed ankle jerk and a sensory loss on the lateral border of the foot.

Investigations
- X-ray may show decreased disc space but it is also useful in excluding other bony disease.
- MRI is useful to show a prolapsing disc.

Differential diagnosis

The differential diagnosis is ankylosing spondylitis, a bone tumour or nerve tumour.

Treatment

Conservative

Heat, analgesia, advice on remaining active and an an occasional benefit from gabapentin or amitriptyline to help with neurological pain. Epidural injection can relieve the pain symptoms in a good proportion of patients.

Surgical

Indications:

- Cauda equina compression.
- Worsening of neurology.
- Failure of conservative treatment after three weeks.

The surgical procedure is a discectomy, an excision of the liquid centre of the disc, the nucleus pulposus.

Complications of epidural injection

- No improvement in condition.
- Epidural haematoma causing acute worsening of neurological symptoms, or even cauda equina compression (a true emergency, presenting as a bilateral neurological deficit with decreased anal tone and urinary incontinence. It must be diagnosed on MRI and the patient returned to theatre for decompression of the haematoma).
- Cerebrospinal fluid (CSF) leak, which may simply result in a headache, worse on vertical posture and better on lying down. This resolves generally with 24-48 hours recumbency. The treatment for a CSF leak is an epidural blood patch; this is an injection at the appropriate level of 15-20ml of the patient's own unclotted blood, which clots (while the patient remains recumbent for two hours after the procedure) 'patching' the leak. However, CSF leak is itself a risk factor for developing meningitis, which requires urgent antibiotic treatment. It presents with severe headache, photophobia, fever, potential alteration of consciousness (unconsciousness in some) and malaise.
- CSF fistula, i.e. persistent leak through the skin puncture wound, which requires re-operation for direct repair of the dura.

Complications of discectomy surgery

- No improvement in the condition.
- Wound infection.
- Haematoma causing cauda equina compression. Emergent surgical decompression is required, as mentioned above.
- Nerve root damage at the time of surgery, resulting in a transient, but sometimes permanent, sensori-motor deficit in the distribution of the affected nerve.
- Dural puncture. Either identified at the time of surgery and repaired directly or presents as a CSF leak as mentioned above. N.B. Risk of meningitis.
- There is a small (in the order of 1 in a 1000), but real, risk of complete paralysis post-operation.
- Very rarely the instrument used to extract the disc material from the nucleus pulposus region accidentally perforates through the anterior disc wall perforating the inferior vena cava, resulting in a potentially life-threatening bleed.

Facet joint dysfunction/osteoarthritis

Presentation

Recurrent episodes of simple (i.e. no associated neurological symptoms) back pain, most commonly lumbar. This can come on spontaneously, after lifting a heavy load, after adopting an unusual position or after sleeping in an odd position. The pain can range from mild to debilitatingly severe with associated lumbar muscle spasm.

Investigations

- Lumbar X-rays are of little value here as the severity of degenerative changes does not (at all) correlate with the degree (or even presence) of symptoms.
- MRI scans can show degenerate disc(s) and facet joint degeneration. They can also reveal any spondylolisthesis or pars defects. MRI can reveal those rare cases of pain secondary to vertebral tumours (there must always be a high

index of suspicion in elderly patients presenting with new onset back pain).

Treatment

- Simple analgesia is often all that is required.
- Physiotherapy and increased gentle sporting activity is of great potential benefit in this condition.
- There is only a small minority of patients presenting with simple backache who undergo surgery. There exists still considerable controversy as to the benefits of spinal fusion surgery (posterior bone graft with instrumentation, i.e. bars and rods locked into pedicle screws) for degenerative back pain. The theory is that fusion and, hence, immobilisation, of the affected spinal segment removes the cause of pain. The problem is that surgery itself is a potential cause of back pain. The benefits may take up to a year to be felt.

Complications

Spinal fusion surgery carries with it the following risks:

- Wound infection.
- Wound haematoma. This can be a simple haematoma, as elsewhere in the body, but it can also be an epidural haematoma that has the potential to cause cauda equina compression, an emergency requiring surgical decompression.
- CSF leak.
- Infection of the implanted metalwork.
- Nerve root injury, e.g. from a misplaced pedicle screw.
- IVC injury, e.g. due to the pedicle screw, or drilling to insert it in the first place.

Spinal stenosis

Presentation

This is a long-term consequence of disc degeneration and osteoarthritis. It causes narrowing of the spinal canal due to hypertrophy of the posterior disc margin and facet joints.

It causes back pain and pseudoclaudication, which is an ache that comes on diffusely in one or both legs,

characteristically after a variable distance and, in contrast to vascular claudication, the pain is not immediately relieved by stopping, but gradually dissipates. The leg pain of spinal stenosis can also come on after prolonged periods of standing, and is relieved by leaning forwards, or by sitting down. It is usually seen in men >50 years of age.

The major differential diagnosis of spinal claudication is, of course, vascular claudication. This is pain felt classically in one (or both) calf(s) that comes on after a predictable walking distance, and is rapidly relieved by rest.

Clinical findings in spinal stenosis are sparse. There tends to be no neurological deficit to identify on formal examination, the patient tends to have palpable pedal pulses and has no signs of limb ischaemia, which differentiates it from vascular stenosis.

Investigations

- The mainstay of investigation is the MRI scan which shows the narrowing of the spinal canal at one or several levels.
- In cases of suspicion of vascular stenosis it is wise to perform an ABPI (Ankle Brachial Pressure Index) of both lower limbs and to ask for a vascular review, which may include an angiogram.

Treatment

- Physiotherapy does not have a great deal to offer in this condition.
- Epidural injection can help a little, but is rarely curative.
- Spinal decompression surgery forms the mainstay of treatment in patients whose symptoms intrude sufficiently with their lives. This is performed through a posterior approach, and the soft tissues that cause the compression are excised. This procedure, performed well, has a good track record in resolution of symptoms.

Complications

Complications of spinal decompression surgery are as follows:

- Nerve root injury.
- Wound haematoma.

- Epidural haematoma (with the potential for cauda equina compression, an acute emergency that requires surgical decompression)
- CSF leak.
- Paralysis (a very low, but very real risk which should be mentioned pre-operatively).

Spondylolisthesis

Presentation

A forward shift of one vertebra on its immediately inferior vertebra, usually at the L5-S1 level.

There are different aetiologies of spondylolisthesis:

- Congenital.
- Isthmic. The use of the word isthmus here refers to the attenuation and eventual fatigue fracture of the pars intra-articularis, of which there are two per vertebra, found in the lamina between the articular surfaces of the facet joints. As these fracture this allows backward slip of one vertebra on another. The reason for this train of events remains uncertain. It classically presents during the adolescent years.
- Degenerative. Seems to occur as a result of chronic disc degeneration and facet joint incompetence allowing progressive slippage of one vertebra on another. This generally presents later in life, after the age of 50.
- Traumatic. Repeated trauma, e.g. in gymnasts performing abnormal manoeuvres involving hyperextension of the back, or as a result of an acute fracture involving the pars intra-articularis.
- Secondary to a pathological bone lesion, e.g. benign or malignant bone tumour, Paget's disease of bone, etc.

Spondylolisthesis can be an incidental finding on X-ray, i.e. causing no symptoms, but it is also a recognised cause of lumbar backache. Spondylolisthesis can vary in severity, i.e. in degree of slip. The most severe version is called spondyloptosis, where the L5 vertebra has effectively 'fallen off' the top of the sacral promontory. As the degree of slip increases, so does the chance that the spinal nerves become trapped as they exit the neural foramina laterally. This produces uni- or bi-lateral radicular symptoms. As the slip is usually at the L5-S1 level, the nerve root involved is usually the L5 nerve root, resulting in weak extension of the great toe and paraesthesiae of the lateral calf and foot.

Investigations

- Plain X-ray of the lumbar spine (lateral view) shows the degree of slip very well; however, seeing the pars defects is considerably harder on plain X-ray.
- MRI scan of the lumbar spine. This is the main investigation of use in spondylolisthesis. It shows alignment of the vertebrae with respect to each other on sagittal views and the pars defects. It can also show other bone pathology, e.g. cysts, tumours, etc. Most importantly, it images the cord, cauda equina, and nerve roots, identifying any compression.

Treatment

- For minor degrees of spondylolisthesis, presenting with mild symptoms, the mainstay of treatment is simple analgesia and physiotherapy if needed. This level of treatment is all that is needed for the majority of patients.
- For more severe and refractory symptoms in patients for whom non-operative measures have failed, or whose imaging shows progression of spondylolisthesis, fusion surgery may be indicated. This is performed through a posterior approach. The posterior elements of the vertebrae are exposed. The surgical options available at this stage are to perform an instrumented (i.e. insertion of pedicle screws joined with rods and bars) or non-instrumented fusion. Fusion is the process of denuding the cartilage from the articular surfaces of the facet joints and the insertion of autologous bone graft posteriorly, resulting in a hard mass of callus that 'fuses' the affected spinal segment preventing movement (and hence pain) at that level. The other surgical choice here is whether to attempt to reduce the degree of slip. It might seem the obvious thing to do, i.e. a return to the normal anatomy for best results; however, this manoeuvre carries a risk of nerve root damage, as well as possible loss of reduction with time despite instrumentation. Many surgeons 'fuse in situ' as a result.

Relief of the painful symptoms from spondylolisthesis can take up to a year postoperatively.

Complications

♦ Nerve root injury.
♦ Wound haematoma.
♦ Epidural haematoma (with the potential for cauda equina compression, an acute emergency that requires surgical decompression)
♦ CSF leak.
♦ Paralysis (a very low, but very real, risk which should be mentioned pre-operatively).
♦ Pseudarthrosis (also called non-union or failure of fusion. This results in persistent pain from spondylolisthesis, which may require re-operation, although having suffered one pseudarthrosis this carries a greater risk of recurrent pseudarthosis).
♦ Failure to eradicate the back pain despite technical success of the surgery, i.e. a good fusion mass visible on X-ray.

The neck

Prolapsed cervical disc

This can occur secondary to a strain or sudden movement (e.g. flexion and extension). However, there is usually a predisposition present (increased nuclear tension), and it can happen in the absence of a precipitating event.

Presentation

A prolapsed cervical disc presents with neck pain, neck stiffness, referred pain to the upper limb, sensory loss in the upper limb and weakness in the upper limb. Lower limb symptoms only occur in frank cord compression, as distinct from root compression.

Treatment

An anterior approach is used for surgery on a prolapsed cervical disc with nerve root involvement. Normally, fusion is performed at this level, an operation termed an anterior cervical disc fusion (ACDF). More recently, disc replacement surgery is also being used.

.
Complications

♦ Nerve root injury.
♦ Wound haematoma.
♦ Epidural haematoma (with the potential for cauda equina compression, an acute

emergency that requires surgical decompression).
♦ CSF leak.
♦ Paralysis (a very low, but very real, risk which should be mentioned pre-operatively).

Note

— Disc prolapse most commonly occurs in association with the C6 vertebra, i.e. there are symptoms present in either the C6 or C7 distribution (because the C6 vertebra has the C6 disc above and C7 disc below it).

♦ Laminectomy of more than one vertebral level carries a risk of spinal instability.

C6 root compression

Presentation

The biceps jerk is lost and there are weak biceps, weak wrist dorsiflexion and sensory changes to the lateral forearm, thumb and index finger (the 'six-shooter' distribution: Figure 7.6).

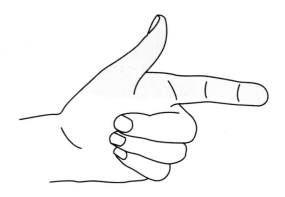

Figure 7.6. The 'six-shooter' distribution (C6).

C7 root compression

Presentation

The triceps jerk is lost and there are weak triceps, weak wrist flexion, weak finger extension and sensory changes in the middle finger.

Investigations

- X-ray changes may show loss of cervical lordosis and decreased disc space.
- MRI is ideal for soft tissues in the neck, i.e. the discs and spinal cord.

Treatment

The mainstay of treatment for cervical root compression is non-operative. Most resolve, or have significantly improved, within six weeks of onset of symptoms. Surgery is uncommon, but indications are progressive motor symptoms, failure of non-operative management and signs of cord compression. Surgery generally is a laminectomy, i.e. a posterior approach to the cervical spinal level, and excision of the posterior elements (left and right laminae and spinous process). This effectively decompresses the cord, which may seem a little counter-intuitive, seeing as the most common cause of cervical root compression is a prolapsed intervertebral disc, i.e. an anterior structure. It is safe surgery and is effective a large proportion of the time. An anterior discectomy is also possible, but it involves an anterior approach to the neck, and is more technically demanding.

Complications

- Wound infection.
- CSF leak.
- Meningitis.
- Discitis.
- Persistent neurological symptoms (?technical error, ?wrong level surgery, ?idiopathic).
- Epidural haematoma causing cord compression (requires urgent surgical decompression).
- Neck pain.

Cervical spondylosis

This is degeneration and flattening of the intervertebral discs and formation of bony spurs (anterior and posterior) from bodies of the vertebrae.

Presentation

Usually seen in patients >40 years old with neck pain and stiffness, often worse on rising in the morning. Neurological involvement is only occasionally seen, secondary to a bony spur irritating the nerve root(s).

Investigations

- X-ray changes show narrowing of one or more of the disc spaces and bony spurs. As previously mentioned though, the severity of degenerative changes does not correlate with severity (or even presence) of painful symptoms.
- MRI shows the soft tissue anatomy in great detail. It will show nerve root compression, cord compression, disc degeneration and most other pathologies.

Treatment

Treatment is by heat and massage to soothe, and a collar is worn during acute attacks. Physiotherapy is the mainstay of treatment, often with the same results as operative treatment. It is, therefore, quite rare for a surgeon to operate for this condition.

Complications

- Analgesics can have side effects, and the patient can become habituated to them.
- The cervical soft collar should not be worn for protracted periods of time (weeks), just during the acute phase of a painful episode, or the neck muscles become atrophied and weak. This is itself another source of pain.

Rheumatoid arthritis of the cervical spine

Presentation

This affects the cervical spine in 30% of patients with rheumatoid arthritis (RA).

There are three common types of cervical disease in rheumatoids:

- Atlanto-occipital joint erosion.
- Atlanto-axial joint erosion.
- Facet joint erosion of the mid-cervical region.

Neurological complications are uncommon.

Investigations

On X-ray, the usual erosive arthritic changes can be shown, with atlanto-axial instability seen on a flexion-lateral view, by a >5mm gap between the back of the anterior arch of C1 and the odontoid peg, which disappears on extension.

Treatment

The decision to proceed towards surgical correction of the complications of rheumatoid arthritis of the cervical spine is truly beyond the remit of this book. It requires an experienced spinal surgeon in conjunction with a rheumatologist. Generally, progressive neurology is the deciding factor in making the decision to operate. However, large degrees of joint erosion and instability seem to be tolerated in this group of patients with surprisingly little amounts of neurological involvement.

Complications

Complications of spinal surgery of the rheumatoid spine are much the same as for non-rheumatoids. The major difference is the poor quality of the bone stock in these patients.

Thoracic outlet syndrome

This is nerve compression syndrome affecting the T1 nerve root, due to a cervical rib compressing thoracic outlet structures against the clavicle (this includes the subclavian vein and artery). It is commoner in women aged 30-50 years.

Presentation

Thoracic outlet syndrome can present with sensory, motor and/or vascular symptoms. Characteristically, there is pain over the ulnar border of the forearm and hand, with associated paraesthesiae (relieved by elevating the arm). A late sign is muscle weakness and wasting. Often there is hyperalgesia in the C8/T1 dermatome. A palpable rib and bruit can be present.

A special test for thoracic outlet syndrome is Adson's test, in which the patient holds the shoulder at 90° of abduction and extends the shoulder backwards. Then they must bend the neck leaning the head towards the affected side. The final aspect of the test is to ask the patient to take a deep breath. In combination these manoeuvres narrow the thoracic outlet and increase the pressure therein. The symptoms are supposed to be reproduced after holding this position for 15-30 seconds. It is thus a provocative test.

Investigations

◆   X-ray to show cervical rib.

Note

−   A proportion of all cervical ribs are cartilaginous, thus an X-ray does not give the complete picture.

◆   Nerve conduction studies are also useful.
◆   An MRI scan shows the cartilaginous portion of the first rib, which, although not seen on X-ray, is capable of being the cause of the condition. It also shows the anatomical positions of important structures (brachial plexus, axillary artery, any abnormal fibrous bands that might be present).
◆   Angiography can show the presence of any aneurysm that could be the origin of the compressive symptoms.

It should be mentioned that due to the dynamic nature of the condition, compared with the static nature of the investigations, negative findings on investigation do not necessarily mean the absence of the condition. This makes the diagnosis of thoracic outlet syndrome problematic. The differential diagnosis is cervical spondylosis, Pancoast's tumour or syringomyelia.

Treatment

Treatment is for the most part non-operative for this condition. It is difficult to diagnose with confidence and controversy exists as to the indications for and the type of surgery to perform. Surgical options include excision of the first rib or accessory rib, and excision of any fibrous band found locally; some also excise the scalenus muscle.

Complications

Complications of surgical procedures in thoracic outlet syndrome include damage to local structures, i.e. brachial plexus, axillary artery. The potential for chronic pain exists, although to be fair, aspects of this condition are similar to chronic pain syndromes even prior to surgery.

Spinal cord injury

The motor cortex of the brain sends fibres via the internal capsule to the corticospinal tracts, which are anterior tracts in the brainstem.

Note

- These pathways decussate (literally cross over) at the level of the pyramids and then lie laterally in the spinal cord, i.e. fibres originating on one side of the brain control the contralateral side of the body.

Sensory pathways in the spinal cord are two-fold:

- Sensory information reaches the spinal cord at the posterior grey horn and enters the spinothalamic tract, the fibres then decussate within the spinal cord to the contralateral anterior or lateral spinothalamic tracts, and ascend via the thalamus to the sensory cortex. The sensory information within the spinothalamic tracts is crude touch, pain, temperature and pressure.
- The other sensory pathway is the dorsal column. Its fibres are ipsilateral until they ascend to the brainstem, where they then decussate. The sensory information within the dorsal column is fine touch, vibration and proprioception.

This difference between decussation at spinal or central levels is responsible for the patterns of neurology seen in certain injury types, e.g. the dreaded Brown-Sequard lesion.

Presentation

Transection of the cord

Loss of function of all motor and sensory pathways, i.e. a sensory level corresponding to the injury, and hypotonia and hyporeflexia initially which, over a period of days or weeks, changes to hypertonia and hyper-reflexia (assuming the transection was above the level of the L2 vertebra, i.e. upper motor neurone pattern).

Brown-Sequard syndrome

The first thing to realise in this syndrome, is that it is due to cord hemisection. Ipsilateral motor weakness and hyporeflexia are seen initially, becoming hypertonia and hyper-reflexia, later. A sensory level is also seen with ipsilateral loss of fine touch, vibration, position sense (dorsal column), and contralateral loss of pain, temperature and crude touch (spinothalamic).

Central cord syndrome

This is a post-hyperextension injury of the cervical spine, if there is pre-existing canal stenosis. There is no fracture or subluxation. Central cord syndrome was originally thought to occur as a result of cord contusion, but now autopsy studies have demonstrated that central cord syndrome may be caused by bleeding into the central part of the cord, leading to a less favourable prognosis. Studies have also shown that central cord syndrome probably is associated with axonal disruption in the lateral columns at the level of the injury to the spinal cord with relative preservation of the grey matter. Thus, it is not a surgically remediable condition. It gives a characteristic motor distribution of symptoms with the upper limbs being markedly weaker than the lower as the fibres to the upper limbs are more superficial and hence are more likely to be involved. Sensory loss is often patchy, with spinothalamic loss at the level of the injury, and preservation below.

Anterior cord syndrome

This occurs as a result of traumatic compression and ischaemic damage to the anterior portion of the cord, at cervical level, generally as a result of pressure from the posterior fragments of the vertebral body on the cord as a result of a fracture.

The anterior column carries motor information from the brain to the muscles via the corticospinal tracts, so there is complete motor paralysis. It also carries sensory information from the periphery to the brain via the spinothalamic tracts, so there is sensory anaesthesia. The posterior columns are spared, and these carry proprioception, vibration, and deep touch from the periphery to the brain. These are thus preserved.

Anterior cord syndrome characteristically presents with greater neurological loss in the lower limbs than the upper limbs. The prognosis for the return of function is poor.

Peripheral nerve injury

Motor symptoms are hypotonia, weakness, hyporeflexia and muscle wasting.

Note

— In mixed nerves, there is sensory loss in the distribution of the nerve (pain or paraesthesia).

Spinal cord injury without radiological abnormality (SCIWORA)

Characteristically, this occurs in children because the skeletal elements of the vertebral column are hypermobile, i.e. spinal cord injury can occur without X-ray changes (subluxation or fracture).

Investigations

Investigation of spinal injuries follow the Advanced Trauma Life Support® (ATLS®) guidelines, as these are generally high energy trauma patients, i.e. the focus is on life-threatening injuries first (airway, breathing, circulation), whilst the C-spine is immobilised and log rolls are performed whenever the patient needs to be moved for any reason.

Standard AP and lateral X-rays of the spine are performed if injury is suspected. Neurological examination will have picked up one or other of the patterns of injury described above, which will prompt a request for an MRI scan to image the level of injury and cord involvement.

Treatment

Treatment is as per the ATLS® guidelines, as mentioned previously.

Spinal injuries are a specialised subject when discussing surgical management. However, you are expected to know the principles of a log roll. Five

people are required for this (including yourself): one to hold the head in line with the spine as the patient is turned; one to hold the chest; one to have one hand on the pelvis and the other hand under the knee (not over the top as one might have thought - this supports the leg); and the last to have both hands under the leg (proximal calf region and under the ankle), also supporting the leg. The person at the head end takes verbal control of the group and instructs all involved in a co-ordinated effort.

The presence of a spinal fracture and a neurological deficit warrants immediate discussion with the local spinal team, continuation of spinal precautions and catheterisation. The decision to proceed to surgery, or not, or even whether surgery is urgent (i.e. progressive neurological deterioration on repeated examinations), lies in the hands of experienced spinal surgeons.

Where indicated, surgery for unstable vertebral fractures is stabilisation of two vertebrae above and below the fractured vertebra by the use of pedicle screws joined by bars and rods. The major benefits of this surgery are prevention of deterioration of neurology (by virtue of stopping further displacement of the fracture fragments into the spinal cord) and greater ease of rehabilitation, as a stabilised spine enables the patient to sit, stand, and be nursed without the restrictions of bed-bound spinal precautions. In the case of the patient who has already suffered complete paralysis, the benefit of stabilisation surgery is, therefore, greater ease of nursing, less pain for the patient, and more rapid rehabilitation, as there is no possibility of worsening the neurological deficit.

Complications

◆ Nerve root injury.
◆ Wound haematoma.
◆ Wound infection
◆ Further cord damage leading to complete paralysis (in those cases of pre-operative partial neurological deficit).
◆ Infected metalwork.

Foot conditions

Pes cavus

Presentation

The incidence is greatest at the age of 8-10 years. It characteristically shows a high arch longitudinally and hyperextension of the metatarsophalangeal joints (MTPJ), commonly associated with claw toes. It results in pain over the MTPJs (metatarsalgia), callosities and, frequently, corns over the toes.

Investigations

Plain X-rays of the foot will show the deformity and the presence or absence of any degenerative changes associated (unusual).

A full neurological examination of the lower limb should be considered as one of the investigations in this condition, as pes cavus can be secondary to a neurological condition (about half are idiopathic, the others result from Charcot-Marie-Tooth disease, Friedreich's ataxia and polio).

Treatment

For the most part the treatment is non-operative (nothing need be done if it is asymptomatic and idiopathic), but footwear can be adapted to help with metatarsalgia, e.g. insertion of a metatarsal bar to offload the MTPJs. There are surgical procedures available for failure of non-operative treatment, the details of which are beyond the remit of this book.

Complications

In broad terms the complications of pes cavus surgery are:

- Failure to fully correct the cavus.
- Overcorrection, i.e. conversion to pes planus.
- Painful gait.
- Neurovascular damage.
- Infection.

Pes planus

Presentation

Also known as flat feet or fallen arches, this is a flattening of the medial arch of the foot. It can be congenital in origin, e.g. congenital fusion of certain of the tarsal bones, or acquired, e.g. rupture of the tibialis posterior tendon, a major contributor to the integrity of the medial arch. It causes foot pain, and patients can be bothered by its unsightly cosmetic appearance.

Investigations

Plain X-rays, as for pes cavus, are unrewarding, but act as a baseline, and can reveal any degenerative changes associated.

In 'rigid' pes planus (i.e. secondary to congenital fusion of tarsal bones), a CT can show the anatomy of the fusion, and provide useful information on the anatomy that will need correction at the time of surgery.

Treatment

If the patient is asymptomatic there is no indication for treatment. The mainstay of treatment for symptomatic pes planus is a medial arch supporting insole. If non-operative measures fail, then surgery might be indicated. Tendon transfer or fusion procedures can be of use in flexible pes planus, i.e. no tarsal bone fusion, and the arch, which is flat when the patient stands, corrects when the patient tip-toes. For tarsal coalitions (fusion) that resist non-operative treatment, then osteotomy of the fusion segments may be indicated.

Complications

The complications of pes planus surgery are:

- Failure to fully correct the planus deformity.
- Painful gait.
- Infection.
- Problems related to prominent metalwork (where used).
- Failure of fusion in arthrodesis procedures.

Hallux valgus

Presentation

Also known as a bunion, the valgus angle at the joint is prominent on the first MTPJ. There is a lateral deviation of the great toe, with a bursa over the joint (the bunion), which is a source of pain in shoes. It is more common in women aged 50-60 years, although it can have a familial element in younger women.

Investigations

X-rays of the foot demonstrate the valgus angle, whether the MTPJ has subluxed or is arthritic. They will also show the state of the rest of the foot anatomy and articular surfaces.

Treatment

Adaptation of footwear may help, but surgery is the only potentially curative treatment. There are various osteotomies of the first metatarsal, and no single operation treats all types or severities of hallux valgus. Important eponymous operations are Mitchell's (distal) osteotomy, scarf osteotomy and Keller's (excision) arthroplasty of the whole joint.

Complications

- Non-union of the osteotomy (results in both pain and failure to correct the original deformity).
- Wound infection.
- Infected metalwork.
- Inadequate correction of the deformity.
- Painful gait.
- Neurovascular damage.
- Avascular necrosis of the first metatarsal head. Over-enthusiastic soft tissue dissection distally can interrupt the metatarsal head blood supply.
- Transfer metatarsalgia. Osteotomy of the first metatarsal can upset the cascade of the metatarsal heads, resulting in greater force through, usually, the second metatarsal head, which becomes painful.

Hallux rigidus

Presentation

This is caused by osteoarthritis of the first MTPJ. It is more common in older men and results in pain on the undersurface of the first MTPJ with or without a callosity, a decreased range of movement and pain on movement.

Investigations

X-rays of the foot demonstrate the presence of degenerative changes at the first MTPJ and also the state of the rest of the foot anatomy and articular surfaces.

Treatment

It is not necessary to treat asymptomatic X-ray findings of first MTPJ degeneration. A 'rocker bottom shoe' can be used to treat early symptoms of pain, which does this by offloading the first MTPJ during the step phase of the gait. After failure of non-operative treatment, arthrodesis of the joint may be considered. In hallux rigidis that has radiological changes of minor joint space loss and a prominent dorsal osteophyte, patients can derive a great deal of benefit from excision of this osteophyte, called a cheilectomy, which is a considerably more minor procedure than arthrodesis. As an aside, there are the first MTPJ arthroplasties on the market, but studies suggest an unacceptable rate of early loosening, and this is not considered conventional treatment.

Complications

- Non-union of the arthrodesis (results in painful movement at the first MTPJ, with much the same symptoms as before the operation).
- Wound infection.
- Neurovascular damage.
- Failure to fuse the joint into an appropriate position can result, in itself, in painful gait. The preferred position is some 10-15° of extension. This enables both stance and toe-off phases of the gait without stressing the fused section too much. If the joint is fused in neutral extension, stance is painless, but as the patient tries to walk, the toe-off phase becomes both difficult and potentially painful.
- Transfer pain, i.e. the great toe interphalangeal joint can become painful now that the MTPJ is fused, or transfer metatarsalgia can occur, as mentioned in the hallux valgus section.

Claw toes

Presentation

This is a flexion deformity of the interphalangeal joints (IPJs) and a hyperextension deformity of the MTPJs. It is either idiopathic or associated with neuropathy (polio, peroneal muscular atrophy or peroneal nerve peripheral neuropathy) and results in metatarsalgia and callosities.

Investigations

X-rays are often performed, but do not generally add to the information available from clinical examination.

Treatment

For the most part treatment is non-operative. Nothing is needed if the condition is asymptomatic. A metatarsal bar can be useful to offload the metatarsal heads in patients complaining of metatarsalgia. For failure of non-operative management, various types of tendon and ligament releases can be performed. This level of detail is not within the remit of this book.

Complications

The complications of soft tissue procedures on the toe, generally speaking, are as follows:

- Failure to correct the claw deformity.
- Wound infection.
- Neurovascular damage (in the rare case of bilateral damage to the digital arteries. This can even result in gangrene and amputation).
- Painful gait.

Hammer toe

Presentation

Identical to Boutonniere's deformity in the fingers. The proximal interphalangeal joint (PIPJ) has a flexion deformity, but the distal interphalangeal joint (DIPJ) and MTPJ have an extension deformity (unknown aetiology).

Investigations

Again, X-rays are often performed, but do not generally add to the information available from clinical examination.

Treatment

For the most part no treatment is required for hammer toes. Better shoewear helps with the problems of corn formation where the prominent PIPJ rubs on the shoe. In cases of failure of non-operative management, then treatment is by surgical excision of the PIPJ, which shortens the toe and straightens it.

Complications

- Failure to correct the hammer deformity.
- Wound infection.
- Neurovascular damage (in the rare case of bilateral damage to the digital arteries. This can even result in gangrene and amputation).
- Painful gait.

Mallet toe

Presentation

As for hammer toe, but this is a flexion deformity at the DIPJ, resulting in a dorsal prominence that can rub painfully on shoewear and cause a corn.

Investigations, treatment and complications are along similar lines as for hammer toe, as it relates to the DIPJ.

The diabetic foot

This is a highly specialised subject and is quite enormous in its scope and, thus, it is not covered here. However, it is important to be aware that in diabetics a diabetic foot can be one of the problems encountered due to peripheral neuropathy, vascular disease, infection and osteoporosis. It results in pain (or numbness), ulceration, gangrene (dry/wet), Charcot's joints and cellulitis.

Talipes equina varus (club foot)

Presentation

Talipes means a talon-shaped foot and equinus means in the style of a horse, the latter being taken to mean the foot is fixed in such a position that the heel and sole of the foot are not in contact with the ground, only the toes and metatarsal heads, or put more simply, the talus points downwards (equinus).

It is more common in boys, the ratio being 2:1. It is a bilateral condition in one third of cases and usually is idiopathic, but it can be associated with spina bifida or arthrogryposis deformity. Risk factors are a positive family history, breech presentation and oligohydramnios.

Investigations

X-rays provide a useful baseline from which later X-rays can be compared, especially after treatment. Further imaging modalities are generally not required.

Treatment

Conservative

Splinting of the foot using tape or Plaster of Paris (POP) changed weekly for six weeks (the Ponseti method utilises serial casting to correct each individual component of the deformity in turn).

Surgical

If conservative treatment fails, the foot requires a posteromedial release, as the major abnormality tends to be overtightness of the soft tissue structures of the joint posteromedially.

Complications

Complications of surgery:

- Wound infection.
- Neurovascular damage.
- Over-correction resulting in a 'rocker bottom' foot.
- Under-correction, i.e. persistent clubbing.
- Stiff, painful and small foot (not necessarily a complication of surgery, as all treated club feet are smaller and stiffer than the norm to some extent).

Bone tumours

Perhaps the most important statement relating to bone tumours is that, numerically, metastases to bone from other tumours are far more common than primary bone tumours. In patients >50 years of age, bony metastases outnumber all other causes of bone tumour added together. For completeness, it should also be noted that infection (e.g. osteomyelitis) can mimic the appearance of bone tumours, and therefore should be considered in the differential diagnosis.

The many and varied primary tumours of bone form a huge subject, the details of which are beyond the scope of this text. However, the principles of recognition of a malignant bone lesion versus a benign one form an important skill that can be tested in exam conditions.

The following is a holistic system for assessing a patient for a possible malignant bone lesion.

History

Pain characteristically presents as a dull ache, at rest as well as at night. These are features worrying of malignant lesions.

Presentation

Look for changes in the overlying skin (swelling, mass, tenderness, lymph nodes). Look for sources of a primary tumour causing a metastasis (breast, thyroid, kidney, lung, prostate).

Note

— The contrived mnemonic for tumours known to metastasise to bone is all the 'B's: Breast, Byroid, Bronchus, Bidney, Brostate.

Investigations

Blood tests

Patients should have routine blood tests done, but these are poor at discriminating metastases from primary tumours, or indeed malignant from benign lesions. The information they provide on the state of health of the patient is nonetheless relevant, as is the ESR or CRP.

Imaging

- X-rays (two films at 90° to each other, termed 'orthogonal').
- A bone scan shows hot spots for many tumours as they have increased bone turnover at that site. One notable exception is multiple myeloma.
- An MRI scan is excellent at delineating the anatomical relations of a tumour and soft tissue involvement.

Biopsy

If a biopsy is indicated, it should be taken through a wound located in the region that a specialist surgeon would choose to excise the whole lesion, should the biopsy result turn out to be malignant. The reason for this is the potential for malignant cells from the biopsy site to 'seed' along the biopsy wound. Therefore, the definitive wound for excision of the tumour (if malignant) will need to incorporate the original biopsy wound, to negate this problem.

The following factors are useful in determining the likely nature of the lesion:

- Age of the patient. Young patients suffer from different tumours than the elderly.
- Solitary or multiple lesions. Multiple lesions in the elderly are more likely to be metastases.
- Site of lesion in the bone. Whether the lesion is epiphyseal at the border of the epiphyseo-metaphyseal border, metaphyseal or diaphyseal is relevant to specific tumour types, as is whether it is central or eccentric within the bone.
- Effect of the lesion on the surrounding bone. For example, high grade malignant lesions will be rapidly destructive of surrounding bone, whereas low grade or benign lesions will not.
- Response of the bone to the lesion. For example, low grade lesions will afford the surrounding bone time in which to react by cortical thickening of the lesion, whereas high grade malignant lesions will not.
- The matrix of the tumour. The appearance of the lesion's core on X-ray, for example, whether it appears to be calcified cartilage, containing stippling, arcs or rings (which would make it a tumour of chondroid origin, i.e. derived from cartilage), or whether it appears more diffuse and fuzzy (in the case of mineralised osteoid, i.e. a tumour of bony, not cartilaginous origin).

Treatment

Clearly, treatment is going to vary on the basis of the diagnosis, surgical resectability of the tumour, life expectancy, likelihood of pathological fracture, attempt at limb salvage and the likely malignant potential of the tumour, as well as other individual factors. It is not within the scope of non-specialist postgraduate exams to test you on this difficult and specialist subject. The basic principles to be aware of, however, can be broadly divided into two:

- The first relates to bony metastases. If a bone has a lytic lesion that is eroding significant amounts of the bony cortex, it is at risk of 'pathological' fracture. There is little doubt that it is easier to nail a bone that has not yet fractured than one that has; this is called 'prophylactic nailing'. The nail is intended to protect the 'whole' bone from fracture, which is straightforward in bones such as the tibia, effectively a straight cylinder, but more difficult in bones such as the femur, which turns a corner at the femoral neck (this problem is solved by specialised nails that allow a locking screw through the nail into the femoral neck and head). Bones that have suffered a pathological fracture should either be nailed, if the fracture is in the shaft (diaphyseal), or be treated with excision and joint replacement, if the fracture is near the joint (metaphyseal). These are broad principles, to which there will be exceptions.
- The second relates to primary bone tumours. These generally require excision, often with a cuff of healthy surrounding tissue, to ensure no malignant cells are left behind, to cause a relapse. This can involve nerve and vessel tissue, and is hence a multidisciplinary type of surgery (involving orthopaedic tumour surgeons, plastic or vascular surgeons in tandem). The bone defects left behind after these excisions are highly problematic, and some of the surgical options available are large endoprosthetic replacements of bone, which can be combined with joint replacement depending on the location of the tumour. Sometimes it is possible to use vascularised fibular strut autograft to replace the removed segment, which incorporates with time. Sometimes, however, the best results are achieved with amputation and a well fitted prosthetic limb.

Complications

Nails for prophylaxis or treatment of established pathological fracture can be complicated by:

♦   Wound infection.
♦   Deep infection.
♦   Neurovascular damage.
♦   There is a significant operative mortality in this patient group, particularly if there is already an established fracture. It is wise to make both patient and family aware of this fact prior to surgery.

Endoprosthetic replacements of bone can be complicated by:

♦   Wound infection.
♦   Deep infection.
♦   Neurovascular damage.
♦   Joint dislocation.
♦   Eventual loosening and need for revision surgery.

Amputation can be complicated by:

♦   Wound infection.
♦   Deep infection.
♦   Neurovascular damage.
♦   Phantom limb pain (pain felt where the amputated limb 'used to be').
♦   Problems with the prosthesis fitting, pain, skin ulceration and neuromas.

Causes of joint pain

There are considerably more causes of joint pain than one initially thinks. All the elements of the following list will be familiar, but it is important to remember this overview when confronted with a patient complaining of pain in a joint.

Joint pain

♦   Joint disease. The arthropathies (especially rheumatoid arthritis and osteoarthritis, psoriatic arthropathy and gout).

♦   Bone disease. Fractures, tumours (primary and secondary), osteochondritis and osteomyelitis, etc.
♦   Soft tissue lesions. Sprain, tenosynovitis, trauma, bursitis and repetitive strain injury.
♦   Arthralgia. The definition is joint pain in the absence of objective evidence of joint disease. Examples of conditions that can cause arthralgia are:
  •   the arthropathies, e.g. polymyalgia rheumatica, systemic lupus erythematosus temporal arteritis, polyarteritis nodosum;
  •   viral infection (influenza is the most common);
  •   bacterial infection and other infections;
  •   drugs;
  •   protein abnormalities (hyperglobulinaemias [IgG, IgM], cryoglobulinaemia).
♦   Referred pain, e.g. shoulder (gallbladder, subphrenic abscess, cardiac, oesophagitic, neurological, apical tumour, pneumothorax, pleurisy).
♦   Psychogenic.

Osteoarthritis

Osteoarthritis (OA) can be primary or secondary. Secondary causes of OA can be the presence of a previous fracture, previous septic arthritis, obesity, congenital dislocation of the hip or avascular necrosis.

There is an equal incidence in males and females, which increases with age (>55 years).

Presentation
OA presents with pain after movement (not worse in mornings), stiffness and deformity. There is bony tenderness, bony swelling, the presence of Heberden's nodes (DIPJs), warmth, erythema, effusion, crepitus and the presence of Bouchard's nodes (PIPJs).

Investigations
X-ray changes:

♦   Loss of joint space.
♦   Peri-articular osteosclerosis.
♦   Subchondral cysts.
♦   Osteophytes.

Treatment

Treatment is by analgesia, physiotherapy, weight loss (if overweight) and surgery, especially on weight bearing joints, e.g. total joint replacement of the hip and knee (only after non-operative treatments have not succeeded). Please see the sections on hip and knee replacement in the 'Operative surgery' chapter for details on surgical technique.

Complications

Complications of joint replacement surgery include:

- Wound infection.
- Haematoma.
- Neurovascular damage.
- DVT/PE.
- Dislocation (in the case of total hip replacement surgery).
- Loosening of the implant and the eventual need for revision surgery.
- Limb length discrepancy (in the case of total hip replacement surgery).
- Intra-operative fracture (rare).

Rheumatoid arthritis

This is a progressive destructive arthritis leading to severe joint deformity and disability. It is a common, widespread chronic polyarthritis, which is bilateral with symmetrical joint involvement.

Pathologically, there is a chronic proliferative synovitis, villous hypertrophy, infiltration of lymphocytes, plasma cells and lymphoid nodules.

The incidence is more common in women aged 40-50 years, with a male to female ratio of 1:3.

The joints affected most commonly are the PIPJs (80%), MCPJs (60%), DIPJs (30%), knees (80%), ankles (70%) and just about any others.

Presentation

Symptoms include morning stiffness, pain on movement, fatigue, general ill health and weight loss.

Signs to watch out for are swollen joints, which are tender, warm, with an effusion, a synovial thickening and erythema, and muscle wasting around the affected joints.

Special signs are ulnar deviation of the fingers at the MCPJ, Boutonniere's deformity (flexion of the PIPJ and hyperextension of the DIPJ), swan neck deformity (hyperextension of the PIPJ and flexion of the DIPJ), a prominent tender ulnar styloid, Baker's cyst, a flexion/valgus deformity of the knees, tender prominent MTPJs on the feet and atlanto-axial subluxation.

The course of the disease can be episodic or have persistent non-articular manifestations, nodules (the elbow is the most common site but they can be anywhere else), tenosynovitis, bursitis, synovial cysts, muscle wasting, ligamentous laxity leading to hypermobility, carpal tunnel syndrome, lymphadenopathy, splenomegaly (rare), pleural effusion, Caplan's nodules (lungs and pleural rheumatoid nodules) and anaemia.

Investigations

X-ray changes:

- Peri-articular osteopaenia.
- Erosions.
- Loss of joint space.
- Bone destruction.

Laboratory tests will show a raised ESR, antinuclear antibody (ANA) is positive, and a latex test is positive.

Treatment

- Relieve pain, adapt lifestyle, suppress disease activity.
- Analgesia, rest, steroid injections intra-articularly, immunosuppressive drugs (e.g. azathioprine, chlorambucil, cyclophosphamide) and biological treatments such as infliximab, which act as an anti-TNF drug.
- Surgery for specific joints (knees, hips, ulnar styloidectomy, etc.).

Complications

The complications of surgical procedures on rheumatoid patients are no different than on non-rheumatoids with the following significant qualifications:

- Rheumatoid bone is softer and hence more easily fractured during orthopaedic surgery.

- Rheumatoid arthritis, being an immune mediated multisystem disorder, has a knock-on effect on the risk of wound infection, which is higher than in the non-rheumatoid population.
- Rheumatoid neck disease makes endotracheal intubation (for any surgical procedure) more risky for the anaesthetist, as it involves forced hyperextension of the neck. This risks fracture and neurological injury, although this is uncommon, as anaesthetists, being aware of the risks, take greater care.

Childhood hip disorders

Most doctors in their surgical training will do a post in orthopaedics, and unusual is a week in which there is not at least one call from the emergency department asking for review of a child with a 'limp; query cause'.

The following is a list of differential diagnoses relating to this query:

- Irritable hip.
- Perthes' disease.
- Slipped upper femoral epiphysis.
- Septic arthritis.
- Developmental dysplasia of the hip.

Irritable hip (transient synovitis)

Presentation
Irritable hip tends to occur in the age range of 6-12 years. Boys are more commonly affected than girls with a 2:1 ratio. The incidence is 3% of children in the above age range.

Symptoms include pain and a limp (pain in the groin, thigh or knee). Symptoms last for 1-2 weeks and then resolve spontaneously, but they may recur months later.

The signs indicate a restriction of movement in extremes, which causes pain and often the hip is held in a flexed position for comfort.

Investigations
- X-ray is normal.
- Blood tests are normal.
- Ultrasound may show a joint effusion.

Treatment
If mild, treatment is by bed rest or protected weight bearing, while symptoms persist. If severe or there is a diagnostic difficulty, the patient should be admitted for observation and advised against full weight bearing.

Note

— If an effusion is seen on ultrasound, aspiration with a EMLA is rapidly therapeutic.

Complications
The major complication of the treatment of irritable hip is having 'missed' a diagnosis of septic arthritis or osteomyelitis of the proximal femur.

Perthes' disease (Legg-Calve-Perthes' disease, 1910)

Presentation
Perthes' disease is avascular necrosis (AVN) of the femoral head, occurring in the age range of 4-8 years, with an incidence of 1 in 10,000. It is more common in boys than girls, with a 4:1 ratio. The cause is unknown; however, it does result in ischaemia, followed by AVN of the femoral head.

Symptoms include pain and a limp, which may last for weeks and can recur.

The signs indicate that the range of hip movement is restricted by pain in all planes.

Investigations
- Diagnosis hinges on X-ray changes. Initially normal, it can show widening of the joint space and asymmetry of the ossific centres.
- A bone scan reveals a void where the femoral head should be.
- Late changes are an obvious increase in the joint space, with flattening and lateral displacement of the epiphysis, and rarefaction and widening of the metaphysis.

- More recently, MRI has been shown to pick up the avascular changes before X-ray changes appear.

Prognostic features

A greater degree of femoral head involvement worsens the prognosis. When the age of onset is <6 years the prognosis is improved. Conversely, an increasing age of onset worsens the prognosis.

Treatment

Conservative
Bed rest and protected weight bearing.

Surgical
Varus osteotomy or an innominate bone osteotomy. Many variations of these procedures exist, and there is little agreement on which is best. This is followed by Plaster of Paris for 6-8 weeks.

The aim of treatment is to alleviate symptoms, maintain shape of the femoral head and prevent development of OA.

Complications
Complications of osteotomy surgery for Perthes' disease include:

- Wound infection.
- Deep infection (osteomyelitis or septic arthritis).
- Neurovascular damage.
- Accidental fracture of the femur or acetabulum.
- Failure to eradicate painful symptoms.
- Failure to stop/slow down progression of degenerative changes.

Note

– OA is the long-term risk of having a dysplastic femoral head as a result of Perthes' disease.

Slipped upper femoral epiphysis (SUFE) (Figure 7.7)

Presentation
The age of onset is at 14-16 years during the pubertal growth spurt. Boys are more commonly

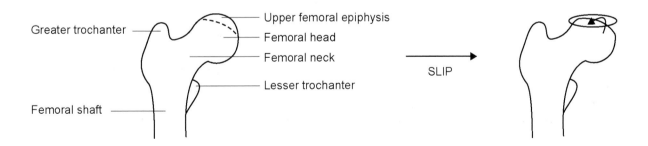

The slip results in asymmetry of the outline of the femoral head that can cause acute pain and predispose to early onset arthritis.

Figure 7.7. Slipped upper femoral epiphysis (SUFE).

affected than girls. Characteristically, it occurs in overweight or very tall children. The cause is unknown, but it seems to be related to a hormonal imbalance. There is often trauma in the history of 30% of cases. The other 70% have a progressive or incremental displacement.

Note

- If the slip is severe, the retinacular vessels are disrupted, which may therefore result in a degree of AVN of the femoral epiphysis.
- Physeal disruption results in premature fusion of the epiphysis.

Symptoms include pain and a limp. The pain is in the groin, thigh or knee.

The signs indicate some external rotation of the knee and shortening of the leg.

Investigations

X-rays (AP and lateral views) of the hip show a 'woolly' and widened epiphyseal plate. Trethowan's sign (Figure 7.8) is a line parallel to the upper neck of the femur which goes above the head (not through it, which would be normal). The lateral view shows the neck tilted posteriorly from the epiphysis.

Treatment

Treatment aims to preserve the epiphyseal blood supply, stabilise the physis and correct any deformity.

Surgical

Surgical treatment is with threaded pins or screws through the femoral neck to the head. The slip is generally not attempted to be reduced back into its anatomical position before being pinned, even though this would seem the logical thing to do. The reason for this is the greater incidence of AVN when the reduction manoeuvre is performed than when the SUFE is pinned *in situ*.

Controversy exists as to whether to prophylactically pin the contralateral (non-slipped) side at the time of surgery, as there is a risk of developing the condition in the other leg. This would prevent the slip.

Complications

- As mentioned, there is a risk of femoral head AVN associated with the condition as well as with the treatment.
- Wound infection.
- Neurovascular damage.
- Further slip (can still happen, either due to a technical error, or to weight bearing too early in a non-compliant patient).
- Contralateral SUFE (not a complication of the treatment, unless you consider not pinning the contralateral side a failure to fully treat).

Septic arthritis of the hip

Presentation

The age of onset is usually under two years. The organism is normally a Staphylococcus. It is caused by a distant focus or directly from osteomyelitis of the femur. Complications include destruction of the cartilaginous head of the femur, therefore causing later osteoarthritis.

Symptoms include pain, a limp and a generally ill child. Signs indicate pyrexia and the child will not move the leg at all, due to the pain.

Investigations

X-ray is of little value. Ultrasound shows an effusion.

Trethowan's sign

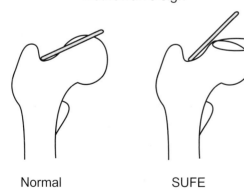

Normal   SUFE

Figure 7.8. Trethowan's sign.

Treatment

Aspirate the pus, administer antibiotics and perform an open arthrotomy with copious washout of the joint. This is urgent as the pus is rapidly destructive of the articular cartilage.

Complications
- Recurrent infection (requires re-operation).
- Missed osteomyelitis, that was the cause of the septic arthritis itself.
- Haematoma.
- Neurovascular damage.

Developmental dysplasia of the hip

Some children are born with a dislocated or dislocatable hip. It is far more common in girls than boys with a 7:1 ratio, and the left hip is more commonly affected than the right because of the left occipitoanterior 'lie' of most fetuses *in utero*. One in five cases is bilateral.

A familial predisposition exists with generalised joint laxity and acetabular dysplasia. The breech position predisposes to developmental dysplasia of the hip. Of the hips that are unstable at birth, 80-90% are fully reduced and stable at three weeks.

Presentation
Clinical signs that may be seen are:

- Asymmetrical skin creases on the thigh.
- Shortened leg.
- Externally rotated leg.

Clinical tests (Figure 7.9) are as follows:

- Ortolani's test for a dislocaTED hip detects a 'clunk' on lateral flexion, as the hip relocates.
- Barlow's test for a dislocatABLE hip. The acetabular head can be levered out of the joint by hip adduction and a vertical load.

Investigations
Ultrasound is the investigation of choice. X-rays are only useful after a minimum of four months, as ossification centres only show up in the femoral head on X-ray at that time.

Treatment

After conservative management, most unstable hips stabilise within three weeks. If the hip is still unstable, however, it will require splinting. The most effective method is by the use of the Pavlic harness, which holds the hip flexed and abducted. If this is ineffective, one may have to consider surgery. Based on an arthrogram (injection of dye into the joint, showing the outline of the cartilage, as well as the bony relations of the joint), it might be appropriate to perform one of the following:

- A closed reduction and plaster.
- An open reduction and plaster.
- An adductor tenotomy.
- A proximal femoral derotation osteotomy.
- A shelf procedure (insertion of a 'shelf' of autograft bone from the iliac crest to a point above the femoral head, effectively containing it better).

Complications
- The Pavlic harness carries the risk of femoral nerve palsy if the hip is splinted at an angle of greater than 90°. This tends to be transient, but could easily be avoided by splinting at a lower flexion angle.
- The Pavlic harness, abduction plaster, with or without open reduction, all carry with them the risk of femoral head AVN.
- The proximal femoral derotation osteotomy carries a risk of non-union, wound infection, deep infection (including of the metalwork, usually a blade plate), and neurovascular damage. It too has a risk of femoral head AVN, although this is minimised by virtue of the osteotomy level being at that of the lesser trochanter, i.e. extracapsular and hence, theoretically, damage to the femoral head vasculature should not occur.
- The shelf procedure carries with it a risk of wound infection, deep infection and fracture of the shelf itself. The surgical approach (anterior) risks meralgia paraesthetica (damage to the lateral femoral cutaneous nerve of the thigh, resulting in a dysaesthetic feeling in the anterolateral thigh. Often it is transient).

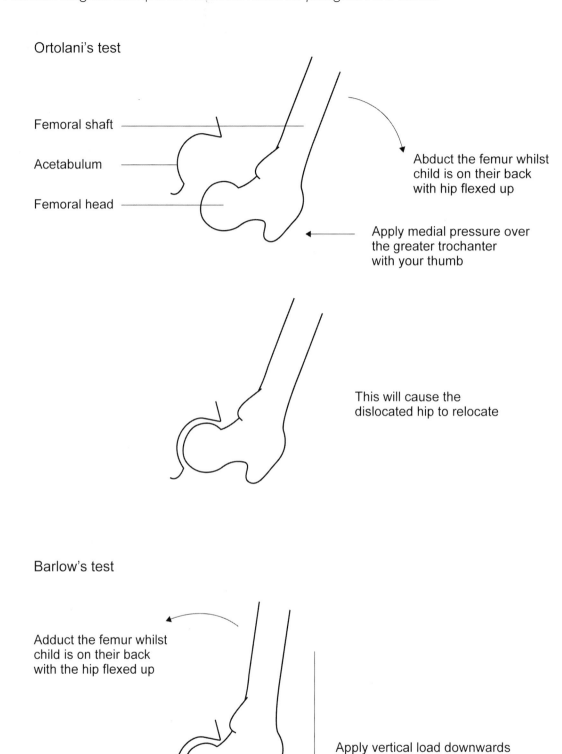

Ortolani's test

Femoral shaft

Acetabulum

Femoral head

Abduct the femur whilst child is on their back with hip flexed up

Apply medial pressure over the greater trochanter with your thumb

This will cause the dislocated hip to relocate

Barlow's test

Adduct the femur whilst child is on their back with the hip flexed up

Apply vertical load downwards on the femur

Figure 7.9. Congenital dislocation of the hip: Ortolani's test and Barlow's test.

Metabolic bone disorders

A brief summary is provided below with the main salient points, as generally, more detail is not required at this stage.

Rickets and osteomalacia

These are both expressions of the same disease: rickets affects children and osteomalacia affects adults. Both are the result of inadequate mineralisation of the bone. It affects areas of high bone turnover in children, i.e. epiphyses and all bone (generally) in adults, which is softened. It is due to a calcium deficiency, hypophosphataemia and a vitamin D metabolism defect, i.e. renal, liver or a congenital enzyme deficiency. Investigations will show a low plasma calcium (and PO_4) and a raised alkaline phosphatase (ALP).

Osteoporosis

This is a disorder where bone is fully mineralised but it is abnormally porous. It can occur as a primary or secondary disorder. Primary osteoporosis occurs mostly in post-menopausal and senile groups. Causes of secondary osteoporosis are hypercortisolism, gonadal hormone deficiency (e.g. post-hysterectomy), hyperthyroidism, multiple myeloma, chronic alcoholism and immobilisation.

Note

- The serum biochemistry in osteoporosis is normal; specifically, the calcium, phosphate and ALP serum levels are normal.

This is poorly taught at medical school in that osteoporosis is not simply the increased porosity of bone, but it is the syndrome of the bony sequelae of this, i.e. vertebral crush fractures, fractured neck of femurs, Colles' fractures, etc.

Paget's disease (osteitis deformans)

This is characterised by enlargement and thickening of bone, with abnormal internal architecture, resulting in brittle bone. This is quite counterintuitive, as to look at the X-ray appearance, you would be forgiven for thinking it would take a great deal of force to break the grossly thickened sclerotic looking bone, but it is more brittle by far than normal bone.

Fractures of Paget's bone are pathological fractures. Paget's disease is due to an overactivity of both osteoblasts and osteoclasts. It is of unknown aetiology, although the finding of inclusion bodies suggests a viral aetiology; this viral aetiology is as yet unproven. It affects both sexes equally, and tends to affect those >50 years. Usually asymptomatic, it presents either incidentally on X-ray or with a pathological fracture.

Note

- There is an increased risk of bone sarcoma with a poor prognosis.

Presentations:

- Nerve compression.
- Fractures.
- Osteoarthritis.
- Bone sarcoma.
- High output cardiac failure, due to increased bone vascularity.
- Hypercalcaemia, if the patient is immobilised.

Management is by treating the fracture, if present. If necessary, calcitonin and bisphosphonates can decrease disease activity when bone turnover is high.

Pathological fractures

These are classified by the causative lesion.

Generalised bone disease

- Osteogenesis imperfecta.
- Post-menopausal osteoporosis.
- Metabolic bone disease.
- Myelomatosis.
- Paget's disease.
- Polyostotic fibrous dysplasia.

Local benign conditions

- Bone cyst.
- Chronic infection.

- Fibrous cortical defect.
- Chondromyxoid fibroma.
- Aneurysmal bone cyst.
- Chondroma.
- Monostotic fibrous dysplasia.

Local malignant tumours

Primary

Chondrosarcoma, osteosarcoma and Ewing's tumour.

Secondary

Metastases spread from tumours in the breast, lung, thyroid, kidney and prostate.

A pathological fracture is abnormal bone giving way, usually as a result of minimal trauma. As mentioned in the section on bone tumours, when dealing with bony metastases that have fractured, these should be nailed (for diaphyseal fractures), taking care to 'protect the whole bone' in case of future lesions. With bony metastases in the proximal or distal parts of the bone (meaning near the joints), it is often better to perform a joint replacement, excising the portion of bone containing the lesion and the articular portion. The best example of this is a fracture of the femoral neck, which can be treated with either a hemi-arthroplasty or a total hip replacement.

The treatment of pathological fractures of primary bone tumours is quite different from that of secondaries. The reason for this is the risk of spread of the tumour at the surgical site. The most extreme example of this is to nail a primary bone tumour, thinking it was a secondary. The reamers and the nail itself carry the malignant cells the whole length of the bone, causing greater spread of what might have been a curable lesion.

Instead, primary bone lesions, even when fractured, still require excision with a cuff of healthy tissue in a specialist bone tumour unit.

Osteomyelitis

Acute osteomyelitis

This literally means inflammation of bone substance. The causes of osteomyelitis can be haematogenous, postoperative, post-open fracture, and post-penetrating injury.

It is more common in those under 21, involving the femur, tibia, humerus and radius in descending order of frequency. There may be an association with diabetes, sickle cell anaemia and immunodeficiency.

The commonest causative organism is *Staphylococcus aureus*, although *Streptococcous pyogenes*, *Streptococcous pneumoniae* and *Haemophilus influenzae* (*Haemophilus influenzae* is more common in childhood osteomyelitis) can all cause it. Haemophilus is seen only rarely now, due to the effectiveness of the HIB vaccine.

Note

– In sickle cell disease, there is a predisposition to Salmonella osteomyelitis, as opposed to the other, usually more common, organisms.

Pathology

The pathological series of events occurring in osteomyelitis occur in the following order:

- Inflammation (influx of inflammatory cells).
- Suppuration (formation of pus).
- Necrosis (death of tissue).
- Reactive new bone formation.
- Resolution and healing.

Presentation

- Pain.
- Fever.
- Inflammation.
- Acute tenderness.

Investigations

- X-rays are normal during the first ten days. Thereafter, they can show a lytic appearance that can appear intramedullary, but can also deform the cortices and occasionally mimic the appearance of a malignant bone tumour.
- The most definitive investigation is by aspiration of pus from the subperiosteal abscess.
- Raised WCC and ESR.
- Approximately 60% of blood cultures are positive.

- MRI. This is the most sensitive investigation. It can show the presence of a Brodie's abscess which is a necrotic segment of bone or tissue found at the centre of the osteomyelitic lesion, which perpetuates the infection, and may require surgery. MRI also shows the extent of the infection anatomically and if there are any soft tissue fluid collections in the region of the osteomyelitic bone segment.

Treatment
- Analgesia.
- IV antibiotics.
- Splintage.
- Surgical drainage.

Complications
- Metastatic infection.
- Suppurative arthritis (joint adjacent to area of bone affected).
- Altered bone growth (in children, obviously).
- Chronic osteomyelitis.

Subacute osteomyelitis

Presentation
This is the milder version of acute osteomyelitis, due to a lower virulence of organism. Rarely is there frank pus in the bone, but usually a cavity with seropurulent fluid. It usually presents in a child with a history of weeks or months of bone pain, with possible swelling, maybe some muscle wasting (locally), and local tenderness.

Investigations
- X-ray may show the cavity, which can be confused with a tumour appearance.
- Isotope scan shows the hot spot.
- MRI. As mentioned previously, the MRI can make the diagnosis and delineate the anatomy, and show any evidence of a Brodie's abscess.

Treatment
Treatment is with six weeks of appropriate antibiotic and immobilisation. If this fails, surgical curettage of the lesion and further antibiotics are needed. Infection is usually caused by *Staphylococcus aureus*.

Complications
The complications of subacute osteomyelitis are as for acute osteomyelitis in the section above, only less common, due to the generally decreased virulence of the organism.

Chronic osteomyelitis

This can follow acute osteomyelitis, but more commonly it follows an operation, open fracture or prosthesis insertion.

Pathology
In chronic osteomyelitis there is a persistent background of chronic inflammation, with necrotic tissue and bone destruction.

Presentation
It presents with pain, local inflammation, a sinus (discharging pus) and pyrexia.

Investigations
- X-ray shows bone resorption/destruction.
- Bone scan shows the hot spot.
- CT and MRI localise the problem in 3D (useful for planning surgery). MRI can show the classic Brodie's abscess.
- Sinogram can be useful.

Treatment
Treatment is with antibiotics and surgical debridement. Antibiotics alone will not eradicate the infection and so the debridement is essential. Insertion of antibiotics into the affected bone can be a useful adjunct to a range of treatments, e.g. insertion of antibiotic-coated gentamycin beads, or a drain through which there is a regular antibiotic infusion.

Complications
The complications of debridement surgery for chronic osteomyelitis are:

- Recurrent infection.
- Neurovascular damage.
- Haematoma.
- Fistula formation.
- Wound breakdown.

Sometimes, despite all best efforts at treatment, chronic osteomyelitis cannot be cured and the choice then has to be made between chronic fistula drainage or curative amputation.

Septic arthritis

Septic arthritis is an infection producing inflammation in a native or prosthetic joint. It can occur *de novo*, after a perforating injury into the joint (e.g. thorn into the interphalangeal joint of the thumb), secondary to osteomyelitis adjacent to the joint, or from haematogenous spread of a septic source.

Presentation

Septic arthritis presents with pyrexia, joint pain and severe stiffness. Patients can have a severe systemic upset if it is left untreated. Examination of the affected joint shows it to be hot. There may be a palpable effusion or overlying cellulitis or redness, and even slight movements (active or passive) can cause severe pain (effectively no range of movement). The joint is generally tender to palpation.

In children, the most common organisms are *Staphylococcus aureus* and *Streptococcus pyogenes*.

In adults of reproductive age, Staphylococcus and Streptococcus are the more common infecting organisms, then to a lesser extent *Neisseria gonorrhoeae*.

In older adults, the most common organism remains *Staphylococcus aureus*, but occasionally a particularly virulent form of septic arthritis is seen secondary to *Streptococcus pyogenes*.

Investigations

- History and examination as above.
- Blood tests show a raised ESR and CRP. The WCC is raised, but not always in the early stage. Blood cultures must be performed for aerobic and anaerobic organisms.
- Needle aspiration of the joint for an urgent Gram stain, and microscopy, culture and sensitivity (MC+S). This is relatively simple in the case of the knee, but is more difficult in the case of the hip or interphalangeal joints in the hand or foot.
- X-ray is not a particularly rewarding investigation in this context, but it must be done. It acts as a baseline picture if later X-rays become relevant. It can show the presence of a foreign body if there has been trauma in the history. It also delineates the normal anatomy of the joint for any planned procedures later.
- MRI. If there is rapid access to an MRI scanner, and diagnostic doubt, then an MRI can image the affected joint. It can also show if there is any underlying osteomyelitis. MRI can also be useful in the recovery phase if the patient continues to complain of pain and pyrexia, despite washout and appropriate antibiotics, again looking for underlying osteomyelitis.

Treatment

It is necessary to wash the joint out surgically. This can be done arthroscopically in the case of the shoulder and knee fairly easily. Other joints, such as the hip, elbow and wrist, can be more problematic with the use of an arthroscope, unless it is in expert hands. If arthroscopic washout is impractical for any reason, then open washout is indicated.

It is very much in this context that the old surgical adage of 'the solution to pollution is dilution' holds true, i.e. large volumes of sterile saline should be used in the washout. In the case of larger limb joints, 3-6 litres is mandatory.

There is some published evidence that repeated aspirations percutaneously (in the knee) with antibiotics have a comparable result with single surgical washout. This should not be the first-line answer in exams, however.

Empiric (broad spectrum) antibiotics should be started after samples have been taken. Once the results of the MC+S have returned it is then possible to convert to a more focused antibiotic regime.

Complications

- Recurrence of the septic arthritis requiring re-operation.
- Haematoma.
- Neurovascular damage.
- Long-term degenerative change (due to damage to the articular cartilage by the pus).

Chapter 8

Vascular surgery

Acute ischaemia

Vascular patients are an unavoidable part of clinical exams. You will see many vascular conditions: chronic ischaemia, venous disease, aneurysms or lymphoedema. Thus, you are very likely to be tested on arterial ischaemia (hopefully not acute ischaemia in the clinical setting, although it is possible it may crop up in viva exams).

Total occlusion of a vessel (Figure 8.1)

Total occlusion of a vessel may occur in the following ways:

- Gradual progression of atheromatous disease.
- Acute thrombus formation (more common), caused by a crack in the atheroma being thrombogenic and the thrombus thus formed occludes the vessel.
- Embolism.
- Other. Thrombosis of aneurysm, dissection, external compression, ligation, trauma.

Note

- The speed of occlusion and the ability to form collateral vessels determine the severity of symptoms (collaterals form over a period of weeks, no faster).
- In advanced ischaemia of a limb, revascularisation can be hazardous due to release of toxic metabolites, e.g. potassium or myoglobin into the circulation. These have dangerous effects on the myocardium and kidneys, most importantly.

The commonest sites for arterial stenosis are:

- Femoral artery.
- Popliteal artery.
- Brachial artery.
- Carotid artery.

Presentation

The six Ps (mnemonic for signs of acute ischaemia):

- Pain.
- Pulselessness.
- Pallor.
- Paraesthesiae.
- Paralysis.
- Perishin' cold.

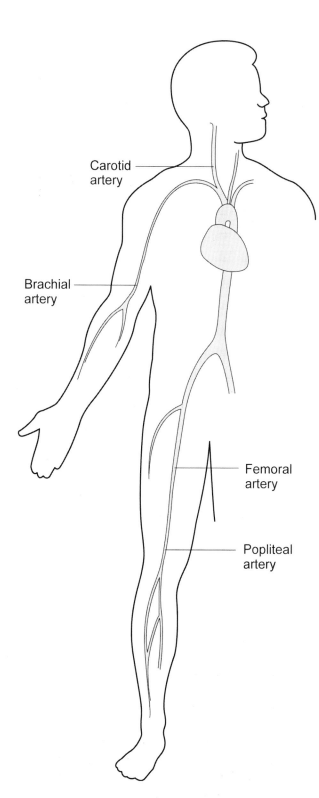

Carotid artery

Brachial artery

Femoral artery

Popliteal artery

Figure 8.1. Total occlusion of a vessel may occur in the marked locations.

Clinical presentation of lower limb ischaemia

Lower limb ischaemia classically presents with claudication. This is the presence of calf pain after walking a certain distance. You will be expected to elicit how far the patient walks before the pain comes on. You also must ask whether the pain is relieved by rest (stopping walking). Classically, claudication pain is rapidly relieved by rest.

Advanced chronic ischaemia also presents with night pain in the calf. You are expected to ask the patient if dangling the leg out of the bed relieves their pain to some extent. Chronic ischaemia classically does show some improvement with this manoeuvre. Smooth hairless skin is also seen in the chronically ischaemic limb. It is also a significant risk factor for the formation of arterial ulcers. These have a classically 'punched out' edge, and do not tend to bleed when pricked with a needle. The absence of palpable pulses in the presence of ulcers is also considered a clue as to the nature (venous vs arterial) of the ulcers.

Because the major differential diagnosis of claudication is spinal stenosis (causing so called spinal claudication), you should be aware of the differences in presentation of the two conditions. Spinal claudication can come on after variable amounts of distance walked. It also tends to come on after prolonged periods of time standing. Some patients notice that spinal claudication tends to come on less if they walk with the aid of a rollator frame, or when they push a trolley (presumably because the forward flexed position adopted opens the spinal canal a little).

Investigations

The Ankle Brachial Pressure Index (ABPI) is the most useful investigation in the clinic setting. See Chapter 13, Examination techniques, on exactly how to perform this test. It basically involves the use of a Doppler probe to compare the systolic pressure of the arm against the leg and is the ratio of these two numbers. In the normal individual the ratio will be 1 (i.e. same pressure in the arm as in the leg), but in an ischaemic limb, the ratio will be less than 0.8 (i.e. lower pressure in the leg). Less than 0.6 is considered critically ischaemic.

Fogarty catheter

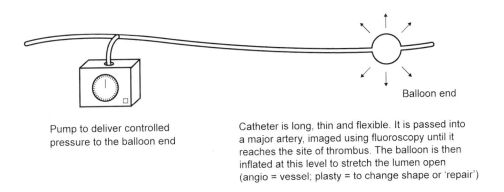

Balloon end

Pump to deliver controlled
pressure to the balloon end

Catheter is long, thin and flexible. It is passed into
a major artery, imaged using fluoroscopy until it
reaches the site of thrombus. The balloon is then
inflated at this level to stretch the lumen open
(angio = vessel; plasty = to change shape or 'repair')

Figure 8.2. Fogarty catheter.

The investigation of choice for ischaemia remains the angiogram (intra-arterial digital subtraction angiogram). This shows the anatomy of the vascular supply to the lower limb in good detail and enables surgical planning.

If surgery is planned (see later section) then it must be remembered that 'arteriopaths' are high risk patients. They must have the usual array of pre-operative blood tests (FBC, U+Es, CS, G+S and a fasting glucose level to look for diabetes), and a chest X-ray and ECG. It is not unusual to pick up other pathologies in this group of patients.

Treatment

Treatment is by angioplasty (for critically narrowed arteries) or fluoroscopically-guided embolectomy (for arteries that have an embolus lodged in an already narrowed segment). Angioplasty is the forced dilation of a balloon catheter (Fogarty type; Figure 8.2) guided angiographically at the site of narrowing. Embolectomy, meaning removal of an embolus, can be performed percutaneously (i.e. fluoroscopically guided) or via an open surgical approach.

Percutaneous embolectomy uses a Fogarty type catheter. First it must be pushed past the embolus, the balloon is inflated and then pulled back, effectively dragging the embolus back out the artery.

Another percutaneous alternative to the above two methods is thrombolysis. This is the intravascular release of 'clot busters' from a fluoroscopically-guided catheter placed just downstream of the blocked section of artery. This can only work on new onset acute-on-chronic thrombus, as the thrombus will not yet have had time to organise, being mostly simple clot. Examples of clot buster chemicals are tissue plasminogen activator (TPA) or streptokinase.

Thrombolysis is the first-line treatment in acute on chronic ischaemia, e.g. thrombus complicating atheromatous disease. Thrombolysis is also useful in proven embolism if the limb is viable, i.e. able to survive ischaemia while the agent works.

If these medical measures are deemed inappropriate, or have failed, then bypass surgery is indicated. This is the formation of a conduit that bypasses the occluded arterial segment. A reversed vein graft can be used (the valves would prevent flow unless reversed) or a synthetic substitute, e.g. Dacron or PTFE. A prerequisite for bypass surgery is the presence of a suitable vessel to plumb the bypass vessel/graft into. If all the distal vessels are too small or too diseased, then bypass surgery simply is not viable. Amputation will then have to be considered.

Amputation is obviously the last resort, but it effectively removes the ischaemic (by now, often painful and useless) limb. Chapter 4, Operative Surgery, provides greater detail on the types of, and techniques for, amputations.

Contra-indications to thrombolysis

Bleeding tendency, peptic ulcer disease, CVA and recent surgery.

Complications

Complications of angioplasty or embolectomy:

♦ Puncture site problems, i.e. haematoma, femoral artery pseudoaneurysm formation, arteriovenous fistula formation.
♦ Problems related to the artery containing the thrombus, i.e. arterial dissection, or dislodging the clot which goes on to embolise further downstream.
♦ Reperfusion compartment syndrome of the limb (requires urgent fasciotomy).

Complications of thrombolysis:

♦ Puncture site problems, i.e. haematoma, femoral artery pseudoaneurysm formation, arteriovenous fistula formation.
♦ Bleeding complications, i.e. intracerebral haemorrhage, or bleeding elsewhere.
♦ Reperfusion compartment syndrome of the limb (requires urgent fasciotomy).

Complicatons of bypass surgery:

♦ Failure of graft on table, e.g. due to inadequate distal vessel run-off to accommodate blood flow though the graft-vessel anastomosis. This requires an alternative site, or even an alternative vessel anastomosis, otherwise

amputation may need to be considered. Patients should be warned of the possibility of amputation prior to surgery.

♦ Graft occlusion.
♦ Graft infection. This is more likely in prosthetic than vein grafts, as they are effectively a 'foreign body'.
♦ Late restenosis.
♦ Distal embolism.
♦ Amputation.

Complications of amputation:

♦ Re-amputation at a higher level for recurrent problems of ischaemia (seen particularly in Buerger's disease).
♦ Wound infection.
♦ Deep infection.
♦ Neurovascular damage.
♦ Phantom limb pain. Pain felt where the amputated limb used to be.
♦ Problems with the prosthesis fitting, pain, skin ulceration and neuromas.

Aneurysms

An aneurysm is a localised dilatation of an artery. This is an essential definition to remember as it may well come up in the exam setting.

Note

– An important semantic point is that if the dilatation is less than twice the original diameter the vessel is considered ectatic, but, if it is more than twice the original diameter the vessel is then considered aneurysmal.

Complications of aneurysms (Figure 8.3)

♦ Thrombosis. A thrombus can occlude the vessel lumen.
♦ Embolisation. An embolus can occlude the vessel lumen.

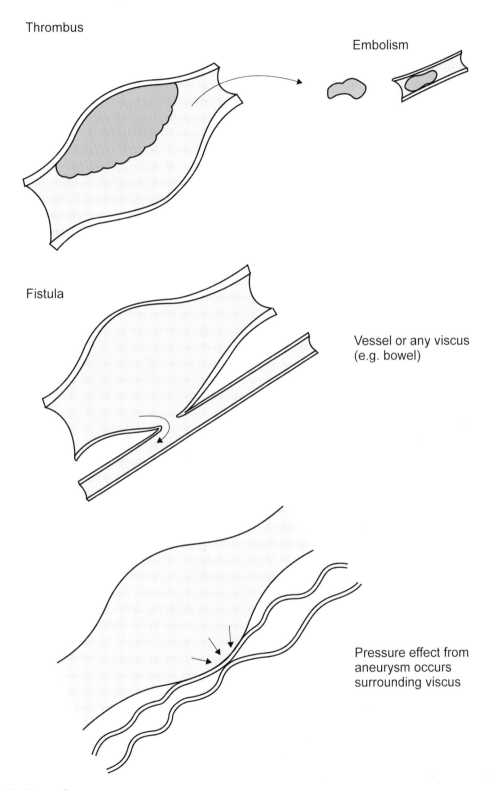

Thrombus

Embolism

Fistula

Vessel or any viscus
(e.g. bowel)

Pressure effect from
aneurysm occurs
surrounding viscus

Figure 8.3. Complications of aneurysms.

♦ Fistulation. A fistula is a tract between two epithelial-lined structures, which would result in high pressure blood loss from the aorta to another viscus, e.g. bowel in an aorto-enteric fistula.
♦ Compression effects on other structures.
♦ Dissection.

Types of aneurysms

Aneurysms can be true or false (Figure 8.4):

♦ True: a dilated artery with normal artery wall structure.
♦ False: the wall of the vessel has been breached and the surrounding structures make up the aneurysm capsule. False aneurysms are generally the result of puncture trauma, e.g. in the hospital setting, the femoral artery can develop a false aneurysm after puncture during an angiogram, or the radial artery can develop a false aneurysm after puncture for arterial blood gas measurement.

True aneurysm

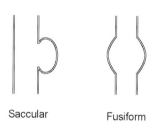

Saccular   Fusiform

False aneurysm

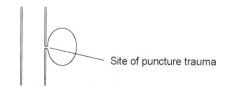

Site of puncture trauma

Figure 8.4. True and false aneurysms.

True aneurysms are subdivided into fusiform (spindle-shaped) or saccular (bulbous from side wall).

Atherosclerosis is the most common aetiological factor in aneurysms; however, syphilis, Marfan's and Ehlers-Danlos syndromes are all rarer causes.

Note

– Mycotic aneurysms can form from a vegetation embolus in bacterial endocarditis (interestingly, mycotic means originating from fungus, but there is no fungal aetiology in mycotic aneurysms; the most common organism is the bacteria *Streptococcus viridans*, or in the case of an IV drug abuser, *Staphylococcus aureus*).

Atrophy of smooth muscle and loss of elastic laminae is seen in aneurysms. These result in weaker walls which the systolic BP can then force into aneurysmal dilatation.

Note

– Mathematically, Laplace's law states that the wall tension increases in proportion to the radius. This induces a vicious cycle of increased pressure as the diameter increases.

Classification of aortic aneurysms (the Crawford classification)

♦ Type I. Thoracic (only) aneurysm.
♦ Type II. Thoracic and abdominal aneurysm.
♦ Type III. Low thoracic and (predominantly) abdominal aneurysm.
♦ Type IV. Abdominal aneurysm (only).

Thoracic aortic aneurysm

These are much less common than abdominal aortic aneurysm (AAA). If it presents asymptomatically in an elderly patient, it is advisable to leave it alone, as complications of surgery are high, but if the patient is young, the aneurysm large, and the patient symptomatic, surgery is indicated.

Complications
- Paraplegia (10-20%), due to vertebral ischaemia.
- Mortality (10-50%).

Abdominal aortic aneurysm (AAA)

The abdominal aorta is the most frequent site of aneurysmal dilatation in the body (found in 2% of post mortems). The aneurysm is usually infrarenal, i.e. located inferior to the renal arteries (the suprarenal incidence is approximately 2% of AAAs). The incidence is greatest in men >60 years who smoke.

AAA is related to atherosclerosis, but why it causes stenosis in some and aneurysms in others is a source of much debate.

Presentation
Most AAAs are asymptomatic. As they increase in size it is possible for the patient to experience some abdominal discomfort. The atheroma in the aneurysm can be the source of emboli to the lower limb, thus, in rare cases the aneurysm can present with lower limb embolic phenomena (digital gangrene, splinter haemorrhages, or even frank acute limb ischaemia).

Aneurysms can rupture and bleed precipitously, leading to presentation to the surgeon with acute abdominal pain, radiating round to the back and cardiovascular collapse (haemorrhagic shock).

Assessment of a patient with an AAA
A clinical examination to find other aneurysms should be undertaken; there is an increased likelihood of the patient having aneurysms at other sites, e.g. femoral and popliteal (most common). This is an important point to raise in clinical exams.

Investigations
Abdominal ultrasound delineates the aneurysm, confirming the diagnosis, and providing an objective measure of the diameter. An angiogram determines whether the renal arteries are involved or not.

If surgery is indicated then pre-operative investigations must include an FBC, U+Es, a CS, Glu, group and cross-match 4-6 units, chest X-ray and ECG.

Note
- The ESR is important because it indicates inflammatory involvement in the aneurysm, which makes surgery difficult, but the aneurysm may respond to steroids, simplifying what could have been challenging surgery.

Treatment
The normal abdominal aortic diameter is 2cm, 2-4cm is ectatic, >4cm is aneurysmal, 4-5cm requires monitoring with serial USS and >5.5cm requires surgical repair electively. It has been shown that the annual risk of rupture when the diameter is >5.5cm is greater than the operative risks of elective repair in these patients, hence the above classification based on diameter.

Note
- Painful or ruptured aneurysms require urgent repair.
- In ruptured AAA, beware of the temptation to overly fluid-resuscitate as this may result in further bleeding (the current school of thought can be summarised as 'keep 'em dry' or, 'the first clot is the best clot').

Complications
Complications of AAA surgery relate to the graft (infection, sinus formation, aorto-enteric fistula, stenosis) or pre-operative sickness of the patient (DVT, MI, MOF, pneumonia, PE).

Other sources of aneurysms

◆ Femoral. Usually asymptomatic and rarely rupture, but they may be a source of emboli.
◆ Popliteal. Most common site of peripheral aneurysm, with an atherosclerotic aetiology. They have associations with aneurysm formation elsewhere. If symptomatic, a bypass or resection with anastomosis is required; if asymptomatic, controversy exists over the need for repair which may carry more risk than benefit.
◆ Ventricular, i.e. in the cardiac ventricle. They occur post-MI with a fibrotic scar.

Carotid artery disease

This forms an important subject and is often asked about in both clinical and viva sections of exams, as it affects large numbers of people and its clinical consequences are serious.

Presentation

Atherosclerosis can affect both intra- and extracranial vessels, i.e. carotid, basilar and cerebral arteries; however, there is a propensity for atherosclerotic disease at the carotid bifurcation. This can present as a complete stroke, transient ischaemic attack (TIA) or amaurosis fugax.

Note

— TIA is a transient ischaemic attack, which by definition is a unilateral weakness lasting less than 24 hours.
— Amaurosis fugax means literally 'creeping blindness', and refers to the transient blindness, over one eye only, descending characteristically like a curtain vertically. It is due to the passage of a shower of small emboli through the arterial vasculature of the retina.

True cerebral hypoperfusion is rare unless bilateral carotid stenotic disease is associated with the Circle of Willis and/or vertebrobasilar disease.

A carotid stenosis characteristically produces a bruit, but do not be drawn into a false sense of security that any further implications can be deduced from the presence of a carotid bruit. Remember instead that severe carotid stenosis can occur without any bruit, and that minimal carotid stenosis can produce truly loud and impressive bruits (not a clinical sign that should be interpreted further).

Investigations

A carotid artery duplex scan is required to delineate stenosis, with or without an intravenous digital subtraction angiogram (IVDSA), intra-arterial digital subtraction angiogram (IADSA) or magnetic resonance angiography (MRA).

Another common exam question relates to the relative advantages and disadvantages of IVDSA versus IADSA. The simple answer is that IADSA requires arterial puncture, less contrast, and produces better pictures. Arterial puncture and passage of a catheter carries a risk of false aneurysm formation and dislodging atheromatous disease as an embolus, and is technically more difficult. IVDSA does not require arterial puncture, requires more contrast, which is more diffuse by the time it reaches the arterial tree, and produces more diffuse (read 'worse') pictures, particularly the more distal the artery required to be imaged, but it does not have the disadvantages of arterial puncture mentioned above.

Obviously, if surgery is contemplated the patient will also need routine pre-operative blood testing, an ECG and a chest X-ray (and others to be determined by their medical comorbidities).

Note

- Duplex is combined Doppler and real-time ultrasound.
- MRA is an MRI using a type of gadolinium-based dye which delineates vascular anatomy in three dimensions when imaged. This is a technique that is gaining greater acceptance, but is limited by the relatively large numbers of patients who would benefit from its use, compared with the relatively small number of scanners in the country.
- A CT of the brain should be done to exclude other causes of CVAs in those patients who have presented with TIA/amaurosis fugax/complete stroke (e.g. bleed/tumour).

Differential diagnosis of TIA

- Multiple sclerosis.
- Epilepsy.
- Stokes-Adams attacks (sudden transient episode of syncope secondary to cardiac dysrhythmia).
- Meningioma.
- Subdural haematoma.

Treatment

If the imaging shows a stenosis to be 70% or greater, then surgery is indicated, even if the patient is asymptomatic. It has been shown in this group that there is a significant reduction of risk of stroke with carotid endarterectomy surgery. This is an open procedure, exposing the carotid artery via an incision based on the anterior border of the sternocleidomastoid muscle and dissecting out the artery's thrombus, taking care not to raise an intimal tear which could go on to progress, called arterial dissection. Symptomatic patients with 50-70% stenosis (i.e. suffering TIAs) also warrant surgery.

Another treatment modality available is carotid angioplasty and stenting. This is performed in patients whose comorbidities make them high risk for open surgery, as it can be done under local anaesthetic. There is little long-term evidence yet for this procedure, but short-term results are encouraging.

Complications

- Stroke (intra-operative risk 1-2%)
- Myocardial infarction.
- Wound infection.
- Recurrent or laryngeal nerve palsy.
- Recurrence of occlusion.
- Death (these patients are by definition severe cardiopaths already prior to surgery).

Carotid body tumours (chemodectomas)

Presentation

- Rare, of an equal sex distribution, with a wide age range, the median age being 50 years.
- Ovoid tumours at the carotid bifurcation, which distort and encase the carotid vessels.

Note

- Only 10% are bilateral.

- Highly vascular.
- Microscopic appearances are unhelpful in determining malignant potential.
- Presents as a mass in the neck, which is pulsatile and occasionally expansile, and there may be a bruit or thrill.
- Clinically, the differential diagnosis is one of the following: lymph node, branchial cyst, neurofibroma, aneurysm.

Investigations

- Digital subtraction angiography.
- Doppler.
- MRA.

Treatment

- Under 50 years - surgical resection.
- Over 50 years - watch and wait policy, radiotherapy.

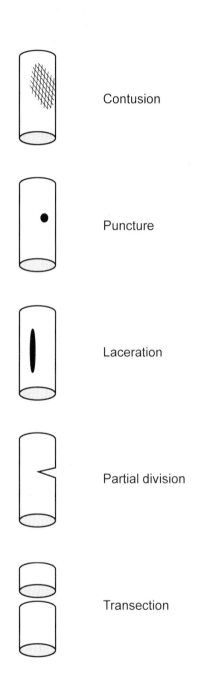

Contusion

Puncture

Laceration

Partial division

Transection

Figure 8.5. Types of arterial injury.

Complications

- Hemiplegia 1-2%.
- Nerve palsy 12-40%.

Arterial injury

Presentation

Arterial injuries will most commonly present in two ways. The first is in the trauma setting, e.g. an arterial bleed associated with a fracture or abdominal injury; the second is in the intra-operative setting, e.g. accidental laceration of an artery in the operative field.

Arterial injuries can be:

- Open or closed.
- Direct or indirect, e.g. secondary to bony injury.
- Traumatic or iatrogenic.

Types of arterial injuries (Figure 8.5) are:

- Contusion (read 'bruising').
- Puncture.
- Laceration.
- Partial division.
- Transection.

Arterial haemorrhage can be:

- Primary (immediate).
- Secondary (when the arteriospasm from the time of surgery has worn off).
- Reactionary (7-10 days post-repair due to infection).

Note

- Bleeding can be concealed, e.g. in the thigh after a femoral fracture.

Investigations

Depending on the circumstances, investigation can take various forms. If an artery has been lacerated under direct vision, then investigation is obviously irrelevant. If presented with a pulseless limb after trauma (e.g. fracture), generally a reduction of any displaced fracture is attempted together with re-examination for a pulse. If the pulse returns, no further immediate action is needed for vascular investigation. If the limb remains pulseless, even using a Doppler probe, an angiogram is required urgently, as well as involving the vascular surgeons on call. Depending on the degree of urgency, an on-table angiogram can be performed using the image intensifier and injection of dye.

If presented with a rapidly distending abdomen after blunt trauma, then investigation again rapidly becomes irrelevant and urgent exploration is indicated.

Treatment

- Local pressure.
- Cross-match.
- Surgical repair.

Types of vascular repair are:

- Simple suture.
- Patch repair.
- End-to-end anastomosis.
- Interposition graft (using vein or Dacron).
- Ligation.

Complications

- Rebleed, i.e. failure of repair.
- Anastomotic failure (this is a variation of the re-bleed, but is important, specifically, where the vascular repair is an anastomosis, rather than any of the other techniques mentioned above).
- Haematoma.
- Reperfusion compartment syndrome (requires urgent fasciotomy).
- Arterial dissection.
- Arterial occlusion.
- Late arterial stenosis formation.

Arterial spasm

Arterial spasm is often associated with intimal damage, requiring urgent arteriography. Surgical exploration of the artery is indicated if it is locally stenosed or occluded on an angiogram.

Arterial occlusion

Arterial occlusion follows severe wall contusion and mural thrombus or intimal tears, but it can happen due to arterial transection.

Arteriography will demonstrate the proximal limit of the occlusion, but cannot show distal vasculature due to the occlusion. This requires surgical exploration, with or without the use of a Fogarty catheter to remove the distal thrombus.

Note

— The Fogarty catheter is something that you may be asked to describe in exams. It is a very thin tube containing one lumen only. The purpose of the lumen is to allow inflation of the balloon at its distal extreme. The catheter is passed down the artery that is blocked by embolus, beyond the embolus, then the balloon is inflated and the catheter drawn back, thus, in theory, dragging back the embolus with it.

If occlusion has been present for 3-4 hours, the limb will require fasciotomies to prevent massive rises in compartment pressure and the consequent risk of ischaemic contracture.

Postoperatively, regular monitoring of distal pulses in the affected limb is required and systemic antibiotics are given to prevent secondary infection.

Arterial dissection

This is a consequence of an intimal tear, resulting in arterial blood entering the intima. It usually does not progress far, as the media is normal. It is seen clearly on arteriography, showing a narrowed lumen and outline of the dissection.

False aneurysm

As has been mentioned before, a false aneurysm is a consequence of an arterial puncture wound, which results in blood leak, haematoma formation and fibrosis, forming a sac in which blood can collect. It is considered to be a false aneurysm, as it does not involve all the layers of the arterial wall.

False aneurysms can be imaged by ultrasound, which is often how the diagnosis is made in the first place. They then should be observed for 24 hours for evidence that they are remaining static or expanding. The most sensible way of doing this, unless it is quite obvious clinically, is by a repeat ultrasound. The reason for this is that there is a risk of rupture of the false aneurysm cavity. If expanding, then the neck of the false aneurysm can be embolised angiographically. The alternative to this is to tie off the neck of the false aneurysm surgically (a higher risk procedure, however).

Note

– Other types of arterial injury are traumatic, arteriovenous fistulae (uncommon) and frostbite.

Types of iatrogenic arterial injury

- Ligation.
- External compression (bandages, plasters, splints).
- Arterial puncture damage.
- Intra-arterial injection of drugs and chemicals.

The vasculitides

Of the following list of vasculitides, far and away the most relevant to the surgeon is, of course, Buerger's disease. You may, however, be asked about temporal arteritis for two main reasons, one, that temporal artery biopsies, although requested by physicians are performed in the main by surgeons, and two, you may save someone's sight by simply starting them on steroids on recognising the condition. Takayasu's disease is rare in this country (the author has only had the privilege of seeing one case).

Buerger's disease (thrombo-angiitis obliterans)

Originally called endarteritis by von Winiwarter, it affects young men aged 20-30 who are nicotine addicts. It affects medium-sized arteries, especially in the lower limb, which become progressively obliterated by inflammation and thrombosis. Collagen is laid down around the vessels, gradually encasing them.

Presentation
Chronic paronychias, poorly healing ulcers, digital gangrene, claudication, superficial and deep vein thrombosis. Rarely, erythema nodosum is seen.

Signs are as follows:

- Absent lower limb pulses beneath the level of the popliteal artery.
- Tender thickened vessels.

Investigations
Arteriography shows a characteristic appearance of corkscrew collaterals.

Treatment
- Stop smoking.
- Sympathectomy (cervical and/or lumbar bypass surgery is very unsuccessful in this disease).
- Antibiotics, footcare, prostaglandins and analgesics are given to tide patients over during periods of ischaemia while collaterals develop.
- Eventually, amputation is required for ischaemia that has progressed to frank gangrene in this group of patients who seem particularly difficult to treat. They often fail to stop smoking, despite the fact that they continue to undergo

increasingly higher levels of amputation for their recurrent episodes of gangrene.

Complications

Complications of sympathectomy include:

◆ Neuropathic pain.
◆ Ureteric damage, either direct trauma at the time of surgery, or fibrotic stenosis noted at follow-up.
◆ Retroperitoneal haematoma or abscess.
◆ Persistent ischaemic symptoms or later recurrence of the ischaemia.

Complications of amputation include:

◆ Re-amputation at a higher level for recurrent problems of ischaemia.
◆ Wound infection.
◆ Deep infection.
◆ Neurovascular damage.
◆ Phantom limb pain (pain felt where the amputated limb used to be).
◆ Problems with the prosthesis fitting, pain, skin ulceration and neuromas.

Takayasu's disease (pulseless disease)

Presentation

Named by Takayasu, after observations of the condition in young Japanese women in 1908. It affects vessels derived from the aortic arch. It causes TIAs, blindness, stroke and arm claudication. It is often associated with pyrexia, malaise, and a raised ESR in the acute stage.

Investigations

Arteriography shows tapering or occlusion of the affected vessels.

Treatment

◆ Surgical bypass.
◆ Steroids.
◆ Azathioprine.
◆ Cyclosporin.

Complications

Complications of surgical bypass include:

◆ Failure of the graft on table, e.g. due to inadequate distal vessel run-off to accommodate blood flow though the graft-vessel anastomosis. This requires an alternative site or even an alternative vessel anastomosis, otherwise amputation may need to be considered. Patients should be warned of the possibility of amputation prior to surgery.
◆ Graft occlusion.
◆ Graft infection. This is more likely in prosthetic than vein grafts, as they are effectively a foreign body.
◆ Late restenosis.
◆ Distal embolism.
◆ Amputation.

Temporal arteritis

Presentation

Described by Jonathan Hutchinson in 1889. Characteristically, it affects women over the age of 60. The male:female ratio is 1:2.

Symptoms are:

◆ Malaise, fever, myalgia (often for several months).
◆ Followed by frontoparietal headache, unilateral, and tender to touch.
◆ Superficial temporal artery may be thickened, tender and non-pulsatile.
◆ Visual loss may occur (30-50% of cases), which is permanent if left untreated.

Investigations

Temporal artery biopsy and ESR.

Treatment

High-dose steroids (60mg prednisolone). Consider azathioprine for steroid conservation.

Note

- Steroids reduce the incidence of blindness.
- Another type of vasculitis not yet mentioned is radiation vasculitis, generally caused by radiotherapy, most commonly seen in the neck and pelvis, as this is where radiotherapy is most commonly applied.

Complications

Complications of long-term steroid administration include:

- Muscle wasting.
- Central obesity.
- Skin fragility.
- Bruising and striae.
- Depression/psychosis.
- Osteoporosis.
- Hypertension.
- Hyperglycaemia.
- Susceptibility to infection.

Arterial vasospasm disorders

This is a group of disorders of uncertain aetiology that appear to be primary conditions.

Note

- There are *secondary* causes of Raynaud's disease.

Raynaud's disease and phenomenon

Named after Maurice Raynaud who wrote a thesis on it in 1862. It is important to know that Raynaud's disease is used to represent the primary condition and that Raynaud's phenomenon is used to represent the secondary condition, i.e. has another aetiological cause. The arteries affected are the digital arteries (digital arteriospasm).

Triggers:

- Cold.
- Emotion.
- Trauma.
- Hormones.
- Drugs.

Phases:

- Local syncope (blanching of digits from arterial spasm).
- Local asphyxia/cyanosis (swollen blue digits, painful, from stagnant anoxia).
- Recovery and reactive hyperaemia (red and tingling fingers due to build up of vasoactive metabolites causing vasodilatation).

Note

- The above order of colour change is best remembered as white-blue-red.

Causes of Raynaud's phenomenon (secondary):

- Connective tissue disorders: scleroderma, systemic lupus erythematosus (SLE), dermatomyositis, polyarteritis nodosum (PAN), rheumatoid arthritis, Sjögren's syndrome.
- Arterial disease: atherosclerosis, Buerger's disease, embolism from cervical rib syndrome.
- Trauma: vibration-induced white finger, frostbite sequelae.
- Blood disorders: cold agglutinins, cryo-globulinaemia, hyperviscocity (polycythaemia).
- Drugs: oral contraceptive pill (OCP), beta-blockers.

Presentation

- 60-90% of sufferers are women, usually young (teens to 30s).
- Chronic paronychia, ulceration, gangrene of digits.
- Wrist pulses are normally present (if absent this suggests it is secondary to arterial disease).
- The neck must be examined to exclude a cervical rib.
- Can use Doppler USS to examine digits after cold provocation.

Investigations

A battery of tests are required to exclude secondary causes: FBC, U&Es, ESR, cryoglobulins, ANA, anti-mitochondrial antibodies, and anti-thyroid antibodies.

Treatment

- Cold avoidance.
- Stop smoking.
- Avoid beta-blockers and ergot-containing drugs.
- Vasodilatory drugs (thymoxamine, reserpine, methyldopa, prazocin, Ca^{2+} channel blockers, [e.g. nifedipine], prostacyclin, PGE1, stanozol, oxypentifylline, and the GTN transdermal patch).
- Cervical sympathectomy, which can either be thoracoscopic or open (provides transient benefit, as the disease tends to return within 1-2 years).

Complications

Complications of cervical sympathectomy include:

- Horner's syndrome. Unilateral pupillary constriction (due to the unopposed pupil dilatory effects of the parasympathetic nerve supply) called meiosis and unilateral anhydrosis, which is decreased sweating (due to interruption of the nerve supply of the sweat glands).
- Gustatory sweating. This is excessive facial sweating when eating foods that would normally cause salivation, e.g. spicy foods.
- Pneumothorax.
- Pleural effusion.
- Chylothorax. Damage to the thoracic duct, resulting in chyle, which is lymph fluid, leaking into the pleural cavity.
- Failure to eradicate, or later recurrence, of the Raynaud's disease.

Other arteriospastic conditions

Note

- All of these are rare, and are included here for interest only. It is worth knowing them, but it would be unusual to be examined on them.

Acrocyanosis

Precipitated by the cold, it affects arterioles (not digital arteries as in Raynaud's). It affects women who should therefore avoid the cold.

Erythrocyanosis frigida

Also known as Bazin's disease it affects healthy young women of stout build with fat hairless legs (yes, really, it does!). Cold weather precipitates painful blotches on the calves, which can ulcerate. The women affected should avoid the cold and lose weight. They can benefit from a lumbar sympathectomy.

Erythromelalgia

Painful, burning, red extremities. It is rare, affecting women more than men, and is worse in the summer months. It is thought to be due to abnormal release of the neurochemical, serotonin (5-HT). Treatment is empirical.

Livedo reticularis

Cyanotic blotchy patches on the lower limbs, which can ulcerate. Cold conditions can precipitate it.

Venous disease

Varicose veins (VV)

Saccular dilatations of veins, often tortuous.

Note

- Varicose veins come up frequently in clinical exams, as they are a common condition, surgically accessible, chronic, and have a number of themes related to them which can be questioned.

Sites of communication between deep and superficial venous systems (Figure 8.6)

- Saphenofemoral junction.
- Short saphenous popliteal junction.
- Thigh perforators (Hunter's canal).
- Medial calf perforators (Leonardo's vein).

♦ Gastrocnemius communicating veins (Cockett's vein).
♦ Lateral calf perforators.

Complications of varicose veins

This is a very common question in exams, so ignore this list at your peril!

♦ Haemorrhage.
♦ Superficial thrombosis.
♦ Lipodermatosclerosis.
♦ Venous eczema.
♦ Venous ulceration.

Aetiology of varicose veins

♦ Incidence of 2% of the population.
♦ The female to male ratio is 4:1.
♦ Incidence increases with age, female sex, obesity, occupation (standing for long periods), heredity.

Secondary causes of varicose veins

♦ Valve damage from previous thrombosis.
♦ Pelvic tumours.
♦ Congenital anomalies (including rare absence of valves).

Note

– Most varicose veins are of undetermined aetiology, i.e. none of the above (the author has often thought of the term 'idiopathic' to mean 'no idiot knows the pathology').

Pathology of varicose veins

The most frequently affected area is in the great saphenous distribution. Histologically, one sees a compensatory hypertrophy of the smooth muscle of the media is present in longstanding cases in association with fibrosis. These changes are characteristically patchy in nature. Macroscopically, the regions where the superficial and deep systems join are where problems start.

Blood travels from the superficial to deep systems along perforating veins, which contain valves. If these valves become incompetent (primary or secondary), backflow occurs causing superficial VVs.

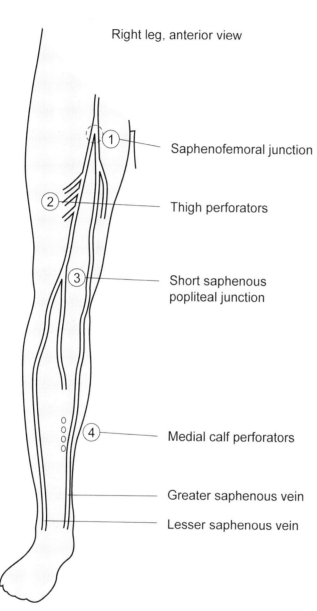

Right leg, anterior view

1 — Saphenofemoral junction

2 — Thigh perforators

3 — Short saphenous popliteal junction

4 — Medial calf perforators

Greater saphenous vein

Lesser saphenous vein

Figure 8.6. Sites of communication between deep and superficial venous systems.

Presentation

Patients present with either a complaint of the cosmetic appearance of the varicosities on their legs, or with an aching discomfort that can come on after periods of time standing.

Clinical examination of varicose veins

This is so likely to come up in clinical exams that it is advisable to become expert in the repeated practice of examination of varicose veins in the run up to exam time.

- Ask the patient to stand.
- Look for pigmentation, oedema, eczema, lipodermatosclerosis and ulceration.
- Look at both the front and back of the legs separately, to see the distribution of varicose veins (basically, the medial calf is the great saphenous distribution, the lateral calf is the small saphenous distribution).
- Feel for small saphenopopliteal incompetence in the popliteal fossa.
- Tap distally while palpating proximally for valvular incompetence. Valves would prevent transmission of the impulse, thus if the transmission is present, the valves must be incompetent.
- The same can be done for saphenofemoral incompetence (the SF junction is located one fingerbreadth medial to the femoral pulsation in the groin skin crease. It is an important definition as it is frequently asked).
- Perform the Trendelenberg test for valvular incompetence: raise the leg, which drains the veins, apply a tourniquet high and ask the patient to stand. If the varicose veins do not fill on standing (with the tourniquet on) this represents saphenofemoral incompetence. If, however, they do fill (despite the tourniquet), then the site of incompetence must be distal to the tourniquet. Releasing the tourniquet, in saphenofemoral incompetence, results in the

veins rapidly filling from above (the opposite of what would happen normally). Thus, it is possible to narrow down the exact location of the valve by repeating the test with incrementally lower tourniquet application, when saphenofemoral incompetence has been excluded.

Investigations

Varicose veins are for the most part a clinical diagnosis, and imaging of the veins themselves is not generally required. It must always be remembered that occasionally these varicosities will be secondary to a pelvic mass (the commonest being pregnancy or a pelvic tumour). It is usually only the history that gives a clue as to the presence of a pelvic mass (sensation of heaviness in the abdomen, change of bowel habit, menstrual/postmenopausal disorder, weight loss elsewhere but increase in abdominal girth). If a pelvic mass is suspected, the patient must be examined and a CT of the abdomen requested.

Treatment

There is variation in an individual surgeon's indications for varicose vein surgery, not simply varying with surgeon choice, but also with local healthcare provider protocols. Some surgeons do not operate for cosmetic reasons alone on varicose veins on the NHS, but some do. The indications for surgery can, therefore, be for cosmetic reasons alone, cosmetic and symptomatic, and purely for symptomatic reasons.

The gold standard operation is the high tie and venous stripping (see the section on varicose vein surgery in Chapter 4, Operative Surgery). More recently, foam injection sclerotherapy has proved itself, at the very least, as an interesting alternative to surgery for varicose veins. It does not have the long-term results of surgery yet, but early results are encouraging.

Complications

- Wound bleeding.
- Persistent wound serous ooze.
- Wound haematoma.
- Wound dehiscence.
- Wound infection.
- Painful scars.
- Recurrence of varicosities.
- Damage to saphenous or sural nerves (closely associated with the veins).

Venous ulcers

Presentation

Venous ulcers often present in patients who have chronic venous insufficiency after an episode of minor trauma in which the skin is broken. The minor wound fails to heal and goes on to form a chronic ulcer.

Note

- Lipodermatosclerosis is a descriptive term to describe the brown, thickened skin changes present in a significant proportion of patients with deep venous insufficiency, i.e. pigmentation and fibrosis.

It is in patients with deep venous insufficiency that ulcers tend to arise. Venous ulcers are terraced simple ulcers with gently sloping edges. These are differentiated from arterial ulcers, as these have a 'punched out' appearance.

Note

- Venous ulcers can undergo malignant change (known as Marjolin's ulcer).

Investigations

Investigation of venous ulcers is singularly unrewarding. Even surface swabs of ulcers do not provide particularly useful information, in that the results will invariably be returned as 'mixed flora'.

Treatment

Treatment is with the use of occlusive dressings - the Charing Cross four-layer compression dressing technique. Clean the ulcer once a week (50-70% heal in 2-3 months, 80-90% in 12 months). If it fails to heal it may need surgical undermining with or without skin grafting.

For episodes of obvious infection, i.e. cellulitis stemming from the ulcer, antibiotics are indicated. These can be oral if the patient is not overtly septic, otherwise they must be IV. Always remember to examine for any clinical evidence of abscess (e.g. fluctuance or leakage of pus), as this will likely require incision and drainage.

The actual aetiology by which venous disease results in skin ulceration/delayed healing has been the subject of much debate of the decades; there is as yet no agreed consensus. A popular theory of the day is that of the activated white cell effect. In this theory the chronic inflammation due to poor venous blood flow and fluid retention due to Starling's forces triggers the immune system to counterproductive effects resulting in poor wound healing and hence ulceration.

Complications

- Complications directly attributable to the bandaging are very rare. At most, because the bandages cover the ulcer(s), they can be accused of masking infection when in the early stages.

- Failure for the ulcer to resolve, which occurs in 10-20% of cases when the bandaging is used for 12 or more weeks.
- Surgical undermining/debridement of the ulcer(s) can be complicated by infection, bleeding, persistence of the ulcer and pain.

Factors affecting venous blood flow

The pumping of the heart establishes a pressure gradient between the arterial and venous systems. Additionally, on the venous side venous return is assisted by:

- Venomotor tone.
- Muscle pumps (calf).
- Respiratory movements.

Note

— Venous return is obviously impeded by gravity. Standing from a seated position causes the weight of a column of blood to act upon calf veins, the valves prevent backflow, the heart continues to pump, thus pressure continues to increase in the lower veins. When this pressure exceeds that beyond the valve immediately above it, then blood flows in the direction of the heart (this too, is a common exam question, in both clinical and viva exams).

Thrombotic events

Deep venous thrombosis (DVT)

Deep venous thrombosis (DVT) is relevant to surgical practice because it can lead to pulmonary embolism (PE), a potentially fatal condition if left unchecked, and also a post-phlebitic limb, which is a chronically swollen discoloured and frequently uncomfortable lower limb. It is important, therefore, to be aware of the risk factors for, and the means of, making the diagnosis of DVT, so that it can be treated, hopefully preventing these two sequelae.

Risk factors for DVT
- Previous DVT.
- Pelvic tumour.
- Obesity.
- Oral contraceptive pill (OCP).
- Clotting abnormality.
- Smoking.
- Cancer.
- Immobility.
- Abdominopelvic surgery.
- Any prolonged surgery.
- Increasing age.

The above may seem a long list, but the question is such a common one in exams that it is worth committing to memory.

Differential diagnosis of DVT
- Ruptured Baker's cyst.
- OA of the knee.
- Ruptured popliteal aneurysm.
- Knee haemarthrosis.
- Cellulitis.
- Ruptured tendo-achilles.
- Osteosarcoma.
- Lymphoedema.
- Ischaemic limb.
- Muscle strain.

Presentation

DVT presents with an uncomfortable swelling of the calf, unilaterally. It can be painless, but it is rarely bilateral (never say never, though). The calf can have a red colour, and occasionally mimic cellulitis, which is its major differential diagnosis.

Clinical examination is notoriously unreliable in making a definitive diagnosis of DVT. In fact, even experienced physicians have been shown to be wrong 50% of the time on clinical grounds alone. Examine for swelling, cellulitis, and tenderness on compression of the calf. Consider performing Homans' test, which is calf discomfort on passive dorsiflexion of the foot. Some feel there is a risk of precipitating embolism of the thrombus by performing this test, and this may come up in the discussion part of clinical or viva exams. The point is difficult to prove one way or the other, but in any case if the patient walked in on their own two feet, this is arguably more of a stimulus to embolism than performing a passive dorsiflexion of their foot.

Investigations

The true gold standard investigation for DVT is the venogram. This involves injection of a dye into a dorsal foot vein. This can be particularly difficult, not to mention uncomfortable, in a patient with an already swollen tender leg and foot. Fortunately, venous Doppler is also very effective at identifying DVTs, especially those in the popliteal vein and the more proximal veins. It has the advantage of being non-invasive and rapid.

A blood test to measure the D-Dimer levels can help in deciding whether thrombosis is present. The normal range for D-Dimers is 0-300ng/ml. If the patient has a normal D-Dimer level, a diagnosis of DVT can be confidently excluded. However, when the value exceeds 500 (different hospitals have different values for this threshold), then DVT is possible. Unfortunately, with a high result this is not very specific, i.e. it is quite possible for recent surgery or trauma to give a raised D-Dimer level and the same is true of infection, e.g. cellulitis.

The question may arise in exams as to what to do, in terms of treatment, if a DVT is suspected, but there is no immediate access to the relevant investigation tool. The answer is to give a treatment dose of low-molecular-weight heparin (LMWH) and continue giving it daily if necessary, until the investigation has confirmed or denied the diagnosis.

Treatment

DVT prophylaxis options
♦   Graduated stockings (thrombo-embolic deterrent stockings [TEDS]).

Note

—   The term 'graduated' refers to the fact that as the stocking becomes more proximal, the actual pressure that it exerts decreases gradually.

♦   Pneumatic calf compression devices.
♦   Intravenous heparin infusion.
♦   Subcutaneous LMWH, e.g. Fragmin, Clexane.

Note

—   Dextran 70*/antiplatelet agents/electrical calf stimulation can also be used, but these all have a lower efficacy.
—   Even with ideal prophylaxis, 5-20% of patients suffer DVT (depending on the type of surgery), and up to 0.2% suffer fatal PE.

*Dextran 70 is a special case in that it is effective in PE prophylaxis but not in DVT prophylaxis.

DVT treatment

Proven DVT is treated by an IV heparin infusion, using APTT to monitor the degree of anticoagulation (although this has unproven accuracy) or subcutaneous LMWH, whilst starting warfarin therapy (for six months), obviously stopping heparin when the INR is high enough (usually considered to be >2).

Note

—   The heparin infusion has been superseded by the advent of low-molecular-weight heparins (e.g. Fragmin), which can be used for treatment while waiting for the INR to be above 2. The advantages are that only one daily dose need be given and there is no need to check the APTR as with the heparin infusion.
—   Sometimes an IVC filter is indicated for the prevention of PE in a patient with DVT, e.g. recent haemorrhagic CVA, acute bleeding duodenal ulcer, etc., as anticoagulation is contraindicated in these patients. Another indication is recurrent PE, despite adequate anticoagulation.

Complications
♦   The major complication of all prophylactic treatments for DVT is that they reduce, but do not eradicate, the risk of suffering a DVT.
♦   Anticoagulant treatments risk operative or postoperative bleeding, i.e. persistent bleeding, haematoma or haemarthrosis, depending on the type of surgery in question.

- Heparin and related compounds can (rarely) cause thrombocytopaenia, termed heparin-induced thrombocytopaenia (HIT).
- Over-anticoagulation, particularly with reference to warfarin treatment for established DVT/PE, can risk bleeding complications, e.g. cerebral bleed, spontaneous haemarthrosis, pretibial haematomas, gastrointestinal bleeds, etc.

Axillary or subclavian vein thrombosis

Originally described by Sir James Paget in 1875. It occurs more commonly in the right arm, particularly after a bout of severe exercise (hence the nick-name 'effort thrombosis'). There is an association with a cervical rib (but not invariably so). It usually presents late in the age range of 35-45 years.

Presentation
Cool, swollen and blue forearm, diminished finger movements and distended subcutaneous veins, visible over the shoulder and chest.

Investigations
- Duplex Doppler.
- Angiography.
- Chest X-ray.

Treatment
If it presents early, treatment is by chemical thrombolysis (e.g. streptokinase), thrombectomy, angioplasty or stent placement. Late presentation is treated by anticoagulation as for DVT (it is effectively a DVT of the upper limb).

Complications
Complications of thrombolysis:

- Puncture site problems, i.e. haematoma, femoral artery pseudoaneurysm formation, arteriovenous fistula formation.
- Bleeding complications, i.e. intracerebral haemorrhage, or bleeding elsewhere.
- Reperfusion compartment syndrome of the limb (requires urgent fasciotomy).

Complications of angioplasty, thrombectomy, or stent placement are:

- Puncture site problems, i.e. haematoma, femoral artery pseudoaneurysm formation, arteriovenous fistula formation.
- Problems related to the artery containing the thrombus, i.e. arterial dissection, or dislodgement of the clot which goes on to embolise further downstream.
- Reperfusion compartment syndrome of the limb (requires urgent fasciotomy).
- Occlusion of the stent by re-accumulation of thrombus.
- Stent infection.

Superior vena cava thrombosis

This is associated with bronchial cancer, retrosternal goitre, mediastinal tumours, thymomas, lymphomas, constrictive pericarditis and mediastinal fibrosis. Patients present with swelling of the face and neck, and shortness of breath.

Presentation
The head and neck are suffused and cyanosed, with distended neck veins (which do not collapse on elevation or with respiration).

Investigations
- Chest X-ray or CT may show the mass which precipitated it.
- Bilateral brachial vein injection of contrast shows the extent of the obstruction.

Treatment
- Radiotherapy to the tumour to shrink it.
- Thrombolysis, angioplasty, or stenting.

Complications
Complications of thrombolysis, angioplasty, thrombectomy, or stent placement are as for axillary or subclavian vein thrombosis above.

Inferior vena cava leiomyomas

Presentation
- Rare.
- Patients present with symptoms and signs of venous obstruction.
- Sometimes palpable as a mass.

Investigations
- MRI shows the soft tissue anatomy of the tumour and any local spread (suggestive of malignant change to a leiomyosarcoma).
- Angiography shows the lumen of the vena cava and the degree of indentation from the tumour.
- CT can be useful in showing any bony invasion (e.g. into the vertebrae), again suggestive of malignant change.
- Abdominal USS gives less information than CT or MRI, but often forms part of the work-up when the diagnosis has not yet been made. It identifies an intra-abdominal mass, leading to further investigations.

Treatment
Resection and vessel reconstruction.

Complications
- Graft occlusion.
- Graft infection (this is more likely in prosthetic than vein grafts, as they are effectively a foreign body).
- Vessel stenosis, late.
- Distal embolism.
- Amputation.

Chapter 9

Ear, nose and throat surgery

Diseases of the external auditory meatus

A summary of the basic conditions of the external auditory meatus is as follows:

- Wax.
- Otitis externa.
- Otomycosis.
- Furunculosis.
- Exostoses.
- Tumours.

Wax excess

Presentation

It is normal to produce wax in the external ear canal and there is a normal distribution of the quantity of wax produced by different individuals. Even large quantities of wax produced, if they do not cause symptoms, do not require treatment. Symptoms that can result from a build up of wax in the ear are hearing loss and an odd sensation in the ear. Occasionally tinnitus can occur if hearing is affected.

Investigations

Otoscopic examination.

Treatment

Treatment is by syringing the wax which may be softened beforehand using oil drops, or microsuction with proper equipment and expertise, due to the risk of damaging the drum.

Complications

Perforation of the drum, when syringing.

Otitis externa

A generalised infection which can involve the whole of the skin of the external canal, in one or both ears.

Hot, humid climates predispose to the condition, as do dust and other irritants and atopic skin types. The most common predisposing environmental factors in the UK are swimming pools and bathwater. Chronic underlying middle ear infection should be excluded in otitis externa.

Presentation

Inflamed bilateral external ears, which are painful and weeping. There is usually no marked hearing loss.

Note

- If the discharge is mucoid, this implies a tympanic membrane perforation as there are no mucus glands in the external ear canal (only ceruminous, i.e. wax producing).

Investigations

Generally, clinical examination and history are really all that is needed to make the diagnosis. A swab can help to identify the organism in recurrent (or fungal) infections, and a CT can help diagnose deep spread (otitis media) if it is suspected.

Treatment

Treatment for otitis externa is as follows:

- Microsuction. Where there exists doubt as to the presence of a tympanic perforation, it is wise to consider the use of ciprofloxacin drops, instead of the usual Gentisone, as Gentisone is potentially ototoxic. (Of note, is that in the UK ciprofloxacin drops are in fact eyedrops, and are not licensed for use in the ear, although they are commonly used as such, and work well.)
- Combined antibiotic and steroid drops (e.g. Sofradex or Gentisone HC).
- Analgesia.

Complications
- Persistent infection.
- Recurrent infection.
- Allergic reaction to eardrops.
- Spread of infection to the middle ear (otitis media).

Otomycosis

Presentation

Otomycosis is fungal otitis externa. It is caused by *Aspergillus albicans*, *Aspergillus niger* or Candida, producing fungal colonies which are white, brown or black.

Investigations

Simple examination of the external auditory meatus with an otoscope is all that is needed.

Treatment

Treatment is with microsuction plus a topical antifungal, e.g. clotrimazole drops, continued for two weeks, otherwise there is a risk of recurrence.

Complications
- Persistent infection.
- Recurrent infection.

- Allergic reaction to eardrops.
- Spread of infection to the middle ear (otitis media).

Furunculosis

Presentation

A furuncle on any part of the body is an infection of a hair follicle; it is no different in the external auditory meatus. Furunculosis can only affect skin at the outer part of the meatus, as there is no hair in the inner part. A pustule forms and the surrounding skin becomes acutely inflamed, swollen and tender. An anterior furuncle results in tissue in front of the tragus becoming inflamed; however, a posterior furuncle may result in the mastoid area of skin becoming inflamed. The meatus can close off resulting in hearing loss.

Note

— In furunculosis, the drum is unaffected. It is the physical obstruction to soundwave progression that causes hearing loss.

Investigations
- Clinical examination and history are all that is needed to make the diagnosis.
- A swab for MC+S can help with identifying the organism in recurrent (or fungal) infections.
- Rarely is imaging indicated unless there is a suspicion of deep spread, e.g. causing otitis media, in which case a CT can be helpful.

Treatment

Treatment for furunculosis is as follows:

- Analgesia.
- If very severe, a broad spectrum antibiotic is required.
- Regular microsuction.
- This is followed by insertion of gauze soaked in ichthammol and glycerine.

Note

— The idea is to keep the meatus rigorously clean, otherwise there is a risk of recurrence.

Complications

◆ Persistent infection.
◆ Recurrent infection.
◆ Allergic reaction to the eardrops.

Exostoses

Presentation

Exostoses are overgrowths of the bony meatus and are common in swimmers. They rarely cause sufficient symptoms to warrant surgical treatment, but if they grow to sufficient size they can obstruct the external auditory meatus, causing recurrent infections due to moisture retention and build-up of squamous debris.

Investigations

Clinical appearance with the otoscope.

Treatment

Burring of the excess bone, termed a 'canalplasty' effectively treats this condition. It is only indicated in symptomatic exostoses. Care is taken to protect the tympanic membrane which is easily damaged in this type of surgery. Occasionally small skin grafts are needed if a broad surface has been exposed by the burr.

Complications

◆ Tympanic membrane rupture.
◆ Infection (otitis externa).
◆ Recurrence, especially if the patient continues swimming frequently.

Tumours of the auditory meatus

These are rarer than tumours of the pinna. Extensive knowledge is not required for examination purposes. Malignant polyps of the middle ear origin can present when they extrude from the meatus. Treatment is by subtotal or total petrosectomy with or without radiotherapy.

Acute mastoiditis

This is now quite rare in the West. It is a complication of acute otitis media and is more common in children than adults. It is the result of extension of infection into the mastoid process.

Presentation

Pain, discharge, high temperature, high pulse rate, hearing loss, tenderness over the mastoid area, oedema over the mastoid area and a perforated drum membrane with visible pus.

Differential diagnosis

It may be difficult to tell between furunculosis, otitis externa and erysipelas, which is an acute streptococcal infection. All have pain, discharge and swelling, and there may be hearing loss.

Note

— Both otitis externa and furunculosis may coexist with otitis media.

Investigations

X-ray of the mastoid region is required, as it shows clouding of the affected cells.

Note

— Full resolution needs to be ensured before stopping antibiotic treatment. This means a return to normal hearing. If any doubt exists, the patient will need surgical treatment, otherwise there is a risk of persistent masked mastoiditis.

Treatment

If treated early, antibiotics can work; if treated later, a cortical mastoidectomy is required to drain the pus.

Complications

◆ Extension of the infection to local anatomic structures.
◆ Hearing loss. This can be conductive, due to the presence of pus or inflammatory liquid in the internal auditory canal, or rarely, sensorineural due to inflammation of the inner ear.

- Chronic osteomyelitis.
- Abscess formation. This can be cerebral, or extend superficially as a subperiosteal abscess, or can be in any of the meningeal layers, and can also result in meningitis.
- Facial nerve palsy. From inflammation in the middle ear and mastoid. N.B. Chronic ear disease is the commonest cause of brain abscess.

The tonsils

Anatomy of the oropharynx

The oropharynx extends from the soft palate to the epiglottis. The fauces at the back of the oropharynx are called palatopharyngeal and palatoglossal arches. The tonsils are, strictly speaking, called the palatine tonsils, because of the lingular tonsils which are in the posterior region of the tongue.

The blood supply is via the palatine branch of the facial artery. Venous drainage is in the form of a plexus, but there is a large vein called the palatine vein, which can bleed a great deal post-tonsillectomy.

Nerve supply is via the tonsillar branch of the glossopharyngeal nerve. Lymph drainage is to the deep cervical nodes.

Acute tonsillitis

A generalised inflammation of the tonsils, with an associated inflammation of the fauces and pharynx. The cause can be bacterial, viral or a combination of both. Causative bacteria are Staphylococcus, Streptococcus and *Haemophilus influenzae*.

Note

- Beta-haemolytic Streptococcus can be responsible for tonsillitis, as well as an associated glomerulonephritis.

The causative viruses are rhinovirus, adenovirus and enterovirus.

Presentation
Sore throat, pain on swallowing, excess secretions, enlarged cervical glands, fever, malaise and headache.

Note

- There can be an associated mesenteric adenitis in children.

The tonsils appear enlarged, reddened, follicular, pustular (tends to occur in bacterial tonsillitis) and oedematous, with a thickened pharyngeal wall.

Differential diagnosis
Glandular fever and Vincent's angina. Look out for a background of AIDS in recurrent tonsillitis.

Investigations
Simple inspection with adequate lighting is all that is required to make the diagnosis.

Treatment
Relative indications for tonsillectomy are:

- Repeated attacks of tonsillitis.
- Peritonsillar abscess (quinsy).

Absolute indications for tonsillectomy are:

- Sleep apnoea syndrome, if this is due to tonsillar size.
- For histology if malignancy is suspected.

The most common technique nowadays is by blunt dissection (blunt with ties, or with bipolar diathermy).

Complications
- Referred ear pain (very common) is frequently misdiagnosed as infection, due to innervation of the throat and part of the ear by the glossopharyngeal nerve.
- Membrane over the tonsillar bed, frequently misdiagnosed as infection.
- Primary haemorrhage. Within 24 hours postoperatively, by definition, but commonly occurs within the first 12 hours. It is due to inadequate or incomplete haemostasis at the time of surgery.

◆ Secondary haemorrhage. Greater than 24 hours postoperatively, by definition, but is usually 5-10 days postoperatively. A membrane develops over the operated site which on sloughing off, results in a bleed.

◆ Sepsis.

Note

— Both primary and secondary haemorrhages are serious, potentially life-threatening, events. Both need haemostasis by direct pressure with pads (hydrogen peroxide or adrenaline soaked), or by ligation under local or general anaesthetic. If left too long, haemorrhage can be fatal.

Quinsy (peritonsillar abscess)

Presentation
This is a complication of acute tonsillitis. The patient is febrile, toxic and unwell, with throat pain, and has difficulty swallowing. The patient may have trismus, spasm of the masseter muscle, making it hard to open the mouth.

Investigations
Simple inspection with adequate lighting is all that is required to make the diagnosis.

Treatment
If treatment is early, soothing gargles and high-dose antibiotics are given. If treatment is late, the abscess needs laying open by lancing or aspiration, usually under local anaesthetic. Definitive treatment can often be done as a 'hot' tonsillectomy (less so in the UK than elsewhere in the world for fear of increased bleeding risk).

Complications
◆ Bleeding, rarely heavy, due to inadvertent perforation of a superficial vessel whilst lancing the abscess.
◆ Recurrence, either due to inadequate technique (missed it), or simple re-accumulation of the abscess.
◆ Systemic sepsis can occur if the abscess is inadequately drained and worsens.

Note

— Lingular tonsils can develop lingular tonsillitis, but this is rarely a problem.

Sinuses

Sinusitis

The sinuses are the maxillary, ethmoidal, sphenoidal and frontal. Sinusitis (meaning an inflammation of the sinus) can affect any of these, e.g. maxillary sinusitis.

Presentation
Following an upper respiratory tract infection (URTI), the patient complains of pain over the cheek (the maxillary sinus is the most commonly affected), which radiates to the frontal region or teeth. The pain is increased by straining or leaning down. A purulent discharge may be absent initially due to obstruction of the natural ostium. The sense of smell is often affected (anosmia), and there is a general malaise and mild pyrexia. Nasal obstruction and rhinorrhoea (anterior or posterior) are usually present.

Aetiology
From an URTI, dental infection or trauma. It can be bacterial or viral. Common organisms are *Streptococcus pneumoniae* and *Haemophilus influenzae*.

Investigations
◆ X-ray may show the fluid level, mucosal thickening and opacification.
◆ A CT scan shows inflammation and fluid in the sinuses with great accuracy, and is particularly useful in imaging chronic sinusitis. It is not, however, necessary to perform a CT scan on someone with an obvious clinical diagnosis of sinusitis.

Complications of maxillary sinusitis
Complications are unusual and include:

◆ Cellulitis.
◆ Osteitis.
◆ Orbital cellulitis.

Treatment

Simple

Treatment includes conservative analgesia, antibiotics (clarithromycin) and decongestant drops.

Recurrent

Surgical treatment includes sinus drainage, meatal antrostomy (middle), functional endoscopic sinus surgery (FESS).

Frontoethmoidal sinusitis

This has the same aetiology, presentation, microbiology, and treatment, but there are different, more serious, complications (due to its anatomical relations). These include orbital cellulitis, eyelid abscess and intracranial sepsis (extradural abscess, subdural abscess, intra-cerebral abscess, meningitis, encephalitis, osteomyelitis).

Treatment

Treatment is now mainly performed by FESS, i.e. using endoscopic means to resect the inflamed sinus tissue and bone.

Complications of sinus surgery

- CSF leak (ethmoidal sinusitis, NOT maxillary). Test the clear fluid nasal discharge for glucose with a conventional dipstick. CSF contains glucose; normal nasal discharge does not.
- Optic nerve damage (ethmoidal sinusitis, NOT maxillary) and, hence, permanent monocular blindness.
- Nasolacrimal duct stenosis.
- Orbital haematoma.

Facial paralysis

Note

- The facial nerve supplies motor innervation to the muscles of facial expression.

Presentation

Facial nerve paralysis is eponymously named Bell's palsy. This is a palsy originating from the intracranial portion of the facial nerve. The importance of this fact is that it has not yet branched out, i.e. all the functions of the facial nerve are affected (not just a unilateral face drop). Patients present with a unilateral face drop, a unilateral inability to close their eye, and a reduced ability to taste. However, tongue movements (trigeminal) and facial sensation (trigeminal) are unaffected. There may be a small area of sensory loss near the ear.

The facial nerve supplies innervation of the sense of taste to the anterior two thirds of the tongue via the chorda tympani. It also innervates the submandibular and sublingual salivary glands, and the lacrimal glands. It has a branch to the eardrum, and a branch to stapedius and to the chorda tympani (a sensory branch of the facial nerve).

The facial nerve emerges from the skull onto the face through the stylomastoid foramen near the origin of the digastric muscle.

Branches of the facial nerve are as follows:

- Temporal.
- Zygomatic.
- Buccal.
- Mandibular.
- Cervical.

Note

- Remember the mnemonic: 'T'wo 'Z'ulus 'B'ullied 'M'y 'C'at for these branches.
- An upper motor neurone palsy of the facial nerve results in the forehead being spared and muscle tone being preserved, as each individual nerve branches late to supply the contralateral half of the frontalis muscle.

Other facial paralysis causes can be divided into intra- and extratemporal.

Intratemporal causes of facial paralysis

- Chronic ear disease.
- Fracture of the temporal bone.
- Postoperative trauma.

- Ramsay Hunt syndrome. *Herpes zoster* reactivation. A herpes rash (i.e. vesicular) is present on the skin and in the external auditory meatus. There is pain and paralysis in the facial nerve distribution. It can also affect the 8th cranial (vestibulocochlear) nerve, causing nausea and vomiting, dizziness and nystagmus.
- Idiopathic: Bell's palsy. There is currently some evidence that *Herpes simplex* may be a possible aetiological agent in Bell's palsy. Treatment is with prednisolone and acyclovir.
- Secondary to a mass, e.g. acoustic neuroma.

Extratemporal causes of facial paralysis

- Trauma (direct or surgical).
- External compression from a tumour, e.g. parotid.

Note

- Facial paralysis can result in loss of the blink mechanism and, therefore, there is a risk of corneal abrasion. The patient may need artificial tears, lateral tarsorrhaphy, with or without injection of botulinum toxin into levator palpebrae superioris to produce transient ptosis.
- It is possible to tape the eye closed as a temporary measure.

Investigations

- The key investigation is, in fact, a careful examination of the cranial nerves, ear and parotid gland: the cranial nerves to accurately identify which nerves are affected, or even if the lesion is central rather than a peripheral nerve in origin; the ear for any evidence of herpetic rash; and the parotid for any evidence of tumour which, if it has affected facial nerve function, is very likely malignant.
- Imaging is not usually required except when there is a suspicion of a compressive lesion, e.g. tumour, or a form of stroke, in which case a CT can be of use.
- EMG studies of the facial nerve are possible, but are rarely performed.

Treatment

Treatment is with prednisolone, acyclovir (for ten days) and eye care, to prevent corneal abrasion as a result of the inability to fully close the eye.

Note

- Acyclovir is frequently used in the treatment of Bell's palsy, although there remains little convincing evidence of its efficacy.

Complications

- Incomplete resolution of the facial paralysis. This occurs in a small proportion of patients. With or without treatment, the majority resolve without incident.
- Persistent altered or absent taste.

Oropharyngeal malignancy

Eighty percent are epithelial (squamous), 15% are lymphomas, and 5% are miscellaneous squamous cell carcinomas (SCCs). The majority present on the tonsil, then a smaller proportion on the posterior third of the tongue, and the rest elsewhere in the oropharynx.

Presentation

Oropharyngeal malignancies can present incidentally, e.g. a lump noticed by an anaesthetist or dentist, that had not caused any symptoms previously. They can cause symptoms such as pain, ulceration and bleeding, dysphagia (difficulty swallowing), referred pain such as otalgia (pain felt in the ear in the glossopharyneal nerve distribution), or 'hot potato speech'.

Investigations

- Routine blood testing (FBC, U+Es, LFTs, ESR, CRP).
- Chest X-ray, looking for any pulmonary metastases.

◆ CT of the soft tissues of the neck delineates the anatomical relations and the presence of local spread or metastasis of the tumour(s).

◆ Biopsy is required for tissue diagnosis (not all oropharyngeal tumours are malignant and, hence, the management can differ significantly based on knowledge of the histology).

Staging

◆ I. Tumour <2cm.
◆ II. Tumour >2cm.
◆ III. Tumour >4cm.
◆ IV. Tumour with a deep invasion, fixed nodes or metastasis.

Treatment

Surgical resection followed by radiotherapy forms the mainstay of treatment for oropharyngeal malignancies. If the tumour is unresectable, then there are chemotherapy regimes available for treatment. The greater the stage the worse the prognosis is after surgery. Stage I has a 90% five-year survival after resection and radiotherapy, whereas Stage IV has only 30%.

Complications

◆ Infection.
◆ Fistula formation.
◆ Postoperative pain, which can become persistent, even long term.
◆ Dysphagia, which can also become persistent.
◆ Pneumonia, e.g. due to aspiration of wound secreta.

Nasopharyngeal carcinoma

This is rare in the UK, but in China it covers 21% of all malignancies. The aetiology is uncertain, but it may involve the Epstein-Barr virus (EBV), as well as having a genetic and environmental predisposition. The male to female ratio is 4:1.

Presentation

Its presentation includes nasal blockage, cranial nerve palsy, sanguinous rhinorrhoea, sometimes frank epistaxis, referred otalgia, conductive hearing loss due to persistent unilateral middle ear effusion, and unexplained cervical lymphadenopathy in the posterior triangle.

Investigations

◆ Examinaion of the nasopharynx under GA.
◆ Plain X-ray of the skull.
◆ CT/MRI.
◆ Examination of the neck for cervical lymphadenopathy.
◆ Biopsy. This gives a tissue diagnosis, confirming malignancy, enabling the oncologist to select appropriate chemoradiotherapy combinations.

Treatment

Standard treatment is radiotherapy alone, for early disease. However, for advanced disease, a combination of chemotherapy and radiotherapy is required. Unfortunately these tumours tend to present late, which invariably means there is already local invasion or metastatic spread at the time of presentation.

Note

— When examining the nasopharynx under general anaesthetic, biopsies must be taken even if nothing is seen, as they may be positive.

Complications

Complications can be attributed to chemotherapy or radiotherapy:

◆ Neutropaenic sepsis (chemotherapy).
◆ Nephrotoxicity (chemotherapy).
◆ Local damage to head and neck structures (radiotherapy), e.g. spinal cord, neck musculature (fibrosis), jaw (trismus, i.e. painful

restriction of the ability to open the mouth),
dental damage.

♦ There is a risk of incomplete treatment of the
tumour, late recurrence or the development of a
'second primary' later.

The salivary gland

Differential diagnosis of parotid gland swellings

Swelling of whole parotid gland
♦ Acute sialadenitis (inflamed salivary gland).
♦ Chronic recurrent sialadenitis.
♦ Sialolithiasis (salivary gland stone).
♦ Sjögren's disease (autoimmune disease of the
exocrine glands, particularly the lacrimal and
salivary glands in this context).
♦ HIV salivary gland disease.
♦ Sialosis (idiopathic swelling of salivary glands).
♦ Sarcoidosis.

Swelling of discrete areas of the parotid gland
♦ Tumours (benign or malignant).
♦ Parotid LN enlargement.
♦ Facial nerve neuroma.
♦ Temporal artery aneurysm.

Extra parotid swellings mimicking parotid swellings
♦ Lipoma.
♦ Dental infection.
♦ Masseter muscle hypertrophy.
♦ Winged mandible.
♦ Transverse process of axis/atlas.
♦ Infratemporal fossa tumours.
♦ Pharyngeal tumours.

Parotid trauma
Classified in three parts:

♦ A. Injury to the parotid parenchyma only.
♦ B. Injury to the duct overlying the masseter
muscle.
♦ C. Injury to the duct distal to the masseter
muscle.

Note
— Parenchymal and duct injuries can result in
cutaneous fistulae. Parenchymal injuries heal
spontaneously, but in duct injuries fistulae
can persist.
— The point of the classification is that Type A
injuries can be managed conservatively,
Type B by primary anastomosis of the duct,
and Type C by transecting the duct at the
site of injury and reimplanting it in the mouth.
— A possible complication of duct injury is a
sialocoele, which is an extravasation of saliva
into the parenchyma.

Acute suppurative sialadenitis

Presentation
This is infection of a salivary gland which can affect
either the parotid or submandibular gland. It is more
common in the submandibular gland because its
secretions are more viscous and, hence, more prone
to stasis.

The aetiology is salivary stasis, secondary to stone
obstruction, duct stenosis or decreased production.
An ascending bacterial infection follows, leading to
suppuration, i.e. the production of pus. The bacteria
involved are *Staphylococcus aureus*, *Streptococcus
pneumoniae*, *Escherichia coli* and *Haemophilus
influenzae*.

Predisposing factors are:

♦ Poor oral hygeine.
♦ Dehydration.

Note
— Mumps is the commonest childhood cause
of bilateral parotid swelling.

Look for pus in the submandibular or parotid
region. Feel for any evidence of stones in either gland,
as this is a risk factor. Palpate for tenderness in either
gland and feel for any swelling and neck
lymphadenopathy.

Investigations

♦ If the patient is displaying any evidence of systemic sepsis, then screening blood tests are of use (FBC, U+Es, CRP, ESR and blood cultures).

♦ Swab the pus for MC+S.

♦ Imaging studies available:
- plain X-ray, which shows presence of stones (80% salivary gland stones are radiopaque);
- sialogram. Injection of contrast into the salivary ducts, which shows if one or more is blocked. This is contraindicated in obstruction;
- CT will show stones, but not ductal anatomy, unless it is combined with a sialogram;
- USS helps differentiate between cystic or solid lesions.

Treatment

Most cases of acute suppurative sialadenitis respond to non-operative treatment, i.e. ensuring the patient is well hydrated and using warm compresses and oral antibiotics (unless systemically unwell, in which case IV antibiotics and fluids are indicated).

If non-operative treatment fails or a large abscess is clearly visible, then incision and drainage is indicated. In cases of recurrent acute suppurative sialadenitis, argument exists as whether to excise the affected gland to prevent further recurrence.

The presence of salivary stone(s) warrants stone excision, either by direct incision, or cannulation of the gland and 'flushing' it out.

Complications

♦ Recurrent infection.
♦ Recurrent abscess.
♦ Bleeding.
♦ Chronically inflamed salivary gland, requiring excision if persistent.

Viral parotitis

This is the commonest teenage cause of parotid swelling.

Presentation

There is discomfort in the parotid region, a severe increase in pain on eating (due to increased secretion of saliva), pyrexia, toxaemia, trismus and cervical lymphadenopathy.

Investigations

♦ Raised WCC, ESR and CRP.
♦ X-ray is usually done, although it is mostly radiolucent. A sialography should never be performed during acute illness.

Note

— TB can cause parotitis.

Treatment

Treatment is with broad-spectrum beta-lactam-resistant antibiotics (e.g. Augmentin), analgesia and mouth washes. Surgery may be needed if the antibiotics fail after 48-72 hours, but ultrasound-guided drainage is sometimes successful.

Complications

♦ Complications of antibiotic treatment are allergy, nausea and vomiting, and potential failure of treatment.
♦ Complications of surgical drainage of the parotid gland are infection, bleeding and fistula formation.

Sialolithiasis

Sialolithiasis is the formation of stones (crystal deposition) in the salivary gland or ducts. This is much more common in the submandibular gland than the parotid gland, because the viscosity of saliva is higher in the submandibular gland, and it usually appears in the 40-50 year age group. It is slightly more common in men than women.

Predisposing factors are:

♦ Reduced salivary flow.
♦ Duct obstruction.
♦ Changes in salivary pH.
♦ Dehydration.

The stone is composed of organic material centrally with calcium salts, phosphates, carbon, ammonium and magnesium.

Note

— People with gout can get uric acid stones.

The submandibular gland has a higher pH and mucus content, and a greater concentration of Ca and PO$_4$ and, therefore, stones are more common here, than in the parotid gland.

Presentation
This depends on the location of the stone. In the parenchyma they can be asymptomatic, but ductal stones present with pain, which is worse on eating.

Note

— Stones can lead to sialadenitis. Sialadenitis is a condition of inflammation of the salivary gland, which can either be acute or chronic. It does not represent infection.

Investigations
♦ Plain X-ray shows the presence of stones (80% of salivary gland stones are radiopaque, but only 30-35% of parotid stones are radiopaque).
♦ Sialogram. Injection of contrast into the salivary gland, which then concentrates in the ducts showing their anatomy, and if one or more is blocked. This is contraindicated in acute infection.
♦ CT will show stones, but not ductal anatomy, unless it is combined with a sialogram.
♦ USS helps to differentiate between cystic or solid lesions.

Treatment

Submandibular
Distal ductal stones can be removed intra-orally; however, gland excision is required if stones are in the proximal duct.

Parotid
Treatment is by duct meatotomy intra-orally if the stones are within 1cm of Stensen's duct (the eponym for the parotid duct). However, if the stones are more proximal, an external incision is required, first identifying branches of the facial nerve.

Note

— A new treatment is the use of specially designed lithotriptors.

Complications
♦ Infection.
♦ Abscess formation.
♦ Bleeding.
♦ Recurrent stone formation.
♦ Chronic inflamed salivary gland, which can require excision if persistent.

Sjögren's disease

Presentation
This is autoimmune damage to the salivary and lacrimal glands, presenting with dry eyes, known as 'sicca' and a dry mouth, with difficulty masticating and swallowing. It is often associated with arthritis.

Sjögren's disease tends to affect the parotid gland more than the other salivary glands, but is capable of causing sialadenitis in any of them.

Investigations
This is a medical (rather than surgical) condition, and the diagnosis is made on the basis of biopsy of the salivary glands (the small ones of the lip often suffice), as well as by serum antibodies (technically auto-antibodies, i.e. circulating antibodies that target the patient's own cells, in this case those of glandular tissue).

Treatment
Treatment of some of the symptoms of Sjögren's disease mentioned here (relating to ENT) offer symptomatic relief in the form of artificial tears, encouraging saliva secretion (e.g. chewing gum) and taking frequent sips of water. There are artificial saliva products available for severe oral symptoms and saline nasal sprays. Good oral hygiene is to be encouraged.

It is rare to have to perform any surgery for Sjögren's disease. Occasionally, recurrent sialadenitis necessitates gland excision.

Complications

Complications of symptomatic treatment are mainly related to times when they are ineffective, through complications of the disease itself, i.e. dry eyes resulting in corneal abrasions, poor oral hygiene resulting in recurrent sialadenitis, dental caries or gingival abscesses.

Salivary gland tumours

Eighty percent are parotid, 10% are submandibular and 10% are in the minor salivary glands (palatal). Benign tumours are more common than malignant. The benign: malignant ratios are as follows:

◆ Parotid 4:1.
◆ Submandibular 2:1.
◆ Palatal 1:1.

Hence, a tumour in a palatal gland is much more likely to be malignant than one in a parotid gland. The only known risk factor for salivary gland tumours is radiation. The most common malignancies are muco-epidermoid, followed by adenoid cystic carcinoma.

Benign salivary gland tumours

The most common tumour is the pleomorphic adenoma.

Presentation

A slow-growing, painless unilateral swelling, with a slightly irregular feel. It does not cause cranial nerve neuropathy; malignancy is suspected if this is present. Diagnosis is made by fine needle aspiration (FNA) and MRI.

Investigations

◆ A tissue diagnosis is vital in determining whether the tumour is benign or malignant. Therefore, a biopsy (e.g. FNA) is mandatory.
◆ Imaging takes the form of either a CT or MRI scan.

Treatment

Treatment is by superficial parotidectomy or full parotidectomy, depending on the location and size of the tumour or excision of the submandibular gland.

Note

— Very longstanding pleomorphic adenomas (benign tumours) may undergo malignant change but this is rare.

Complications

◆ Tumour recurrence tends to occur because of incomplete excision of the tumour margins.
◆ The parotid gland contains the facial nerve, so facial nerve paresis may occur postoperatively, although it often resolves with time. However, permanent damage to the facial nerve can occur.
◆ Salivary fistula formation (rare and self-limiting).
◆ Gustatory sweating (Frey's syndrome) can be treated with topical antiperspirants.
◆ Infection or abscess formation.
◆ Bleeding.

Malignant salivary gland tumours

This is uncommon (1-2 in 100,000). It is more common in women in the 40-60 year age group. The only known risk factor is radiation exposure. Histologic grade determines the aggressiveness of the tumour's behaviour.

The most common malignant tumours are the muco-epidermoid and adenoid cystic tumour. The muco-epidermoid is more common in the parotid gland.

Adenoid cystic tumours arise most frequently in the parotid glands. However, in the submandibular glands they represent a higher proportion of all neoplasms (~20%). They are the most common malignant tumour of minor salivary glands.

Note

— Lymphomas can occur in the parotid LNs and *de novo* in the gland, although this is rarer.

Presentation

Usually presents as a painless mass within the substance of the gland (as opposed to generalised swelling of the gland), but there can be pain.

The presence of a nerve palsy (e.g. facial nerve in a parotid tumour) is highly suggestive of malignancy.

Investigations

- Again, a tissue diagnosis is vital. FNA biopsy is indicated. USS guidance can be helpful.
- CT or MRI imaging are both excellent at identifying tumour location, invasion and other features.
- USS scans are helpful in guiding biopsy providing detailed information, compared with CT or MRI, but they are particularly useful in identifying solid or cystic masses.

Treatment

Treatment is by excision with a generous margin of healthy tissue, or excision of the entire gland. An attempt should be made to spare the facial nerve in the parotid, but if it is invaded it requires excision. There is always the option of postoperative radiotherapy if the tumour is close to, but not invading, the nerve.

Note

— The parotid gland contains (from superficial to deep) the facial nerve, retromandibular vein and external carotid artery (which is the source of arterial blood to the gland). The nerve supply is from the otic ganglion.

Note

— The floor of the mouth is made up of the mylohyoid muscle in two halves meeting in a central raphe. It is the base on which the tongue muscles are fixed.

Complications

The complications of parotidectomy for malignancy are in fact the same as for benign tumours, as listed on the previous page.

Swallowed foreign body

Presentation

Foreign bodies can cause problems by virtue of their size causing obstruction called a 'swallowed food bolus', or as a result of their shape, specifically if they are sharp, i.e. swallowed sharp foreign bodies. The history will show swallowed meat or a fish bone (young children swallow anything!) with subsequent dysphagia.

In cases of obstruction (with swallowed food bolus, which generally gets caught at the level of the cricopharyngeus), the patient presents with drooling (inability to swallow their own saliva) and if given a glass of water to drink, they immediately regurgitate it.

In the case of a swallowed sharp foreign body, patients present with pain on swallowing. This symptom does not, however, differentiate between a sharp foreign body that is stuck in the orophaynx or one that has caused a superficial mucosal laceration, but has already passed. To be sure of the diagnosis a quick endoscopic assessment can sometimes be required. In most cases an X-ray of the soft tissues of the neck can exclude a bony foreign body in the throat. It can also exclude surgical emphysema, in the highly rare case of perforated oesophagus by a sharp foreign body.

Investigations

An X-ray of the soft tissues of the neck and a chest X-ray should be conducted to exclude surgical emphysema (very rare), which is indicative of oesophageal perforation.

Treatment

Treatment is removal of the foreign body. Small perforations of the oesophagus heal with conservative treatment (IV antibiotics, NBM and parenteral feeding). Larger lacerations cause systemic upset, shock, and can be rapidly fatal. Therefore, this requires drainage, diversion and primary repair.

Complications

- Iatrogenic perforation of the oesophagus, with all the potential sequelae that can follow on from this, i.e. bleeding, mediastinitis, generalised sepsis, potential for further surgery.
- Incomplete removal of the foreign body, resulting in persistent symptoms, and the potential need for re-operation.

Epistaxis

The nasal cavity is supplied by both internal and external carotid arteries. The majority of bleeding comes from the anterior septum, at the confluence of arteries known as Little's area (Kiesselbach's plexus). The plexus is the anastomosis of the sphenopalatine artery (from the maxillary artery) with the superior labial artery and greater palatine artery, and the anterior ethmoidal artery.

Most bleeds are arterial in origin and arise from the nasal septum. They frequently occur in young children and in the elderly.

Causes of epistaxis (general or local)

Note

— Hypertension does not predispose to epistaxis in the general population, but does seem to make it worse when it happens.

Local causes of epistaxis
- Idiopathic and trauma (nasal picking, other or surgical).
- Inflammatory and allergic conditions (causing crusting and bleeding) and tumours.

General causes of epistaxis
- Bleeding dyscrasias (Christmas disease, haemophilia, von Willebrand's disease, lymphoma, leukaemia, drugs [warfarin, aspirin], liver failure, ITP).
- Hereditary haemorrhagic telangiectasia (Osler-Weber-Rendu syndrome).
- Pregnancy and cellulitis.

Presentation

Epistaxis presents with bleeding from either nostril or down the posterior pharynx (if swallowed). A specific ENT examination should only be done after the general observations are completed. Look for purpurae, bruising and swollen joints.

Investigations

Most cases of epistaxis are self-limiting; however, in those that are severe and require admission for emergency treatment, the investigations required are as follows:

- FBC.
- CS.
- G+S.

Treatment

Treatment depends on the severity of the bleed, and ranges from simple advice (local pressure, i.e. pinch the alar cartilages onto the nasal septum, use of Naseptin or Bactroban cream) to more invasive treatments generally requiring a hospital environment:

- Cautery. Silver nitrate stick.
- Nasal packing (e.g. with Merocel®; this is a nasal tampon that expands on contact with fluid, forming an effective pack). This can be combined with lignocaine and oxymetolazine (adrenaline analogue) for analgesic and vasoconstrictive actions.
- Balloon catheters to apply pressure posteriorly.
- Septal surgery.
- Endoscopic arterial ligation (sphenopalatine artery or anterior ethmoidal artery).
- Embolisation.
- Other treatments, e.g. replacement of clotting factors, platelets, vitamin K, etc.

Complications

- Re-bleed.
- The balloon catheter inflation, or packing, can result in vagal stimulation and hence a vasovagal syncope.

- Prolonged pressure in the nasal cavity (e.g. balloon catheter or packing) can result in septal perforation due to pressure necrosis.
- The balloon catheter or packs can become dislodged, allowing a re-bleed.
- Bleeding into the posterior oropharynx can be a risk factor for aspiration into the lungs.

Eye and orbit

The following represents a list of conditions to be aware of relating to the eye and orbit. The finer points of ophthalmology are not required knowledge, and the following section introduces an overview and simple definitions only. Should you encounter one of these conditions in normal practice, the key is to recognise those that represent an emergency and to refer them on to a specialist ophthalmologist.

External eye disease

- Diseases of the lids. Trauma, a stye (eyelash follicle, hence these lesions are external to the lid), meibomian gland cysts (secretes grease from a gland, hence these lesions are internal to the lid), and tumours.
- Diseases of the conjunctiva. Conjunctivitis (bacterial/viral) and trauma.
- Diseases of the cornea. Abrasion and ulcers
- Diseases of the lacrimal apparatus.

Acute painful visual loss

There are two main conditions that can cause pain and loss of vision. The first is acute closed angle glaucoma, raised intra-ocular pressure, which, if untreated, can result in permanent optic nerve damage from pressure effects. The closed angle refers to the anatomical reason for the rise in intra-ocular pressure. Aqueous humour is secreted into the eye from behind the pupil, and then drained through Schlemm's canals. These are microscopic channels where the pupil joins the sclera, separating the aqueous from vitreous cavities, and thus forming an angle. If this angle is narrow, the canals are effectively closed cutting off the outflow, but not affecting inflow of aqueous humour; this raises the intra-ocular

pressure. The second condition is uveitis: any inflammation of the 'middle layer' of the eye, i.e. the iris, the vitreous cavity, or the retina and choroid.

Painless visual loss

Acute

- Retinal artery occlusion. This is embolic occlusion of the retinal artery (monocular visual loss, complete) or one of its branches (monocular visual loss, incomplete, e.g. peripheral field loss), initially a reversible lesion if treated emergently by an ophthalmologist, but after 90-100 minutes, it becomes permanent.
- Retinal vein occlusion. This is spontaneous thrombosis in the retinal vein, associated with diabetes, hypertension or hypercoagulable states. It can cause gradual visual loss and haemorrhage into the vitreous cavity.
- Vitreous haemorrhage. This is bleeding into the vitreous cavity of the eye. Obviously it can occur secondary to direct trauma, but there are other, more common, non-traumatic causes. The most common is breakthrough bleeding after macular degeneration, but bleeding can occur due to an ocular tumour, or after retinal vein occlusion. It results in a painless blurring of vision, with or without 'floaters'.
- Retinal detachment. This is the physical detachment of the retina from the underlying choroid layer. The patient complains of floaters preceeding visual field loss. This is an emergency requiring referral to an ophthalmologist for reattachment, usually by laser therapy or intra-ocular gas to tamponade the retina.

Chronic

- Cataract. This is opacification of the lens, caused by denaturation of the lens proteins, which can be multifactorial in origin, e.g. congenital, radiation damage, prolonged UV exposure or secondary to diabetes.
- Chronic open angle glaucoma. This is prograssive occlusion of the Schlemm's canals with time, but without the narrowing of the angle between the lens and sclera seen in closed angle glaucoma, thus there is only a

gradual rise in intra-ocular pressure and gradual painless visual loss.

- Macular degeneration. The macula is the small region in the centre of the retina that contains a high concentration of cone-photoreceptors, which are responsible for our high acuity colour vision in the centre of our visual field. Macular degeneration is an age-related condition where these cells degrade and the patient suffers central field visual loss, being left with only poor acuity peripheral field vision.

Extra-ocular eye disease

- Enophthalmos. The recession of the eyeball into the eye socket, e.g. blow-out fracture of the orbit.
- Exophthalmos. The opposite of enophthalmos, i.e. the anterior bulging of the eyeball out of the eye socket. This can occur in peri-orbital cellulitis and Graves' disease, which is autoimmune hyperthyroidism with goitre.

Swellings in the neck

A lot of the knowledge from this chapter will be useful when asked for the differential diagnosis of a swelling in the neck in exams. The following represents a means of organizing your answer, based on pathological cause. You can of course subdivide the neck into anatomical regions, e.g. anterior and posterior triangles, if you wish, and organize your answer in this fashion. See the 'Triangles of the neck' section in Chapter 3, Anatomy, for the appropriate lists.

Swellings in the neck can be due to the following:

- Congenital.
- Tumour.
- Lymph node.
- Glandular.
- Diverticulae (pouches).
- Trauma.
- Thyroglossal cyst.

Congenital

- Thyroglossal cyst: a midline neck lump, which moves with protrusion of the tongue.
- Dermoid cyst: a cyst containing hair or hair follicles, and sebaceous glands.
- Epidermoid cyst: inclusion cyst of epidermal tissue, not a sebaceous cyst.
- Cystic hygroma: a lymph fluid-filled swelling, from a fetal developmental failure of lymph ducts to join to veins to allow drainage of the lymph into the venous blood.
- Branchial cyst: a failure of normal obliteration of the second branchial arch during fetal development, resulting in an involucrum of epidermal tissue, hence a lateral neck swelling.

Tumours

- Salivary tumour.
- Thyroid tumour.
- Sarcoma, fibroma, lipoma, etc.
- Chemodectoma. A slow-growing tumour of the carotid body at the carotid bifurcation.

Lymph node enlargements

If you do identify cervical lymphadenopathy on clinical examination, or are asked about it as a subject, you must have an organized means of presenting your answer. Here then are the main causes of lymph node enlargement:

- Primary malignancy. Lymphoma and leukaemia.
- Metastatic malignancy. Skin, mouth, nasopharyngeal, oesophageal, thyroid, infraclavicular malignancy, e.g. lung, breast, gastrointestinal tract (GIT).
- Lymphadenitis:
  - non-specific, e.g. upper respiratory tract infection (URTI);
  - specific, e.g. Epstein-Barr virus (EBV), human immunodeficiency virus (HIV) and TB.

Glandular

The major cause of neck lumps due to glandular enlargement are from the salivary glands (submandibular or parotid) or the thyroid gland:

◆ Salivary gland, e.g. sialolithiasis, sialadenitis, benign or malignant tumours.
◆ Thyroid gland, e.g goitre, benign or malignant tumours.

Diverticulae/pouches

A laryngocoele is a rare condition resulting from high pressure within the larynx forcing the laryngeal mucosal lining through a weak point in the thyrohyoid membrane, resulting in a lateral reducible neck mass that recurs on sneezing or coughing.

A pharyngeal pouch is a diverticulum which forms between layers of the inferior constrictors of the pharynx, the thyropharyngeus and the cricopharyngeus, usually in the elderly, resulting in cough, halitosis and regurgitation. It can cause aspiration pneumoniae.

Trauma

Sternocleidomastoid 'tumour'; this is not a tumour in the malignant sense of the term. It is, in fact, a post-traumatic haematoma with subsequent fibrosis, causing a swelling in the SCM muscle, giving the appearance of a soft tissue mass within it.

Thyroglossal cyst

The thyroglossal tract (Figure 9.1) is a remnant which marks the descent of the thyroid gland, from

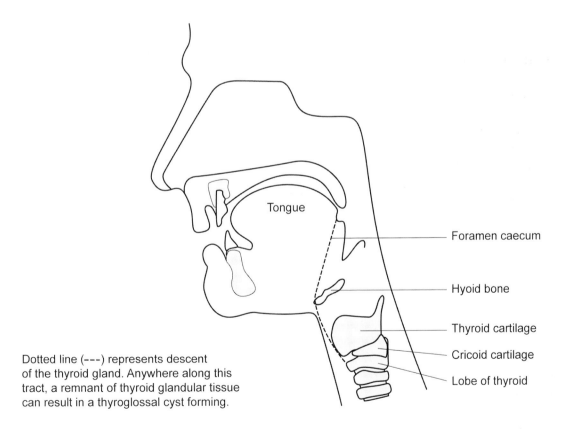

Dotted line (---) represents descent of the thyroid gland. Anywhere along this tract, a remnant of thyroid glandular tissue can result in a thyroglossal cyst forming.

Figure 9.1. Thyroglossal tract.

the fourth fetal week of life. Through the developing second branchial arch, the tract solidifies and then involutes.

Persistence of this duct results in a thyroglossal cyst. Ectopic thyroid tissue can also grow anywhere along this tract, typically as the pyramidal lobe of the thyroid, but it can become a lingual thyroid.

Presentation

This is predominantly seen in the first decade of life, although it can present at any time. It appears in the midline 75% of the time, with an equal male to female ratio.

The cyst will rise on protrusion of the tongue in theory, because of the remnant tract attaching it to the tongue, but in practice any structure above the hyoid will move upwards on moving the tongue.

Investigations

Ultrasound is the investigation of choice to image the cyst and exclude the differential diagnosis of ectopic thyroid glandular tissue.

Treatment

The thyroglossal cyst (and tract) is excised surgically by Sistrunk's operation. This involves a horizontal incision over the sinus, following the tract upwards and excising the middle one third of the hyoid bone. In doing so the tract must be fully excised.

Complications

A possible complication of this procedure is the formation of a thyroglossal sinus, which is an opening that intermittently drains seropurulent fluid requiring re-operation.

Otherwise complications of neck surgery follow those mentioned in Chapter 11, 'Endocrine surgery':

- Hoarse voice, due to recurrent laryngeal nerve palsy (or superior laryngeal nerve).
- Hypocalcaemia, due to proximity of the parathyroid glands whilst operating.
- Haematoma, which can result in stridor if it compresses the larynx, leading to respiratory compromise and respiratory arrest, then death, unless the pressure is relieved. Pressure relief takes the form of removing the neck wound clips and releasing the haematoma.
- Wound infection.

Chapter 10

Breast surgery

Benign conditions of the breast

Fibroadenoma

Presentation

A fibroadenoma is not a true neoplasm; it is considered more an aberration of development, appearing more commonly in the 15-25 age group. It is well circumscribed, smooth, mobile, firm and may be multiple and bilateral. They can increase in size; however, most do not and they disappear after 2-3 years.

Investigations

The clinical diagnosis is often wrong and, therefore, the patient should have ultrasound and fine needle aspiration (FNA) to exclude malignant causes of breast masses.

Treatment

Fibroadenomas can be observed or removed after diagnosis; all above 4cm in diameter should be removed. Malignant change is very rare.

Complications

Excision of fibroadenoma carries the same local risks of excision of all superficial type masses:

- Wound infection.
- Dehiscence.
- Incomplete excision of mass.
- Recurrence of mass.
- Haematoma formation.
- Damage to local structures.

Supernumerary breasts

Presentation

These occur in the milk line which is found by joining a line from the axilla to the groin; however, they are most common under the axilla.

Investigations

Supernumerary breasts generally do not require investigation.

Treatment

The majority are small and unobtrusive. Of course if the patient finds them cosmetically unacceptable, it is possible to excise them, swapping the mass (breast) for a scar.

Complications

As for all excisions of superficial masses, the specific complications are:

- Wound infection.
- Dehiscence.
- Incomplete excision of mass.
- Haematoma formation.
- Damage to local structures.

Note

- An extra breast is termed polymazia.
- An absence of breast is termed amazia.

Prepubertal breast development

Presentation

Development of breasts before the age of eight years, but in the absence of any other pubertal symptoms, is diagnosed as prepubertal breast development.

The important differential diagnosis here is that of precocious puberty, which presents with early breast development, as well as pubic or axillary hair, swelling of the vulva mucosa and vaginal discharge/bleeding.

The reason to identify the one condition from the other is that precocious puberty can be secondary to hormone-secreting tumours, whereas prepubertal breast development is generally a normal variant.

Investigations

- Serial height charts, looking for evidence of pubertal growth spurt.
- Left hand and wrist X-rays, with comparison to the standards of Greulich and Pyle. Advancement of greater than two standard deviations above the norm suggests precocious puberty.
- Pelvic ultrasound, looking for evidence of pubertal development of the female reproductive organs.
- Plasma gonadotrophin levels (follicular stimulating hormone [FSH] and luteinising hormone [LH]), before and after infusion of gonadotrophin releasing hormone (GnRH).
- Cranial imaging, CT or MRI, if a pubertal pattern of gonadotrophins is detected, looking for pituitary or hypothalamic tumours.

Treatment

Details are fortunately beyond the remit of this book, but to summarise, prepubertal breast development needs no treatment. Precocious puberty, where no underlying hormone-secreting tumour has been identified, may require no treatment, but gonadotrophin suppressive (GnRH antagonists) therapy may be used in specialist hands to help prevent early fusion of the epiphyseal growth plates and resultant short stature. In hormone-secreting pituitary tumours, there is a potential indication for surgical excision.

Complications

You are not expected to know the potential complications of GnRH antagonist therapy.

Complications of pituitary surgery are:

- Damage to normal pituitary tissue, resulting in the interruption of secretion of pituitary hormones, thus replacement therapy becomes necessary (thyroid hormone, cortisol, growth hormone, oestrogen or testosterone [if the production of LH or FSH is interrupted]). This occurs in 5-10% of cases.

Other rarer complications include:

- Damage to the posterior pituitary causing diabetes insipidis (polyuria and polydipsia).
- Damage to the carotid artery, resulting in stroke or death.
- Postoperative haematoma results in compression on the optic chiasma with visual loss.
- CSF leak can result in meningitis.

Cyclical breast pain

Presentation

Pain in one or both breasts that comes on in the premenstrual phase of the cycle.

It occurs in the absence of a palpable breast lump on examination, although nodularity can be a feature of cyclical breast pain.

Investigations

Generally unnecessary if there are no worrying features in the history and examination.

Treatment

Evening primrose oil (also known as Efamast), danozol, or bromocryptine generally treat this condition. Surgery is not indicated.

Complications

You are not expected to know the complications of medical therapy for cyclical breast pain.

Non-cyclical breast pain

Presentation

The sources of non-cyclical breast pain are the breast itself or the chest wall. Costochondritis (also known as Tietze's syndrome) is an inflammation of the junction between the bony and cartilaginous components of a rib. This presents with a background aching pain and acute exacerbations on deep inspiration, coughing or sneezing. It generally (although not invariably) comes on after a cough, cold or sore throat.

Non-cyclical pain arising from the breast itself should prompt a search for other features of breast lesions, e.g. an abscess (also presents with pyrexia, a fluctuant tender breast mass, with or without discharge), or a breast tumour (see the section on 'Breast cancer' for more detail). Non-cyclical breast pain in the absence of any breast mass is not generally attributable to malignancy and thus, the patient can be reassured.

Investigations

Tests for costochondritis are unrewarding: inflammatory markers are not always raised and the chest X-ray is normal. The diagnosis is a clinical one.

Painful breast masses must be investigated thoroughly to exclude malignancy (see the section on 'Breast cancer'). Masses presenting as abscesses may benefit from aspiration to confirm the presence of pus, but generally one should proceed to treatment (see the section on 'Breast abscesses').

Treatment

Costochondritis is treated most effectively by simple analgesics, preferably NSAIDs, if the patient has no contra-indications (acid indigestion, reflux, asthma or a specific allergy).

Breast abscess and breast tumour treatment is covered in depth later in this chapter.

Complications

See later sections on 'Breast abscesses' and 'Breast cancer'.

Breast cysts

Presentation

Most commonly occur in the 38-53-year-old group, particularly in perimenopausal women. The pathology of a cyst is a distended and involuted lobule. A cyst presents clinically as a smooth and painful discrete breast lump, and can be both fluctuant and non-fluctuant.

Investigations

The patient should have a mammogram and fluid aspirated to confirm the cystic nature.

Note

— If the fluid aspirate is blood-stained, it must be sent for cytology.

All cysts should be fully drained. Things to look out for are:

- Refilling of the cyst more than two times.
- A palpable lump after cyst drainage.
- Blood-stained cyst aspirate.

These suggest malignancy.

Treatment

Aspiration alone treats a large proportion of breast cysts.

Underlying breast masses, after aspiration, should be investigated as for breast tumours, especially if the cyst later reaccumulates.

Complications

Aspiration, being a percutaneous procedure, obviously carries with it a small risk of infection, i.e. a small risk of cellulitis or abscess formation.

As previously mentioned, there is a risk of reaccumulation of the cyst, or of there being an underlying tumour.

Duct ectasia

Presentation
Duct ectasia is most common in the 40-50-year-old age range. It can present with nipple discharge (characteristically brown), breast pain, inversion of the nipple, a lump or thickening near the nipple.

It is a condition of a normal variant of involution of a breast duct, which subsequently fills with liquid containing cellular debris.

This is not a malignant condition and is often self-limiting, requiring no treatment. However, when persistent symptoms are present, it may be necessary to excise the ectatic duct(s) surgically.

Investigations
- Ultrasound, to look for solid or cystic masses.
- Mammogram, to look for any microcalcification indicative of malignancy.
- Histological analysis of the discharged fluid, to look for any evidence of malignant cells.

Treatment
Infection of the ectatic duct results in abscess formation or cellulitis, both of which can potentially be treated by antibiotics, although the abscess may require aspiration or incision and drainage.

Persistent discharge or pain is unusual, and the patient can be offered excision surgery via a peri-areolar incision.

Complications
The complications of doing nothing are of having a persistent discharge, persistent pain, abscess formation and the potential for the patient to worry about the presence of malignancy because of these symptoms.

The complications of excision surgery are:

- Infection (cellulitis or abscess formation).
- Fistula formation.
- Recurrence of the duct ectasia.

Breast abscesses

Presentation
Breast abscesses can be lactating or non-lactating.

Lactating breast abscesses
These are related to cracks in the nipple and invasion by (usually) *Staphylococcus aureus*, but occasionally by *Staphylococcus epidermidis*.

Non-lactating breast abscesses
- Usually peri-areolar (in young women).
- Can have an associated fistula.
- Often caused by anaerobes, e.g. Bacteroides or some Streptococci.
- A hot fluctuant mass, which causes pain and nipple discharge, and nipple retraction appears in cases of repeated infection.

Note
- There are also peripheral non-lactating breast abscesses, which are less common than peri-areolar abscesses.

- Peripheral non-lactating breast abscesses are often caused by *Staphylococcus aureus*.

Note
- Look out for malignancy which can occasionally underlie this.

Investigations
Often no investigation is necessary when the presentation is clinically obvious (red, hot, fluctuant and tender mass in the breast). However, in cases of clinical doubt, an ultrasound will show a fluid-filled cavity which can subsequently be aspirated, showing pus, confirming the diagnosis.

Treatment
Breast abscesses, both lactating and non-lactating, can be treated in one of two ways: either needle aspiration and antibiotic cover with repeat aspirations as required, in an attempt to avoid surgery; or surgical incision and drainage, which theoretically obviates the

need for antibiotic administration, but patients should be treated on a case by case basis.

Complications
♦ Abscess recurrence is a risk of either form of treatment.
♦ Fistula formation and haematoma.
♦ There exists a small risk of wound dehiscence in surgical incision and drainage.

Duct papilloma

Presentation
A duct papilloma is a benign condition of the breast. It is a neoplasm of the lactiferous duct that can result in nipple discharge (characteristically blood-stained) and a small mass near the nipple, which can be tender.

Blood-stained discharge, a mass and pain are worrying symptoms of malignancy, and this is the important differential diagnosis. As duct papillomas tend to present in 40-50-year-olds, the same demographic as for breast cancer, this warrants careful assessment and investigation.

Investigations
♦ Ultrasound.
♦ Mammogram.
♦ Biopsy and histological analysis.

Treatment
Surgical excision of the affected duct (when malignancy has convincingly been excluded), termed a microdochectomy, is the treatment of choice.

Complications
♦ Wound infection or abscess formation.
♦ Haematoma.
♦ Loss of nipple sensation.
♦ Very rarely, nipple loss.

Nipple discharge

Nipple discharge is a common presenting condition. It is worthwhile knowing this list of causes of nipple discharge for exam purposes. It invariably comes up as a simple introductory question for the many different pathologies, benign and malignant, of the breast. A list of causes of nipple discharge are as follows:

♦ Duct papilloma.
♦ Duct ectasia.
♦ Pregnancy.
♦ Periductal mastitis.
♦ Epithelial hyperplasia.
♦ Galactorrhoea.
♦ Breast cancer.

Lipoma of the breast

Presentation
Breast lipomas are no different from lipomas found anywhere else in the body. They can mimic the appearance of a breast tumour and thus this warrants their inclusion as a separate entity in this chapter. They present as smooth, soft, non-tender, untethered masses. They are generally found in the superficial fat of the breast, but occasionally can be located deeper.

Investigations
In any case of doubt these must be investigated as for malignant breast lesions, i.e. an ultrasound, mammogram and biopsy with histological analysis.

Treatment
Breast lipomas, as for other lipomas elsewhere in the body, do not necessarily warrant surgical excision. This is only performed for cosmetic reasons if the patient requests it, or if doubt exists as to the benign nature of the diagnosis despite investigation.

Breast cancer

Epidemiology of breast cancer

♦ There is a peak incidence at 45-75 years of age.
♦ It is more common in nulliparous women in developed countries.

- It is likely related to oestrogen exposure, early menarche and late menopause.
- There is no proven link with the oral contraceptive pill (OCP).
- Obese women have an increased incidence. It is postulated that this is due to peripheral androgen to oestrogen conversion in subcutaneous fat.
- Hereditary breast cancer represents a small proportion of the national total. There are two identified breast cancer genes, which, when inherited, lead to an increased predisposition to developing breast cancer (in women, but also in men with the gene). These genes are BRCA1 and BRCA2; this stands for BReast CAncer. These genes can be tested for in high risk individuals, i.e. those in whom breast cancer has occurred in at least three first or second degree relatives.

Presentation

- Lump (hard irregular, fixed to breast tissue, skin or muscle).
- Secondary nodal masses.
- Skin ulceration.
- Skin tethering.
- Nipple retraction.
- Paget's disease of the nipple (eczematous change in the nipple).
- Cancer en cuirasse (infiltration of skin of the breast, chest, back and neck).

Note

- A cuirasse is a French term for a type of body armour that protects the thorax, known as a breast plate.

- Peau d'orange (localised oedema, dimples due to tethering of hair follicles, and breast suspensory ligaments of Astley Cooper).

Note

- Astley Cooper was the second ever President of the Royal College of Surgeons of England, after John Hunter.

- Mastalgia (painful breast).
- Nipple discharge (bloody or serous).

Staging of breast cancer

TNM or Manchester staging systems.

TNM staging of breast cancer

- T1. 2cm.
- T2. 2-5cm (nodes may be palpable but mobile).
- T3. >5cm (axillary nodes involved).
- T4. Any size with fixation to the chest wall or skin ulceration.
- N. Nodes I - III.
- M. Metastases 0 or I.

Manchester staging of breast cancer

- Palpable tumour/lump confined to breast (corresponds to TNM stage I).
- Axillary nodes enlarged but mobile (corresponds to TNM stage II).
- Tumour and/or nodes fixed to surrounding tissues (corresponds to TNM stage III-IV).
- Distant metastases (corresponds to TNM stage IV).

Pathology of breast cancer

The cells in the breast are derived from a lobule or a duct (hence lobular carcinoma or ductal carcinoma). If the carcinoma is not invasive it is termed carcinoma *in situ,* hence lobular carcinoma *in situ* (LCIS) or ductal carcinoma *in situ* (DCIS). DCIS is seen as microcalcification on mammography. These are pre-malignant conditions. Most actual breast cancers are invasive ductal cancers. The prognosis is worsened by the increasing number of axillary nodes found positive for malignant change.

The tumour grade is also a good prognostic indicator (tubule formation, pleomorphism, mitotic activity). This is the basis of the Bloom and Richardson classification for breast cancer.

Investigations

◆ Take a history.
◆ Examine the four quadrants, axilla, nipple and areola.
◆ Assess the liver for enlargement, implying metastasis.
◆ Mammography (showing the symptomless breast as well).
◆ Aspirate any dominant lumps. If cystic and blood-stained, send for cytology; if there is a residual lump, FNA is required.

Note

— USS-guided techniques can be used for obtaining a histological sample.

◆ CXR.
◆ LFTs.

The presence of disease in axillary nodes signifies the likelihood that micrometastases are present already by haematogenous spread, i.e. lymphatic spread to nodes implies there has also been haematogenous spread elsewhere.

These micrometastases can take years to decades to become clinically apparent; however, they are of relevance when considering hormone or chemotherapy.

The triple assessment

The triple assessment is an important concept to remember for exam purposes.

It comprises:

◆ The surgeon.
◆ The cytologist.
◆ The radiologist.

This is a team that are all in one clinic dedicated to the investigation of women presenting with breast disease. Each specialist grades the woman's findings from 1-5 (where 5 = malignant).

This gives a maximum score of 15.

The cytology score is as follows:

◆ 1. Inadequate aspirate.
◆ 2. Benign.
◆ 3. Atypia, but probably benign.
◆ 4. Suspicious, probably malignant.
◆ 5. Malignant.

The higher the score, the greater the likelihood of malignancy. The surgeon scores from 1-5 depending on the size, fixity to local structures, presence of axillary nodes and their fixity. The radiologist scores from 1-5 depending on USS appearance (in younger women) and mammography (in older women).

Note

— Be aware of the concept of sentinel node biopsy. This can be used to determine the need for adjuvant radiotherapy or axillary clearance.

Treatment

Criteria for operable breast cancer

T1 - 3, N0 - 1, M0 or Manchester 1 - 3. The current trend is for breast-conserving surgery, with or without adjuvant therapy.

Note

— Always emphasise that even though breast-conserving surgery is attempted, it is excision of the entire tumour mass with safe margins that is the first priority, followed by consideration of breast conservation.

It used to be the case that radical mastectomy was performed in the hope of eradicating all the tumour. However, the results are no better, in terms of survival and tumour recurrence, if a well executed lumpectomy is performed, taking care to excise a circumferential cuff of healthy (fatty) tissue. This is what is meant by breast-conserving surgery. Breast-conserving surgery, where the axillary lymph nodes test positive for disease, is generally followed by a course of radiotherapy.

Controversy exists between axillary lymph node clearance (or sampling) followed by radiotherapy in node-positive patients, even down to the method of sampling; random or sentinel node biopsy.

Sentinel node biopsy is performed by injection of a dye (methylene blue) or radio-active isotope (technetium99) around the tumour, and identifying the first lymph node it reaches (the one that is blue, when the dye is used at the time of surgery, or the one that causes the hand-held Geiger counter to react, when the isotope is used). This first node, the sentinel node, has been shown to reliably contain micrometastases when the disease is node-positive, and not when it is negative, obviating the need to sample any of the other nodes surgically for staging reasons.

Recently, it has been found that axillary clearance carries no survival (or disease recurrence) benefit, compared with adjuvant therapy, but axillary clearance does have significant side effects (pain, lymphoedema, risk of wound infection). Treatment algorithms vary from department to department and it will serve you well to quote your local department's policy in exams, but also be aware of the other possibilities as explained above.

Axillary node clearance

This has three levels (relating to pectoralis minor):

- I. Inferior to pectoralis minor.
- II. At the level of pectoralis minor.
- III. Superior to pectoralis minor.

Thus, a level III clearance involves a great deal more dissection than does a stage I.

Note

– Thoracodorsal and long thoracic nerves are at risk of damage in axillary node dissection/clearance (this is a common exam question).

The long thoracic nerve supplies the serratus anterior muscle and the thoracodorsal nerve supplies the latissimus dorsi muscle.

Adjuvant therapy for breast cancer

- Tamoxifen. A useful drug in post-menopausal women, it reduces mortality by 16%.
- Anastrazole. An aromatase inhibitor that inhibits the conversion of androgens to oestrogens in the peripheral circulation, reducing the oestrogen levels as a result, thus it reduces the risk of recurrence of breast cancer. It is an alternative to tamoxifen, and may have improved results in oestrogen receptor-positive breast cancer.
- Chemotherapy. CMF (cyclophosphamide, methotrexate, fluorouracil). In pre-menopausal women, chemotherapy reduces mortality by 17%. This and the 16% figure above are quoted from a ten-year study by Peto referring to women with node-positive disease.
- Radiotherapy. A dose of radiation is calculated to be able to reach the depth of the axillary lymph nodes. The beam is tangential to the thorax, i.e. avoids damaging the thoracic contents, passing through breast and axillary soft tissues only.

Complications

Chemotherapy can be complicated by the following:

- Acute toxicity:
  - bone marrow;
  - gastrointestinal;
  - alopecia.
- Long-term toxicity:
  - carcinogenesis;
  - gonadal damage.
- Bladder:
  - fibrosis;
  - haematuria.

Axillary radiotherapy can be complicated by the following:

- Skin:
  - inflammation and desquamation.

- Bone marrow:
  - bone marrow suppression.
- Lymph tissue:
  - lymphoedema.

Complications of breast cancer surgery (lumpectomy or mastectomy) are:

- Wound infection.
- Haematoma.
- Seroma.
- Shoulder ache and stiffness.
- Lymphoedema (ipsilateral arm).
- Insensate nipple (or even loss of the nipple, due to vascular interruption, particularly in centrally located breast tumours).
- Long thoracic and/or thoracodorsal nerve damage.

Breast reconstruction

Despite the term breast-conserving surgery, the patient can be left with a cosmetically unacceptable disparity in breast size and shape. This can be addressed when all the cancer treatment has been completed, and the operated breast has recovered from the initial surgical insult, preferably six months or more down the line.

Various options are available to the cosmetic or breast surgeon at this point. Fundamentally, the choice of options are:

- Breast implant surgery to the affected side in order to match the original.
- Breast implant surgery to both breasts, so that they match.
- Musculocutaneous graft surgery, e.g. a latissimus dorsi graft taken with its vascular pedicle and a predetermined sized overlying patch of skin.
- Nipple reconstruction, if indicated.

The decision as to which surgical modality to use in these emotionally sensitive cases is beyond the remit of this book, but it is as well to be aware of the options.

Chapter 11

Endocrine surgery

Anatomy and physiology of the thyroid and parathyroid glands (Figure 11.1)

The thyroid is an endocrine gland, overlying the inferior aspect of the thyroid cartilage, and the cricoid cartilage. It is responsible for hormone secretion that regulates metabolic rate as well as calcium homeostasis. A normal thyroid gland weighs 20-40g.

Thyroxine (T4) and tri-iodothyronine (T3) are the iodine-based hormones secreted by the thyroid gland. T4 is less metabolically active than T3; there is peripheral conversion of T4 to T3. Both these hormones are bound to protein in the blood, called thyroid binding globulin. Hormone that is not bound is metabolically active.

T4 and T3 are secreted from the thyroid in response to thyroid stimulating hormone (TSH), which is itself released from the anterior pituitary gland. TSH is secreted in response to thyrotrophin releasing hormone (TRH) from the hypothalamus. This system is regulated by a negative feedback loop, i.e. raised levels of T3 inhibit TRH secretion from the hypothalamus, resulting in reduced TSH and hence decreased T4 and T3 secretion from the thyroid. Other hormones that are involved in feedback at the hypothalamic and pituitary level, are somatostatin, glucagon, oestrogen and testosterone.

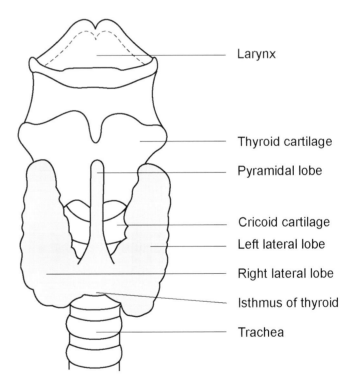

Larynx

Thyroid cartilage

Pyramidal lobe

Cricoid cartilage

Left lateral lobe

Right lateral lobe

Isthmus of thyroid

Trachea

Figure 11.1. The thyroid gland.

Calcitonin is a hormone secreted from the parafollicular cells of the thyroid. Calcitonin has effects on renal tubules and bone to lower calcium. Its exact physiological role is unclear.

The parathyroid glands are located on the posterior surface of the thyroid gland. They secrete parathyroid hormone (PTH), which is the main governor of calcium concentration. Calcium homeostasis is important as both raised or low levels of calcium in the serum have significant effects on the cardiac and nervous systems. The parathyroid glands can detect a drop in the serum calcium level and will therefore secrete more PTH. The PTH in systemic circulation is responsible for stimulating osteoclasts to resorb bone which results in release of calcium into the blood, raising its level. PTH also has an effect on the gastrointestinal tract (as well as the kidneys) resulting in increased calcium absorption (it acts in concert with vitamin D, in this respect, and PTH is necessary for vitamin D activation).

Congenital abnormalities

As with other organs, the thyroid gland is subject to congenital abnormalities. These range from asymptomatic incidental findings, through to congenital hypothyroidism at the more severe end of the scale:

- Lingual thyroid. Usually symptomless (many are actually hypothyroid), although the tissue can be subject to any of the normal thyroid disorders. It only very rarely causes obstructive symptoms.
- Thyroglossal duct. Persistent remnant of the path the thyroid gland took when migrating from its position in the orpharynx (in the fetus) to its postion in the neck. Thus, a duct remnant is present through the base of the tongue.
- Thyroglossal cyst. A cyst associated with a persistent thyroglossal duct which presents as a lump in the midline of the neck. It can vary in size. It rises on protrusion of the tongue. Unless large, it rarely causes symptoms, but is capable of causing dysphagia or becoming infected.
- Congenital hypothyroidism leads to cretinism if severe (learning difficulties, failure to thrive, delayed milestones).

Goitre

This is a non-specific term indicating enlargement of the thyroid gland. Clinically, it can be diffuse or nodular. Physiological goitre is a result of physiological demand for TSH, causing thyroid hyperplasia, e.g. at puberty, pregnancy, lactation.

Pathological goitre occurs with iodine deficiency, benign or malignant nodules, goitrogens and genetic disorders. Goitrogens (drugs or food that are implicated in goitre formation) are chemicals which inhibit thyroid hormone synthesis, resulting in reflex stimulation of TSH and hence goitre.

Clinical classification of goitre

- Diffuse.
- Nodular:
  - solitary;
  - multiple;
  - dominant.

Presentation

All goitres present with a similar pattern:

- Cosmetic.
- Discomfort/pain.
- Tracheal/oesophageal compression.
- Retrosternal extension.
- Suspicion of malignancy.
- Hyperthyroidism.
- Hypothyroidism.
- Hoarse voice.

Risk factors that a nodule is not benign (bearing in mind that the majority of thyroid disease is indeed benign) are:

- Age (increased risk if <20 or >50 years).
- Sex (increased risk if male).
- Size (lump greater than 4cm at presentation).
- Lump continuing to increase in size.
- Hoarse voice.
- Family history.
- Therapeutic or accidental radiation exposure.

Nodular goitre

Clinically, this may present as solitary, multiple, or dominant nodule(s). Pathological changes associated with nodular goitre are fibrosis with associated inflammatory changes (infarction, haemorrhage, fibrosis, calcification, colloid cyst formation, and areas of nodular hyperplasia). This results in new follicle formation with inelastic fibrous stroma. These nodules can function independently of TSH control.

Thyroid neoplasms

Benign

Practically all of these are follicular adenomas, encapsulated solid lesions of thyroid tissue.

There is a problem in that FNA cannot distinguish between follicular adenoma (benign) and follicular carcinoma (malignant). Therefore, a cytologically proven follicular lesion will usually be removed, e.g. by thyroid lobectomy.

Malignant

It is important to emphasise that malignant disease of the thyroid is rare. A primary care physician will see one new case approximately every 15 years and it represents less than 1% of cancer deaths overall. Risk factors for malignant thyroid disease are history of radiation exposure (e.g. medical radiotherapy to the neck), family history (e.g. MEN II, [multiple endocrine neoplasia Type II]).

Presentation

Thyroid cancer presents with a lump in the neck. It is not necessarily painful, although it can be (pain is a sign of locally invasive disease). A worrying presentation is a goitre with voice change; this is rare in benign disease.

Clinical findings to look out for in malignancy are as follows:

- A hardness and fixity to structures is a suspicious finding.
- Associated lymphadenopathy is also suspicious.
- The presence of multiple nodules does not exclude malignancy. (In fact thyroid malignancy can present either as unilateral or bilateral goitre.)
- Concomitant hyperthyroidism makes malignancy less likely, but it does not exclude it.
- The sole presentation of thyroid cancer may be an enlarged cervical node, or cervical lymphadenopathy.

Investigations

- TSH level, if abnormal, then free T4 and T3 levels should be obtained, as well as thyroid antibodies.
- USS. This identifies suspicious features of a nodule, e.g. hypoechoic signal, punctuate calcification, irregular outline, abnormal vascular signals, and is good for looking at the lymph nodes.
- FNA biopsy is performed for a cytological diagnosis, in patients with euthyroid goitre. The cytology should be taken in context of the clinical risk factors.
- CT/MRI scan. This can delineate anatomy in patients with stridor, retrosternal goitre and malignancy.
- Routine pre-operative bloods (FBC, U&Es, CS, G+S, and calcium levels, chest X-ray).
- ECG.
- Laryngoscopy.

Note

- The only definitive means of completely excluding malignancy is by thyroid lobectomy. Clearly, this is not indicated in all cases. But if there is any diagnostic uncertainty, with presence of risk factors, then a thyroid lobectomy is indicated.

Types of thyroid cancer

♦ Differentiated:
  • papillary;
  • follicular.
♦ Medullary.
♦ Anaplastic.
♦ Lymphoma.

Differentiated thyroid cancer

Papillary thyroid cancer

This represents 80% of all thyroid cancers. Key points to remember are that it is usually multifocal and spreads to the lymph nodes.

Follicular thyroid cancer

This represents 20% of thyroid cancers. Key points to remember are that it is solitary, encapsulated, angioinvasive, and spreads to bones.

Treatment of differentiated thyroid cancer

For papillary microcancer (<1cm in diameter), often incidental, a thyroid lobectomy is sufficient in most patients. For most patients with differentiated thyroid cancer there is controversy as to whether a thyroid lobectomy or total thyroidectomy is indicated. The author's preferred treatement is a total thyroidectomy.

Lymph node dissection is considered for some patients with papillary thyroid cancer.

Post-surgical treatment with radio-iodine is used for ablation of residual thyroid tissue. This then permits postoperative surveillance with serum thyroglobulin levels (a sensitive marker of recurrent disease) and diagnostic scans, e.g. a diagnostic radio-iodine scan. Thyroxine is given at a dose to suppress TSH, which is itself a potent growth factor for differentiated thyroid cancers.

Most patients with papillary thyroid cancer have an excellent prognosis. Patients with follicular cancer for the most part have a good prognosis.

Adverse risk factors for a poorer prognosis are: increased age, male sex, lesion size, extrathyroid invasion and the presence of distant metastases.

Medullary thyroid cancer

This arises from parafollicular cells (C-cells) which secrete calcitonin, a sensitive marker of medullary thyroid cancer (MTC). MTC is genetically determined in 25% of cases (multiple endocrine neoplasia [MEN] Type IIa, IIb and familial medullary thyroid cancer [FMTC]). Even if there is no preceding family history, genetic screening for the RET-mutation is mandatory in all MTC. Prior to performing thyroid surgery for MTC, every patient must have a biochemical test to exclude phaeochromocytoma.

MTC presents as a thyroid mass, with lymph node metastases, and in patients with systemic disease, with diarrhoea.

Note

— Syndromes that include medullary thyroid cancer are:
  • MEN IIa - MTC 100%, phaeochromocytoma 50%, and hyperparathyroidism (rare).
  • MEN IIb - MTC 100%, phaeochromocytoma 50%, mucosal ganglioneuromas (mouth and tongue), marfanoid appearance.
  • FMTC - MTC alone.

Treatment of medullary thyroid cancer

Treatment is by radical surgery, a total thyroidectomy and lymph node dissection. Postoperative replacement thyroxine is given. TSH suppression is not required. Radioactive iodine ablation is not used. Calcitonin levels are monitored to detect residual or recurrent disease.

Anaplastic thyroid cancer

This carries the worst prognosis of all thyroid cancers. The mortality is almost 100% at six months. It has an increased incidence in areas of high endemic goitre. It almost always presents in elderly patients and always presents late.

Treatment of anaplastic thyroid cancer

Surgery is only really of use in relieving obstructive symptoms, i.e. usually palliative.

Lymphoma of the thyroid

Presents typically as a patient with Hashimoto's thyroiditis and a sudden increase in thyroid size. It is usually a B-cell type.

Treatment of lymphoma of the thyroid

The treatment of lymphoma of the thyroid is medical, not surgical. The lymphoma must be staged according to lymphoma protocols. Diagnosis is confirmed with a core or incisional biopsy. Treament with hydrocortisone is very effective for patients who present acutely with airway obstruction prior to chemotherapy.

Other causes of malignant tumours of the thyroid

Metastases to the thyroid are more common than sarcoma. Both are rare presentations of malignant thyroid masses.

Hyperthyroidism

Sixty percent of all hyperthyroidism is caused by Graves' disease (see below).

Other causes of thyrotoxicosis are:

- Toxic multi-nodular goitre (MNG - Plummer's syndrome). This is treated by either radio-iodine or surgery, depending on surgeon/physician preference.
- Hyperfunctioning adenoma. This is treated by either radio-iodine or surgery, depending on surgeon/physician preference.
- Overdose of thyroxine.
- Subacute/acute thyroiditis.
- Functioning thyroid carcinoma.
- TSH-secreting tumours (choriocarcinoma, hydatiform mole, testicular cancer, pituitary tumours).
- During iodine-131 therapy.
- Struma ovarii (a rare, benign, tumour of the ovary, containing thyroid tissue).

Graves' disease

This is an autoimmune-mediated thyrotoxicosis, because patients produce TSH receptor antibodies which stimulate the thyroid gland to secrete T3 and T4. It is more common in women (10:1) with a peak incidence at 20-40 years of age, although it can occur at any age.

Presentation
- Weight loss, despite a healthy (if not increased) appetite.
- Fine tremor.
- Heat intolerance.
- Emotional instability, a tendency to nervousness that may not have been present before.
- Exophthalmos (bulging eyes in which the sclerae are visible cicumferentially). This is known as thyroid-associated ophthalmopathy (TAO). In isolation, surgical treatment of Graves' disease does not affect TAO.
- Goitre.

Investigations
Free T3, free T4 and TSH levels should be measured. The differential diagnosis is toxic MNG or hyperfunctioning adenoma. An isotope scan will help tell the difference between the three (if required). Thyroid microsomal antibodies can be tested. All patients require treatment.

Treatment

Medical (anti-thyroid drugs).

Beta-blockers are used prior to biochemical control of thyroid function to treat the sympathetic symptoms. Carbimazole (standard treatment) or propylthiouracil can render the patient euthyroid. The standard treatment is to give the patient anti-thyroid drugs for one year. When the medication is stopped, 60% of patients relapse. If they do relapse they are offered radio-iodine or thyroidectomy.

Note

— The side effects of carbimazole are nausea, dyspepsia, and agranulocytosis (always preceded by a sore throat). It is important to be aware of this, as agranulocytosis (a dangerous decrease in the level of granulocytes, i.e. white blood cells) can result in a rapidly fatal septicaemia. It is easily identified on FBC testing. The carbimazole must be immediately stopped and the patient referred to a medical specialist.

Radio-iodine

This is direct radioactive damage to the follicular cells. The advantages are that it is cheap, simple and safe. The disadvantages are that it is contraindicated in pregnancy and lactation, and there is a risk of late hypothyroidism. An important restriction placed on patients after radio-iodine treatment is that they are not to come into contact with children, most especially not to cuddle, as they are radioactive over short distances.

Surgery

The patient must be rendered biochemically euthyroid. Not all patients need to be beta-blocked. Lugol's iodine can be used pre-operatively to reduce thyroid vascularity. The operation is a total, or near-total, thyroidectomy.

Complications

The complications of thyroidectomy are as follows:

♦ Voice change due to recurrent laryngeal nerve palsy (or superior laryngeal nerve, although this gives a voice that tires, which is relevant for professional singers or telephonists, or people who need to talk for long periods of time for their job). It is usually transient, but can be permanent. There is a 1% risk of permanent palsy.

♦ Bilateral recurrent laryngeal nerve palsy, which is fortunately a rare complication. It results in paralysis of both vocal cords causing stridor and respiratory distress, or poor cough reflex, or aspiration. The vocal cords can be paralysed in one of two positions resulting in different clinical entities: they can be paralysed when the cords are together in the midline, i.e. closed, which blocks the airway and the patient cannot breathe; or, they can be paralysed with the cords away from the midline, i.e. open, as a result the patient can breathe, but there is a high aspiration risk.

♦ Hypocalcaemia, usually due to surgical trauma to, or inadvertent removal of, the parathyroid glands, especially in bilateral thyroid surgery. This is the reason calcium levels are checked 24-48 hours after surgery. There are symptoms of paraesthesiae in the hands and feet and peri-oral numbness at their most mild, but this can progress to laryngospasm or even cardiac arrest at the severe end of the spectrum.

♦ Haematoma. It is not purely a mass effect from the haematoma that causes the complications, it is in fact a combination of lymphatic and venous obstruction causing subglottic oedema. This airway oedema is potentially life-threatening, and is difficult to intubate. The neck wound is closed with a single continuous suture so that in the event of a haematoma causing respiratory compromise, the single suture can be rapidly removed on the ward, permitting decompression of the haematoma (this can be a life-saving manoeuvre). The patient may still need an emergency tracheostomy if intubation is impossible and respiratory distress still persists.

♦ Thyroid storm. This is a rare postoperative complication, rare nowadays because pre-operative chemical induction of a euthyroid state prevents it (surgery is not contemplated until the patient has been successfully rendered euthyroid). If a patient is hyperthyroid in the pre-operative state, then manipulation of the thyroid at the time of surgery can release toxic doses of thyroid hormones, resulting in hyperpyrexia and severe tachycardia.

♦ Wound infection (uncommon).
♦ Hypothyroidism. Around 30% of patients after thyroid lobectomy become hypothyroid and need permanent thyroxine replacement therapy.

Plummer's syndrome

Presentation

This is hyperthyroidism in MNG due to development of one or more independently functioning nodules. Hyperthyroidism, as a result of one of these nodules producing thyroid hormones independently of the normal feedback mechanisms, is called Plummer's syndrome.

Note

— Hoarseness can be due to distortion of the larynx by goitre, or by recurrent laryngeal nerve palsy, which may suggest malignancy.

Investigations
♦ Thyroid function tests.
♦ Thyroid microsomal antibodies.

Treatment

Medical
Physiological goitre does not require treatment. The investigations mentioned are intended to sift out those patients who require either surgical management or those who can safely be discharged.

Surgical
The indications for thyroid surgery in benign thyroid disease are:

♦ A diagnostic lobectomy and isthmectomy.
♦ Treatment of a symptomatic or retrosternal goitre, e.g. mechanical or obstructive symptoms.
♦ Cosmetic reasons.
♦ Treatment of thyrotoxicosis.

Complications
As outlined previously on p348.

Hyperparathyroidism

Eighty-five percent of primary hyperparathyroidism (HPT) is caused by enlargement of a single parathyroid gland (adenoma), 10-15% multiple gland hyperplasia, and 1% cancer.

The three causes of hyperparathyroidism can be summarised as:

♦ Primary HPT.
♦ Renal HPT (secondary or tertiary).
♦ Familial.

The pathology can be:

♦ Adenoma (single or multiple).
♦ Hyperplasia (may be asymmetric).
♦ Carcinoma.

It should be mentioned that these different causes of HPT have different biochemical patterns seen on testing. In primary, tertiary and familial HPT, elevated levels of serum corrected calcium and PTH are seen. In secondary HPT, serum corrected calcium is normal, but the PTH is grossly elevated. Remember, secondary HPT is caused by renal failure (the patient is usually on dialysis) or vitamin D deficiency. Tertiary HPT occurs in patients who have had a successful renal transplant.

A little aide memoire for the above is that secondary, tertiary and familial causes of HPT result in multiple-gland disease.

Presentation

♦ Asymptomatic (very common, i.e. only found on routine biochemical testing), the so called mild hypercalcaemia.

Note

— Other causes of hypercalcaemia include malignancy with bony metastases (e.g. lung, breast), TB, sarcoidosis, familial hypocalciuric hypercalcaemia, drugs (e.g. thiazide diuretics), Paget's disease, thyrotoxicosis, Addison's disease.

These presenting symptoms and signs are mainly due to the systemic effects of hypercalcaemia:

- Bone disease (bone pain, pathological fractures, pepperpot skull, Brown tumours).
- Renal disease (stones, polyuria, haematuria, polydipsia).
- Gastrointestinal tract (GIT) disease (peptic ulcer disease - hypercalcaemia stimulates gastrin and, hence, increased gastric acid secretion. Hypercalcaemia can also be a cause of acute pancreatitis. It can also present with constipation).
- Hypertension.
- Psychiatric and neuromuscular symptoms.

Investigations

- Raised serum corrected calcium (which 'corrects' for the amount of calcium that is protein bound to albumin). Remember that a consequence of the blood albumin level increasing is that the 'corrected' calcium level will fall, which helps in the interpretation of blood results in these patients.
- Check serum PTH levels which are raised in HPT.
- USS and SestaMIBI localise 60-80% of abnormal parathyroid glands.

Treatment

Conventional surgery (four gland exploration) will cure the hypercalcaemic state in >95% of patients, without the need to resort to pre-operative USS or SestaMIBI, but, only when performed by an experienced surgeon. These scans are mandatory when a minimally invasive surgical technique is planned. At surgery, only enlarged glands are removed. Patients with multiple gland disease affecting all the glands can be treated with a subtotal parathyroidectomy or a total parathyroidectomy and autotransplantation, e.g. re-implantation into the forearm, brachioradialis muscle.

A minimally invasive approach includes videoscopic parathyroid surgery, small incision (focused) parathyroidectomy, or unilateral open neck exploration.

Complications

- Haematoma, with a consequent risk of stridor and respiratory distress.
- Wound infection, actually very unusual in thyroid surgery.
- Voice change from recurrent laryngeal nerve palsy, usually unilateral.
- Hypocalcaemia, usually due to surgical trauma to, or removal of, the parathyroid glands. Calcium levels must be checked 24-48 hours after surgery. Symptoms are paraesthesiae in the hands and feet and peri-oral numbness at their most mild, but can progress to laryngospasm or even cardiac arrest at their most severe.

Hypoparathyroidism

Hypoparathyroidism can be congenital or acquired. Acquired is post-surgical and is the most common cause. Congenital can be as a result of Di George syndrome, which is thymic hypoplasia with hypoparathyroidism and cardiac defects.

Presentation

This is much more commonly seen as a postoperative complication of parathyroid surgery or thyroidectomy, or other neck surgical procedures. Low PTH levels result in low circulating levels of calcium. Calcium levels need to be monitored postoperatively.

Symptoms are of tingling in the fingers or lips, and carpopedal spasm. Trousseau's and Chvostek's signs are positive. Trousseau's sign is brought on by the use of a tourniquet on an upper limb inflated to greater than the patient's systolic pressure, and observation of contraction of flexor muscles resulting in a flexed wrist and fingers. Chvostek's sign is elicited by tapping the facial nerve anterior to the tragus of the ear, and observing twitching/contraction of the muscles of facial expression.

Severe hypocalcaemia can be associated with cardiac arrhythmia. Chronic hypocalcaemia is associated with cataracts and bone demineralisation with deterioration in mental function.

Note

— 'Hungry bones' are a cause of postoperative hypocalcaemia in patients with severe hyperpituitarism treated by parathyroidectomy (or after thyrotoxicosis surgery), where the bone cells devoid of the high PTH to which they have become accustomed act to absorb circulating calcium into the bones.

Investigations

♦ Check serum calcium and corrected calcium levels which are low in hypoparathyroidism.
♦ Check serum PTH levels which are low in hypoparathyroidism.

Treatment

In patients with mild, or asymptomatic hypocalcaemia, treatment is with oral calcium, and sometimes vitamin D replacement.

In patients with severe hypocalcaemia, treatment is with a slow IV bolus, or an infusion, of calcium chloride, or calcium gluconate in normal saline.

Complications

♦ Calcium replacement in the long term is a risk for calcium kidney stones.

The adrenal disorders

There are normally four parathyroid glands (but the number is variable). They are located posterior to the thyroid gland, anterior to the thyroid and cricoid cartilages. They are responsible for calcium homeostasis. They achieve this thanks to calcium receptors that stimulate release of PTH when low calcium is detected. PTH results in increased blood calcium by stimulating increased osteoclast activity in bone (increased bone resorption and, hence, calcium release). It also activates vitamin D which stimulates increased gastrointestinal absorption of calcium, and stimulates increased reabsorption of calcium from the kidneys.

Normal adrenal glands secrete glucocorticoid (cortisol) from the adrenal cortex (which is the outer layer of the gland, representing 90% of its weight), mineralocorticoid (aldosterone) and sex steroid precursors. Noradrenaline, adrenaline and dopamine are secreted from the adrenal medulla, which is the inner layer of the gland, representing 10% of its weight.

Cortisol metabolism

Cortisol is a steroid molecule, the archetypal 'corticosteroid' which is 90% bound to the specific carrier protein, cortical binding globulin or albumin. When bound, it is not metabolically active; it is only active when free.

Cortisol has a classic hypothalamus-anterior pituitary-adrenal negative feedback mechanism, i.e. high cortisol inhibits hypothalamic corticotrophin releasing hormone (CRH) and anterior pituitary adrenocorticotrophic hormone (ACTH) secretion.

Actions of cortisol

Cortisol increases gluconeogenesis, and reduces glucose uptake and utilisation. In the liver cortisol causes an increase in protein synthesis, elsewhere it has catabolic effects.

Excessively raised levels of cortisol are associated with an increased rate of lipolysis and redistribution of body fat. Central nervous system actions include altered sleep and mood. On musculoskeletal tissue there is osteopaenia, vertebral body collapse and growth retardation in children. Other signs of excessive cortisol are muscle wasting, thin skin, poor wound healing and bruising. Cortisol also has an immunosuppressive and anti-inflammatory action.

It is a hormone with a broad range of actions, but the easiest way to remember the important functions is by summarising them as catabolic, anti-anabolic and diabetogenic.

Cushing's syndrome

Presentation

Named in 1932 after Harvey Cushing, a neurosurgeon, Cushing's disease is caused by a pituitary adenoma. Cushing's syndrome is effectively all other causes of a syndrome of cortisol excess in non-pituitary disease.

Excess cortisol causes muscle wasting, central obesity, skin fragility, bruising and striae, and can also cause depression/psychosis, osteoporosis, hypertension, hyperglycaemia and susceptibility to infection, buffalo hump and moon face.

Note

— Cushing's syndrome is four times more common in women than men.

Hypercortisolism is either ACTH-dependent or ACTH-independent.

Pituitary dependent:

♦ Pituitary adenoma Cushing's disease (causes bilateral adrenal hyperplasia).
♦ Ectopic ACTH-secreting tumours, e.g. bronchial carcinoid or oat cell, pancreatic, ovarian, stomach, medullary thyroid cancer, cause bilateral adrenal hyperplasia.

ACTH-independent:

♦ Adrenocortical tumours (adenoma or carcinoma - unilateral).
♦ Macronodular adrenocortical hyperplasia (often bilateral).
♦ Iatrogenic steroid administration (bilateral small adrenals). Strictly speaking this is a Cushingoid condition.

Note

— An adrenal tumour in an adult is more likely to be benign than malignant.

Investigations

To determine the cause of hypercortisolism the cortisol excess must first be confirmed (a and b). Then the loss of the ACTH feedback must be confirmed (c). Finally, whether it is ACTH-dependent or independent disease is identified:

a) Loss of diurnal variation of cortisol serum levels.
b) Elevated urinary-free cortisol.
c) The overnight 1mg dexamethasone suppression test (low-dose dexamethasone) is a screening test. If it is abnormal, 48-hour low-dose dexamethasone is administered and ACTH is measured. This will identify it as ACTH-dependent or independent.

The results are interpreted as follows: if cortisol excess is confirmed and ACTH is suppressed, the adrenals are examined with either CT or MRI (a cortisol secreting tumour from the adrenals will result in inhibition of ACTH); if ACTH is not suppressed, or even increased, the pituitary or the chest is examined with MRI and a chest X-ray, looking for a pituitary or ectopic (lung tumour) source of ACTH, to account for this. In pituitary ACTH-secreting tumours, petrosal sinus sampling can also be performed, which will help locate the side of the pituitary disease. This will be helpful in identifying which half of the pituitary to excise, as this will leave behind healthy pituitary tissue whilst still treating the condition.

A high-dose dexamethasone test is used to separate pituitary from non-pituitary disease.

Treatment

Medical

To switch off excess production of cortisol. Metyrapone or ketoconazole can be used, but usually these are temporary treatments.

Surgical

- Pituitary adenoma:
  - trans-sphenoidal microsurgical dissection and excision of the basophil adenoma;
  - radiotherapy of the pituitary (the effects can take several years to manifest);
  - a bilateral adrenalectomy can be offered for persistent disease or relapse.
- Ectopic ACTH-secreting tumour:
  - excision/debulking, e.g. pancreatic or chest tumour.
- Adrenocortical adenoma:
  - unilateral adrenalectomy.
- Adrenocortical carcinoma (very poor prognosis):
  - unilateral adrenalectomy;
  - radical surgery if advanced.

Note

- 60% of adrenocortical carcinomas are hormone secreting, and 40% are non-functioning.
- Nelson's syndrome occurs in patients with a pituitary tumour after bilateral adrenalectomy, and is a syndrome of hyperpigmentation. It is caused by very high levels of ACTH stimulating melanocytes.

Note

- Adrenalectomy can be performed by either open or laparoscopic means. The consensus is that laparoscopy represents the gold standard as the complication rate is significantly lower.

Complications

For both laparoscopic and open adrenalectomy the complications are:

- Bleeding at the surgical site. If the bleeding is uncontrolled, a conversion to open surgery may be required. However, the transfusion requirement is low.
- Damage to local structures, e.g. pancreas, diaphragm, pneumothorax, renal artery and the IVC.
- DVT/PE.
- Wound infection (in open) and port-site infection (in laparoscopic). Port-site infection is considerably less common.
- Incisional hernia/pain/laxity of abdominal muscles (in open); very rarely seen in laparoscopic surgery.
- Fragmentation of the adrenal gland. This increases the risk of recurrence. Intra-operatively, this is more common in laparoscopic than open surgery.
- Patient death, secondary to steroid deficiency, termed an Addisonian crisis. An Addisonian crisis can either be due to acute, or chronic, steroid insufficiency. This is because, in removing the unilateral adrenal adenoma that was secreting excessive cortisol, the other adrenal gland would have been hypofunctioning over a long period, and would not immediately secrete enough cortisol to meet the patient's needs. The patient would therefore need peri-operative steroid cover and subsequent maintenance hydrocortisone therapy until recovery of the hypothalamic-pituitary-adrenal axis. However, in the specific case of bilateral adrenalectomy, patients require both glucocorticoid (e.g. hydrocortisone) and mineralocorticoid (e.g. fludrocortisone) replacement therapy to prevent deficiency.

Addison's disease (hypoadrenalism)

There are three causes of hypoadrenalism. Dr. Thomas Addison, a British physician in 1855, only actually named the tuberculous cause.

These causes are:

- Primary - adrenocortical disease (described by Addison).
- Secondary - hypopituitarism.
- Tertiary - CRH deficiency.

The most common cause is autoimmune disease, followed (worldwide) by TB.

Presentation

This is an adrenocortical insufficiency, usually the result of an autoimmune destruction of adrenal cortical tissue. Cortisol deficiency leads to anorexia, fatigue, lethargy, a high secretion of ACTH (due to decreased feedback inhibition), resulting in skin pigmentation (due to melanocyte precursor protein preceding ACTH synthesis), poor tolerance of stress, fever, loss of female secondary sexual hair, weight loss and hypoglycaemia.

An Addisonian crisis is seen most commonly in surgical practice as a result of a patient who usually takes exogenous corticosteroids or has done so in the last year (e.g. for inflammatory bowel disease), suddenly ceases, resulting in a severe acute adrenal insufficiency. This potentially fatal condition can present with severe abdominal as well as upper and lower limb pains, with vomiting, diarrhoea and consequent dehydration. Also, hypoglycaemia, hypotension and convulsions may present.

To prevent those patients who have taken oral steroids long term from suffering an Addisonian crisis in the peri-operative period (where the body's steroid requirements are increased, but the adrenals cannot react appropriately due to long-term suppression by exogenous steroid administration), they should be given hydrocortisone IV/IM for the immediate postoperative period and for the subsequent 48 hours. A standard dose is 100mg IV three times daily.

Investigations

- Because adrenocortical insufficiency can be primary (autoimmune destruction of the adrenal cortex) or secondary (failure of the pituitary to secrete enough ACTH), a test to distinguish between the two should be performed - the Synacthen test. This stands for synthetic ACTH. The test requires the administration of ACTH and measuring the subsequent cortisol levels to see if the ACTH prompts an increase in the cortisol plasma level (occurs in secondary Addison's disease, as the otherwise normal adrenal responds to ACTH by secreting cortisol) or whether the administration of ACTH has no effect (occurs in primary Addison's disease, as the adrenals have largely been destroyed by the autoimmune process and are

incapable of secreting any more cortisol than they already are).
- Low serum sodium (hyponatraemia).
- Low serum glucose (hypoglycaemia).
- Raised serum potassium (hyperkalaemia).
- There may be a lymphocytosis (raised white cell count).

Treatment

Treatment of an acute Addisonian crisis is by IV administration of hydrocortisone, dextrose and saline.

Treatment of adrenocortical insufficiency is with oral hydrocortisone and fludrocortisone (mineralo-corticoid). In secondary adrenocortical insufficiency, where ACTH secretion is low, only hydrocortisone is required.

Hyperaldosteronism

Hyperaldosteronism can be either primary (adrenal adenoma, termed Conn's syndrome) or secondary (e.g. to renal artery stenosis, or chronic renal failure).

Excess aldosterone results in excess salt and water retention, and loss of K^+ (hypokalaemia) and H^+ (alkalosis) from the kidney.

Primary hyperaldosteronism
- Adrenal adenoma (most common, 85% of cases).
- Bilateral hyperplasia.
- Adrenal carcinoma (rare).

Note

– An adrenal adenoma is termed Conn's syndrome, after Dr. Jerome Conn, 1955.

Presentation

It can occur at any age, but the peak incidence is at 20-40 years old. Adenomas are more common in females than males. It causes hypertension, cardiac dysrhythmias, headaches, hypokalaemia, muscle weakness, cramps, polyuria, polydipsia and nocturia.

Investigations

- Elevated plasma aldosterone.
- Suppressed plasma renin activity.
- Hypokalaemia.
- High K^+ in urine (in the presence of hypokalaemia).
- MRI/CT can identify the adrenal lesion. In Conn's syndrome most lesions are <3cm in diameter. When there is doubt about which adrenal gland is abnormal, selective catheterisation of either the left or right adrenal vein is performed to measure aldosterone levels and lateralise the hormonal abnormality.

Treatment

Medical
Spironolactone (an aldosterone antagonist) and K^+ replacement with or without amiloride.

Surgical (unilateral adrenalectomy)
Laparoscopic resection of unilateral adrenal adenoma. After surgical treatment 60% of patients are still on antihypertensives, but less drugs are needed, and the pressure is easier to control.

Causes of secondary hyperaldosteronism
- Severe hypertensive chronic renal failure.
- Severe hypertensive cardiovascular disease.

Note

— This is due to chronic stimulation of renin secretion, and hence high aldosterone (as opposed to low renin in primary aldosteronism).

Complications
For both laparoscopic and open adrenalectomy the complications are as listed on p353 (section on Cushing's syndrome).

Congenital adrenal hyperplasia (CAH)

Presentation
CAH has a variation of severity of presentation from mild to severe. This is a deficiency of a variety of hydroxylase enzymes in cortisol synthesis. Consequently, there is a low cortisol level and, therefore, a high ACTH (trying to stimulate more cortisol). The adrenal gland expands (adrenal hyperplasia), resulting in increased secretion of androgenic steroid precursors which cause signs of virilisation. It is very rare.

In males, it causes short stature (early physeal fusion) and the phenotype of 'mini-Hercules'. In females, it causes masculinisation (pseudohermaphroditism, clitoral enlargement). In both, there is impaired aldosterone secretion; therefore, there is a raised urinary salt loss and, hence, hyponatraemia, vomiting and a failure to thrive (in the newborn).

Investigations
- 17-hydroxyprogesterone is elevated on serum analysis.
- Androstenedione is also elevated.
- Urinary steroid profile is also deranged.
- Raised serum potassium (hyperkalaemia).
- Low serum sodium (hyponatraemia).
- One may see a low serum glucose (hypoglycaemia).

Treatment
Treatment is by corticosteroid replacement.

Complications
You are not expected to know the complications of treatment of congenital adrenal hyperplasia. This section is included for completeness in disorders of the adrenal glands and occasionally questions relating to your awareness of the topic may arise.

Phaeochromocytoma

Presentation
Named by Pick in 1912, this is a functioning tumour of chromaffin cells; 80-90% occur in the adrenal gland, 10% are extra-adrenal.

Note

— Rule of 10s with phaeochromocytomas:
  - 10% are bilateral;
  - 10% are malignant;
  - 10% are extra-adrenal.

Familial phaeochromocytoma (30% in adults) occurs in a variety of syndromes:

- MEN IIa.
- MEN IIb.
- Neurofibromatosis Type I.
- von Hippel-Lindau syndrome.
- The succinate dehydrogenase mutation (known as familial paraganglioma syndrome).

Thus, all patients under the age of 40 require genetic screening.

Phaeochromocytoma is the great mimic due to a wide variety of symptoms: hypertension (constant or variable), headaches, sweating, palpitations, tachycardia, angina, arrhythmias, MI, CVA, LVF, cardiomyopthy, flushing, pallor, pupillary dilatation, Raynaud's, fever, tremors, nausea, weight loss, heat intolerance, vertigo, anxiety, feeling of impending doom, generalised abdominal pain, ileus, pseudo-obstruction, glucose intolerance, hyperglycaemia.

Investigations

The diagnosis needs to be proven and the tumour localised.

Investigations are as follows:

- 24-hour urine collection for fractionated catecholamines, metanephrines and normetanephrines.
- CT/MRI scan.
- 1,2,3-MIBG (meta-iodobenzylguanidine; a metabolite only taken up by high-catecholamine-secreting tissue).

Treatment

Surgical

An alpha-blocker (e.g. phenoxybenzamine) should be started at diagnosis and increased in the pre-operative phase until side effects occur. Routine beta-blockade is not indicated. Patients should only be given beta-blockers if they are already on alpha-blockers and tachycardia develops.

An ECG, central line, arterial line, and potent antihypertensives and anti-arrhythmics are required on hand during surgery.

Excision of the adrenal gland, an adrenalectomy, represents the surgical treatment of phaeochromocytoma. Surgery entails a laparoscopic adrenalectomy.

Note

- Urinary catecholamines can be measured four weeks postoperatively to confirm cure.

Complications

- Intra-operative hypertension can occur with manipulation of the adrenal, releasing a bolus of catecholamines. This carries with it a risk of CVA and MI. This is minimised by pre-operative alpha +/- beta-blockade.

Otherwise, complications of adrenalectomy for phaeochromocytoma are similar to those mentioned previously in this chapter:

- Bleeding at the surgical site. If the bleeding is uncontrolled, a conversion to open surgery may be required. However, the transfusion requirement is low.
- Damage to local structures, e.g. pancreas, diaphragm, pneumothorax, renal artery and the IVC.
- Recurrence of adrenal tumour.
- DVT/PE.
- Wound infection (in open) and port-site infection (in laparoscopic). Port-site infection is considerably less common.
- Incisional hernia/pain/laxity of abdominal muscles (in open); very rarely seen in laparoscopic surgery.
- Fragmentation of the tumour is associated with a risk of seeding within the peritoneal cavity.

Incidentalomas of the adrenal gland

These are adrenal tumours found on cross-sectional imaging in patients undergoing a scan for an unrelated reason.

Investigations

A protocol for biochemical testing to exclude a hyperfunctioning adrenal gland is outlined previously. The absence of any symptoms in patients in whom an incidentaloma is identified on scanning does not exclude a biochemical abnormality, e.g. a functioning adenoma.

In patients with a history of malignancy, an adrenal metastasis will explain the incidentaloma in 50% of cases.

Biopsy of the adrenal gland should never be performed until phaeochromocytoma has been excluded by biochemical testing. It is potentially fatal.

Treatment
This should be treated as previously set out.

Chapter 12

Urology

Prostatic disease

Benign prostatic hypertrophy (BPH)

Presentation

The aetiology of BPH is unknown, but it has been postulated to be related to local androgen imbalance.

In BPH, the detrusor muscle becomes hypertrophied to overcome the outflow obstruction of the enlarged prostate, which can result in detrusor muscle irritability and hence symptoms of urinary urgency, i.e. a feeling that one needs to urinate right now, or one will lose continence.

There is a variety of symptoms caused by BPH and these are collectively termed as lower urinary tract symptoms (LUTS): hesitancy (difficulty initiating the flow of urine), poor stream, intermittency, dribbling and nocturia (having to repeatedly get up at night to urinate). BPH can also present with acute urinary retention in the emergency setting. The patient presents with a history of being unable to initiate the flow of urine, followed by increasing lower abdominal discomfort that becomes an acute and severe pain, associated with the desperate need to urinate.

It appears, counter-intuitively, that the size of the prostate and severity of obstructive symptoms may be unrelated.

Hypertrophy of the detrusor will eventually not be able to overcome bladder outflow obstruction (BOO), and back pressure results in incomplete voiding, bilateral hydronephrosis and eventually renal failure.

Chronic retention of urine, as a clinical entity separate to the symptoms mentioned in BPH, presents as painless, dribbling overflow incontinence, with a lower abdominal mass and often with symptoms of renal failure (high pressure chronic retention). Often it is due to chronic BOO, secondary to BPH, but it can be due to cauda equina syndrome.

Other causes of acute urinary retention

BPH is the commonest cause of acute urinary retention in men over the age of 55 years, but other causes are:

◆ Urethral stricture, after instrumentation use (e.g. catheterisation or urethroscopy), urethritis, or rarely from a urethral stone.
◆ Traumatic urethral rupture.
◆ Spinal cord injury (spinal shock).
◆ In children, congenital urethral valves (at the level of the verumontanum, which is the small crest in the urethra where the seminal ducts enter).
◆ Postoperative retention (pain, recumbency, detrusor irritability secondary to anaesthesia). This can be on a background of prostatic symptoms, drugs, e.g. tricyclics.

Investigations

- Digital rectal examination (DRE) is mandatory in men presenting with LUTS or retention. It is important to note the size and consistency of the gland. A hard prostate should raise the suspicion of prostate cancer.
- Urine dipstick, looking for blood, leukocytes and nitrites (evidence of infection).
- Urinary MC+S if infection is suspected.
- USS of kidneys, ureters, bladder (KUB) and prostate, looking for hydronephrosis, bladder distension, post-micturition residual and prostate size.
- Blood tests: FBC, U&Es (looking for renal failure).
- Prostate-specific antigen (PSA) test. This should be offered only after appropriate counselling to the patient. PSA is not cancer-specific and can be elevated with infection, inflammation, instrumentation of the prostate, urinary retention and BPH.

Treatment

Acute urinary retention

Catheterisation of the bladder, via the urethra, rapidly resolves this acute condition (to the great relief of the patient). If the bladder contains more than 1L of urine, it is wise to admit the patient under the care of the on-call urology team, with a venous cannula for rehydration. It is mandatory to measure serum creatinine and electrolytes, looking out for any evidence of renal failure. In patients with impaired renal function, the urine output should be measured hourly to rule out pathological diuresis, as this requires fluid replacement. Remember the normal maximum capacity of the urinary bladder is around 500ml. This can gradually increase in chronic BOO, to reach values in excess of 1.5L.

BPH

Medical treatment:

- Alpha-blockers decrease the sympathetic stimulation of the bladder neck sphincter and also the smooth muscle fibres within the prostate gland. Tamsulosin and alfuzosin are in common use.
- 5-alpha-reductase inhibitor. Finasteride inhibits the conversion of testosterone to dihydrotestosterone (more potent than testosterone), thus, shrinking the size of the prostate gland.
- Combination of an alpha-blocker and a 5-alpha reductase inhibitor (combination therapy) has been shown to be superior to monotherapy alone in the relief of symptoms and progression of BPH.

Surgical treatment:

- Transurethral resection of the prostate (TURP).
- Retropubic Millin's prostatectomy (via a transabdominal incision, called a Pfannenstiel incision, which means bucket handle in German). Only the enlarged lobes of the prostate gland are removed and this approach is used occasionally when the prostate gland size is more than 80-100g. This operation should not be confused with retropubic radical prostatectomy where the entire prostate gland is removed for localised prostate cancer.
- Laser prostatectomy.
- Transurethral needle ablation (TUNA) of the prostate and thermotherapy are not particularly effective.

Complications

- Infection.
- Bleeding (prostate capsular perforation may result in haemorrhage from the vein plexus, requiring transfusion or even conversion to open surgery).
- Clot retention
- Retrograde ejaculation.
- Impotence.
- Incontinence due to damage to the external urethral sphincter.
- Urethral strictures.
- Urgency.
- A rare complication is transurethral resection (TUR) syndrome. This is fluid intoxication secondary to the irrigation fluid (which is a glycine solution) getting into the circulation via the venous plexus. This results in metabolic complications and confusion, with or without coma, requiring ITU treatment. The risk factors include prolonged resection time, a large vascular prostate and the weight of the tissue resected.

Carcinoma of the prostate

Aetiology

The cause is unknown. The incidence increases with age. It is present in about 60-70% of men over 80 years on autopsy. However, not all men with prostate cancer in this age group will die of prostate cancer.

Presentation

Presents with:

◆ BOO symptoms or acute retention.
◆ Renal failure.
◆ Sclerotic bone metastases (characteristically to vertebrae, ribs and pelvis) causing pain.
◆ Haemospermia/back or perineal pain.
◆ Rectal obstruction.
◆ In the developed nations, most often the diagnosis is reached due to PSA screening for prostate cancer.

Pathology

The most common type of prostate cancer is adenocarcinoma, which has an acinar (berry-shaped termination to a gland) architecture. Transitional cell carcinomas and epidermoid carcinomas can also arise from large prostatic ducts.

Staging

TNM (2002) staging classification

◆ Tx: primary tumour cannot be assessed.
◆ T0: no evidence of original tumour.
◆ T1: clinically unapparent tumour, not detected by DRE or visible by imaging:
  • T1a: tumour is an incidental histological finding in 5% or less of tissue resected;
  • T1b: tumour is an incidental histological finding in more than 5% of tissue resected;
  • T1c: tumour is identified by needle biopsy, e.g. performed because of raised PSA.
◆ T2: intracapsular (contained within the capsule), distorting anatomy of the gland:
  • T2a: tumour involves one half of one lobe or less;

• T2b: tumour involves more than one half of one lobe but not both lobes;
  • T2c: tumour involves both lobes.
◆ T3: extracapsular, i.e. extends through the capsular wall:
  • T3a: extracapsular extension, unilateral or bilateral;
  • T3b: tumour invades the seminal vesicles.
◆ T4: tumour is fixed or invades adjacent structures other than the seminal vesicles, e.g. bladder neck, rectum, levator muscles and/or pelvic wall.
◆ Nodes and metastases:
  • N0: no positve nodes:
  • N1: positive nodes;
  • M0: no metastases;
  • M1: metastases.

Grading

Tumour grade is a reliable prognostic indicator of cancer progression and the likely response to treatment. Grading can be taken to mean the microscopic appearance of the tumour. Factors that affect tumour grade are degree of cellular differentiation, number of mitoses, appearance of the nuclei (normal or pleiomorphic, meaning abnormally shaped), and cellular variation.

A different way of grading a prostatic tumour is the Gleason classification, which ranges from I-V, and is based on the degree of glandular differentiation. The Gleason score is now the standard in reporting prostate cancer.

Note

— Different parts of the prostate may have different grades. In this system, the two most common grades are added together, i.e. I + III = IV. Because two such scores are made for the 1st and 2nd most common pattern and are added together, the maximum score is therefore 10 (i.e. 5 in two separate sections of the gland).
— It is not, however, expected of you to know the details of the Gleason classification for exams.

Investigations

- PSA.
- Tissue diagnosis from transrectal ultrasound (TRUS)-guided prostate biopsy.
- Blood test: bone profile for alkaline phosphatase and calcium levels, both of which would be high in prostate cancer.
- Bone scan (performed if PSA >20, the total Gleason score is >7, alkaline phosphatase is raised or in patients with bony pain).

Treatment

Treatment depends on various factors such as the patient's age, comorbidity and also staging of the prostate cancer.

Prostate cancer can be broadly divided into localised (confined within the prostate gland), locally advanced (invading locally into surrounding tissue or spread to local lymph nodes) and metastatic prostate cancer.

Localised prostate cancer

In men younger than 75 years (i.e. with a life expectancy of >10 years), the options available are surgery, radiotherapy and active surveillance. The choice of treatment depends upon the prognostic factors of the cancer detected (i.e. level of PSA, Gleason score) and also the patient's choice. The surgery performed for localised prostate cancer is a radical prostatectomy. Radiotherapy is via external beam radiotherapy or brachytherapy. Active surveillance is advocated in patients with good prognostic markers for prostate cancer, where regular DRE and PSA measurements are taken with a view to intervene with radical treatment if there is a suggestion of progression of cancer.

Locally advanced prostate cancer

Neoadjuvant radiotherapy has been shown to improve survival, although it carries an associated morbidity. Hormone therapy may also be considered in this group of patients.

Metastatic prostate cancer

Hormone therapy is the mainstay of treatment in this group of patients. Androgen deprivation therapy has shown to decrease the rate of progression of cancer and also morbidity associated with the spread of cancer. However, hormone therapy has the drawbacks of inducing hot flushes and impotence.

Hormone therapy

Because the prostate cancer is androgen-dependent, suppressing the production of testosterone (or blocking its receptor) induces tumour regression. This can be achieved by bilateral orchidectomy, synthetic gonadotrophin releasing hormone (GnRH) or anti-androgen drugs and oestrogen administration. GnRH analogues and/or anti-androgens are the first-line drugs in the current management of metastatic prostate cancer.

Palliation

- Radiotherapy for bone pain.

Note

- Poor response to chemotherapy.

Surgical

- Radical prostatectomy. This is performed through one of two possible surgical approaches:
  - open retropubic approach or a perineal approach;
  - minimally invasive laparoscopic or robotic-assisted approach.

Complications of radical prostatectomy

- Impotence.
- Incontinence.
- Contracture of the bladder neck.
- Wound infection (and possible dehiscence).
- Haematoma.

Renal tumours

Renal cell carcinoma (also known as Grawitz tumour or hypernephroma)

Hypernephroma is a misnomer as it was thought to arise from the adrenal gland ('hyper' in this case meaning 'above', i.e. above the kidney is the adrenal gland).

Classical clear cell carcinoma of the kidney arises from the cells of the proximal convoluted tubule of the kidney. It accounts for 90% of all adult renal malignancy and is usually unilateral, but in 2% can be bilateral.

Risk factors
- Smoking.
- Genetic predisposition, e.g. 65% of patients with von Hippel-Lindau syndrome develop multiple/bilateral renal cell carcinoma.
- Chronic dialysis.

Epidemiology
The male:female ratio is 3:1, occurring in older individuals of 60-70 years.

Presentation
Patients presenting with the classic triad of haematuria, an abdominal mass and loin pain is seen less often these days. Other possible presenting symptoms include weight loss, fever, night sweats and malaise. A particular sign to look out for is acute presentation with a left-sided painless varicocoele, occurring as a result of obstruction of the opening of the testicular vein into the renal vein by the tumour thrombus arising from the renal cell carcinoma. More than 50% of renal cell carcinoma today is picked up on a routine ultrasound scan of the abdomen for other unrelated symptoms.

Macroscopic appearance:

- A tumour greater than 3cm diameter is most often a renal cell carcinoma rather than a benign lesion.
- Variegated appearances with golden yellow, grey and brown areas of coloration.
- Tendency to invade the renal vein.

Microscopic appearance:

- Papillary, solid, cystic and sarcomatoid patterns.
- Granular, clear and eosinophyllic cells.
- Contain glycogen and lipids.
- Contain vascular stroma.

Note

- Most renal cell tumours should be regarded as malignant; benign renal tumours are less common.
- Renal cell carcinoma represents 90% of all tumours of the kidney.
- Renal cell carcinoma can arise from a complex renal cyst.
- In children, Wilms' tumour (nephroblastoma) can occur, which is hereditary or sporadic. It is only bilateral in 5-10% of cases, presenting as an abdominal swelling with or without haematuria and pyrexia. Treatment is undertaken in specialist centres by nephrectomy with or without radiotherapy and chemotherapy, depending on the stage of the tumour.

Investigations
- FBC and U+Es, looking for anaemia and renal function.
- Serum calcium, as renal cell carcinoma can cause hypercalcaemia as a paraneoplastic syndrome.
- LFTs, looking for hepatic metastases.
- ESR, often raised in renal cell carcinoma.
- Urine sample for cytology, looking for evidence of malignant cells (note that urine cytology is performed only if there is a suspicion that the tumour is a transitional cell carcinoma from the renal pelvis).
- A CT scan is used to stage the tumour and also to rule out metastatic spread to the lymph nodes, liver and lungs. It can also delineate the anatomy, showing what structures are involved with the tumour and also invasion of the renal vein.
- Bone scan. Particularly useful in cases of suspicion of bony metastases, which shine as 'hot spots'.

Treatment

Medical

Renal cell carcinoma, when advanced and metastatic, may benefit from chemotherapeutic or biological therapy. The two can be used in combination. You are not expected to know much detail of the actual agents involved, but you should be aware that renal cell carcinoma is an immunologically active tumour, and as such can respond to immunotherapy (also called 'biologic' therapy), for example, interferon-alpha or interleukin-2.

Surgical

Radical nephrectomy is the operation of choice for large tumours (if less than 4cm, a partial nephrectomy can be performed). This entails removal of the entire kidney, the perinephric fat and its capsule. In cases where the tumour has spread locally to bowel, spleen or the psoas muscle, the *en bloc* removal can include these structures.

The surgical approach is generally via an oblique incision in the flank, although there are other approaches depending on the tumour's position, size and other involved structures. A thoraco-abdominal approach is used if the tumour is large and occupying the upper pole, there is a suspicion of involvement of the IVC or if excision of a solitary pulmonary metastasis is considered.

For tumours less than 7cm, laparoscopic radical nephrectomy is considered the gold standard. Some specialist centres use the laparoscopic approach for larger tumours as well. There is no difference in the oncological outcome with the laparoscopic approach but it has significant advantages over open surgery, i.e. less painful, earlier discharge from hospital and less wound complications.

Complications

Complications of radical nephrectomy
- Ileus (transient).
- Bleeding.
- Wound infection.
- Damage to local structures, e.g. spleen, liver, pancreas, bowel, duodenum.
- Basal atelectasis with consequent risk of pneumonia (usually on the operated side).

Oncocytoma

An oncocytoma is a well differentiated eosinophillic granular cell renal tumour. The appearance is due to a cytoplasm that is packed with mitochondria. It can behave in an entirely benign fashion and has uncertain malignant potential in some cases.

Presentation

Oncocytomas can present with haematuria, or pain felt within the flank. They can simply present as an abdominal mass with no other symptoms. Most often they are identified incidentally as a renal mass when imaging is performed for another reason.

Investigations
- CT or MRI show the mass and its anatomical relations very well.
- USS does not give such good detail as a CT or MRI, but often forms part of the baseline investigations that show the abdominal mass, after which further imaging is performed.
- Percutaneous USS-guided biopsy is not usually helpful as it is extremely difficult to differentiate this tumour from a chromophobe variant of renal cell carcinoma.

Treatment

It can be difficult to successfully establish the diagnosis of oncocytoma (as opposed to renal cell carcinoma, which it resembles in many ways) prior to excision of the solid renal mass. As a consequence the safe course of action is to perform a partial nephrectomy if amenable or, indeed, a radical nephrectomy.

Complications
- Ileus (transient).
- Bleeding.
- Wound infection.
- Damage to local structures, e.g. spleen, liver, pancreas, bowel, duodenum.
- Basal atelectasis with consequent risk of pneumonia (usually on the operated side).

Embryoma of the kidney or Wilms' tumour

Presentation
Max Wilms characterised this tumour in 1899. It is the most common malignant neoplasm of the urinary tract in children. It is rare after the age of seven years and the peak incidence is between 3-4 years. It is responsible for 10% of childhood tumours and 15% of patients have other congenital anomalies. One in ten Wilms' tumours are bilateral. An association between Wilms' tumour, aniridia (absence of the iris) and hemihypertrophy (overgrowth of limbs on one side of the body) is recognised.

These are tumours of mesodermal origin, microscopically an admixture of epithelial and mesenchymal components. Spread is by direct invasion, but haematogenous spread is known.

Children often present with abdominal pain or the parent has appreciated an abdominal mass. They may also present with haematuria as a consequnce of invasion into the renal pelvis, but this is a poor prognostic sign as this occurs late. Children with Wilms' tumour may also present with fever (because of tumour necrosis) and anaemia.

In general, tumours of less than 5cm diameter are not known to metastasize. There are exceptions and very small tumours can invade into the renal vein and give rise to distant metastases via this route.

The pathological grading is complicated in this tumour, and you are not expected to know it. There are four grades based on the nuclear characteristics:

- Grade I. Round uniform nuclei, difficult to distinguish from the norm.
- Grade IV. Multilobed nuclei and heavy chromatin clumps within the nucleus.

Investigations
- Ultrasound is a very useful investigation.
- CT and MRI are necessary to evaluate the extent of the tumour.

Treatment
Treatment is by a multidisciplinary combination of radical nephrectomy followed by six weeks of chemotherapy. This combined approach can achieve an 80% cure rate in unilateral disease.

Complications
Complications of radical nephrectomy are outlined previously (see page 364).

Complications of chemotherapy are:

- Cardiac parenchymal damage.
- Renal failure (can result in a type of Fanconi syndrome that causes vitamin D loss and, hence, rickets).
- Hepatic damage.
- Testicular damage.

Bladder tumours

Bladder cancer

This is the second most prevalent urological malignancy in middle aged and elderly men after prostate cancer. It is 2.5 times more common in men than in women. More than 90% are transitional cell carcinomas (TCC); however, 2-5% are squamous cell carcinomas (SCC) and 2% are adenocarcinomas.

Aetiology
- Occupational risk factors. Exposure to urinary nitrosamines found in the chemical industry is a significant risk factor.
- Cigarette smoking. It increases the risk four-fold and is the most common aetiological association in the Western world.
- Bilharziasis (parasitic infestation of the bladder) and chronic cystitis.
- Pelvic irradiation.
- Oncogenes (a gene that, when a mutation occurs in it, can lead to cancer; the opposite of a tumour suppressor gene).

Presentation
Bladder cancers grow as either papillary tumours (nipple-like appearance) or as solid infiltrating growths. There are often no associated symptoms or signs for long periods of time. They may be picked up incidentally as microscopic haematuria on dipstick testing. Otherwise the patient presents with macroscopic (frank) haematuria, which is

characteristically painless. Bladder cancers can cause irritative voiding symptoms such as urinary urgency or urinary frequency.

Note

— A field change results in the possibility of multiple urothelial primaries.

Investigations

- Mid-stream urine (MSU).
- Urine cytology (microscopic examination of a urine sample looking for malignant cells shed from the tumour).
- Ultrasound KUB. This can detect any solid lesion in the kidney; it can also pick up hydronephrosis and may pick up papillary lesions within the bladder.
- IVU. This can pick up other TCCs in the ureter or renal pelvi-calyceal system.
- Flexible cystoscopy.
- A CT or MRI scan is usually reserved for staging investigations in invasive bladder TCC.

Types

- Superficial. Limited to the epithelium and lamina propria. Carcinoma *in situ* (CIS) is a flat lesion limited to the mucosa. Although superficial, it is a high-grade lesion that has the potential to become an invasive form of bladder cancer.
- Invasive. Invading the muscle and deeper tissue.

Remember that 50% of invasive TCCs may have micrometastases at the time of presentation.

Grade

- G1. Well differentiated.
- G2. Moderately differentiated.
- G3. Poorly differentiated.

Treatment

Management is by cystoscopic resection (transurethral resection of bladder tumour [TURBT]) of the bladder tumour and establishing the grade and stage of the disease. If superficial, then regular cystoscopic surveillance is sufficient. In recurrent

cases and those with high-grade superficial TCC, intravesical chemotherapy in the form of BCG or mitomycin C is needed. CIS of the bladder requires intravesical BCG therapy.

Invasive cancer requires definitive treatment. Radical cystectomy, with formation of an ileal conduit or a neobladder, is preferred in those who are fit for major surgery. Cystectomy takes place through a midline abdominal incision. There is an increasing trend in younger patients towards construction of a neobladder (new bladder) and attaching it to the urethra after the bladder has been removed. The neobladder is formed using a segment of the ileum. Radiotherapy is also a recognised option in the treatment of invasive bladder cancer. Radiotherapy is not indicated if there is associated CIS changes.

The cure rate with surgery is 50% and with radiotherapy it is more in the region of 35-40%. Metastatic TCC is managed with systemic chemotherapy with a response rate of 15-20%.

Complications

Early
- Urine leak.
- Lymphatic leak.
- Ileus (transient).
- Wound haematoma.
- Wound infection.

Late
- Problems of recurrent urinary tract infections (UTIs).
- Urinary strictures.
- Parastomal herniation.
- Renal stones.
- Stoma retraction.
- Hydronephrosis.

Upper tract TCC

Upper tract TCC is less common (mostly a papillary type). The risk factors are similar to bladder TCC. Diagnosis is usually established with IVU findings, retrograde studies and selective cytology. Tissue diagnosis is obtained by ureteroscopy (rigid or flexible). The treatment is usually by nephro-ureterectomy. However, in patients with poor renal function and a solitary kidney, conservative resection by endoscopic, percutaneous or surgical means is possible.

Note

- Patients who present with a bladder TCC have a 2-4% risk of going on to develop an upper tract TCC, i.e. in the ureter or renal pelvis, mostly in high-grade disease. Patients presenting with an upper tract TCC subsequently have a 40% risk of going on to develop a bladder TCC.

Haematuria

The term haematuria can be interpreted to mean either microscopic, i.e. visible under the microscope or on dipstick analysis, or macroscopic, i.e. frank, visibly blood-stained urine. Dipstick haematuria should be confirmed on microscopy as there are many factors contributing to false positive results.

The two findings have different implications. Asymptomatic microscopic haematuria can be, and often is, entirely normal, e.g. after sporting activity. It can also be associated with disease, e.g. UTI, pyelonephritis, glomerulonephritis, nephropathies, prostatitis, prostatic malignancy, renal stone disease, renal or bladder malignancy, bacterial endocarditis, or other systemic diseases.

As you might expect, these diseases come with their own characteristic cluster of symptoms which will be associated with microscopic haematuria, e.g. pyrexia, urinary frequency and dysuria in UTI, dribbling incontinence and nocturia in prostate disease or, severe flank pain in renal stone disease.

Macroscopic haematuria can present in a different fashion related to the urinary stream: at the start of the stream this suggests prostatic pathology or urethral pathology; if it occurs throughout the stream, this is suggestive of bladder or renal pathology (malignancy must be excluded); or, if it occurs at the end of the stream, this is suggestive of schistosomiasis (a helminthic infection of the bladder which is rare in the UK). However, this is not a rule.

Do not forget to look for warfarin in the drug history of macroscopic haematuria. It does not exclude malignancy as a cause, but it can afford a little reassurance.

Patients presenting with macroscopic haematuria or microscopic haematuria (with risk factors such as age, smoking, occupational exposure to dyes, urinary symptoms) require thorough evaluation and this is often done through a one-stop haematuria clinic. In this clinic, an ultrasound, flexible cystoscopy and urine cytology are performed. If these investigations are normal, then an IVU may be performed to complete the haematuria work-up.

The take home message for haematuria, especially macroscopic, is that malignancy must be excluded. (See the sections on renal and bladder malignancies for more detail.)

Renal stone disease

Aetiology

This is more common in men than women (ratio of 4:1) and appears more in the summer than winter. This is presumed to be because of increased concentration of the urine with the heat and less fluid intake.

The stones form due to precipitation of the salt from which they are made when it reaches a threshold concentration in the urine. There are various types of stone (see below).

Pathology

It is not simply the case, in urine, of salts reaching a certain concentration, then precipitating out causing a renal stone. There exist certain crystallisation inhibitors in normal urine, the most important of which is citrate. This forms a complex with calcium, one of the stone-forming ions, resulting in calcium citrate, which does not precipitate out. Other inhibitors are mucoproteins, glycoproteins and magnesium.

The pH of urine is also key to stone formation in certain disorders. The more acidic the urine, the greater the chance of uric acid stone formation.

Note

— A raised plasma uric acid concentration is not necessary to develop uric acid renal stones.

The presence of a UTI (specifically Proteus and Klebsiella) is implicated with an increased incidence of stone formation. Stone formation occurs as a result of urease activity, an enzyme that splits urea into ammonia, alkalising the urine. This increases the likelihood of staghorn calculus formation, a truly huge type of stone that can take on the shape of the renal pelvis surrounding it.

Calcium stones form from a combination of raised urinary concentration of calcium, a deficiency of inhibitors and matrix initiation. Calcium can form salts of oxalate and phosphate.

Note

— Hypercalcaemia symptoms can be remembered by the mnemonic 'bones, stones, abdominal groans and psychic moans'. It certainly increases the risk of renal stones and hence renal colic (accounting for the stones and abdominal groans).

Stones of mixed origin can also form in a reaction called epitaxy. A small, pure crystal of one chemical origin forms, and acts as a framework on which other salts can crystallise out, increasing the size of the stone.

If for any reason urine becomes stagnant in the urinary system, then the risk of stone formation increases, e.g. anatomical anomalies (pelvi-ureteric junction obstruction or horseshoe kidney).

Stones, when formed, can either lodge within the renal pelvis or migrate down the ureter. If <4mm they may pass spontaneously with no symptoms, but often cause renal colic. If they grow to sufficient size they can obstruct the ureter, and hence cause pelvicalyceal dilation, which if present long enough can result in obstructive atrophy of the renal parenchyma. Stones can also become colonised with bacteria and be the source of UTIs.

Presentation

Classically, renal stones in the kidney or ureter cause renal colic. The clinical presentation of renal or ureteric colic cannot be reliably differentiated. Both shall be referred to by the term renal colic in this chapter.

It is important to remember that renal stones can also be asymptomatic (the incidence of which is difficult to determine) and are only found incidentally on investigations for other reasons.

Renal colic presents as an emergency with acute severe flank pain, radiating to the groin, often associated with vomiting. Characteristically, the patient with colic cannot find a position of comfort, and either adopts a fetal position or paces around the examination room in obvious pain. They may be tender on palpation of the flank, and possibly round from the flank down to the groin.

An important differential diagnosis list (from which it can actually be quite difficult to tell the difference, clinically) is appendicitis, biliary colic, bowel obstruction, aortic aneurysm, and ruptured ectopic pregnancy. Other renal pathologies that can also present with acute pain are pyelonephritis or a perinephric abscess.

An important clinical sign to note is the change of nature of the pain from an initial colic to a constant pain. This can be associated with renal obstruction.

Note

— In patients above the age of 50 years, it is very important to rule out the presence of a leaking AAA (abdominal aortic aneurysm), as ruptured aneurysms often present with symptoms suggestive of renal colic.

Investigations

◆ A urinary dipstick should show up microscopic haematuria. More importantly, if there is any suggestion of nitrites, leukocytes and/or protein, an infected and obstructed stone should be considered. This makes the case a real emergency, as this can rapidly cause severe sepsis and renal damage.

◆ The following blood tests should be conducted: FBC looking for a raised WCC in infection; U&Es looking for any evidence of renal failure, but also acting as a useful baseline; and an ESR/CRP looking for indirect evidence of infection.

◆ An X-ray KUB (Kidneys, Ureters, Bladder type of abdominal X-ray) can be performed, as a proportion of stones are radio-opaque (90%). When present in the ureter, the stones should show up along a line tracking along the lateral edges of the lumbar vertebral transverse processes until the pelvic brim is reached. However, with CT being the investigation of choice, an X-ray KUB does not add much more to the information.

◆ A CT KUB (without contrast) is the gold standard investigation for patients presenting with renal colic. It has a higher sensitivity and specificity than an IVU and has the advantage of picking up other intra-abdominal pathologies that are giving rise to the patient's symptoms.

◆ An IVU can be performed in centres where CT is not available; such centres most often perform single-shot IVU (plain X-ray KUB followed by injection of contrast and another X-ray 20 minutes later).

Whenever an infected urinary stone is suspected, the patient should be referred from the casualty setting to the care of the on-call urology team. A CT KUB or an IVU is performed to confirm the diagnosis. An obstructed infected stone is an emergency and to prevent acute pyonephrosis and gram-negative septicaemia, a nephrostomy is placed by an interventional radiologist using ultrasound or an image intensifier to delineate the pelvicalyceal system. A nephrostomy is a drainage tube (often a single J stent) placed into the renal pelvis through a puncture wound on the loin of the patient. This allows the kidney to continue producing urine without the back pressure of the blockage, and not to become a stagnant collection of infected urine, which can cause pyonephrosis.

Treatment

The most useful piece of information is that the majority of stones <4mm pass spontaneously within a few days. The severe pain seems to be most effectively treated by the administration of diclofenac (it is more effective than morphine in this context). Recently, alpha-blockers such as tamsulosin or alfazosin have been tried with good success.

An anti-emetic (metoclopramide, cyclizine, prochlorperazine) is useful when the patient is vomiting. However, for those stones that do not pass spontaneously, there is a need to remove them. This can be done by non-operative means for the most part but, rarely, open surgery is required.

Extracorporeal shock wave lithotripsy is the use of a focused shock wave in combination with localisation of the stone using imaging either with ultrasound or an image intensifier. The stone becomes fragmented into numerous smaller stones, which can then pass spontaneously. Possible complications include haematuria, flank bruising, flank pain, renal haematoma and obstruction of the ureter by these small fragments.

For a large renal stone (>2cm) it may be necessary to perform a percutaneous nephrolithotomy (PCNL). A needle, radiologically guided, is used to form a tract that can be expanded for passage of a grasping tool, which can then be used to grab the stone (if small) or break it into smaller fragments under the direct vision of a nephroscope. Complications include bleeding, haematuria, transient urinary leak, pyelonephritis and a perinephric abscess.

Ureteroscopy (via a transurethral insertion) can be used to grasp ureteric stones from as high as the mid to upper ureter with a basket attachment. Stones, if large, can also be fragmented using energy sources such as LASER.

In the case of large renal stones, it is occasionally necessary to perform an open (or laparoscopic) operation for removal and, very rarely, if associated with a non-functioning kidney, a nephrectomy may be required.

Depending on the cause of the stone in the first place, there is a place for medical management in the prevention of recurrence. To prevent urinary concentration the patient should remain well hydrated. The pH of urine can be rendered alkaline by regular sodium bicarbonate ingestion in uric acid stone formers. Occasionally if the above measures are insufficient to prevent recurrence of uric acid stones, there is some evidence that allopurinol may contribute to a decreased recurrence rate in patients with uric acid stones. UTIs should be treated with the appropriate antibiotics.

Complications

Complications of ureteroscopy

Complications include ureteric perforation (usually self-limiting), haematuria and late ureteric stricture (regarded as secondary to traumatic ureteroscope insertion).

Complications of nephrectomy

- Ileus (transient).
- Bleeding.
- Wound infection.
- Damage to local structures, e.g. spleen, liver, pancreas, bowel, duodenum.
- Basal atelectasis with consequent risk of pneumonia (usually on the operated side).

Renal injuries

Presentation

Most commonly seen in high energy blunt abdominal trauma, e.g. a road traffic accident. The patient can present with a variety of signs and symptoms along a spectrum of severity, i.e. from the least severe, simply complaining of abdominal pain having walked into the department, to the most severe, an obtunded patient in shock with a bruised and distended abdomen.

Signs to look out for are:

- Cardiovascular compromise.
- Microscopic haematuria.
- Macroscopic haematuria.
- Flank bruising.
- Boggy sensation on palpation of the flank.
- Guarding on palpation of the flank.
- Fractured lower ribs posteriorly.

Grades of renal injury

- I. Contusion or non-expanding subcapsular haematoma.
- II. Cortical laceration less than 1cm deep, without extravasation of urine.
- III. Laceration extending more than 1cm into the cortex without urinary extravasation.
- IV. Laceration extending through the corticomedullary junction and into the collecting system. Thrombosis of a segmental renal artery.
- V. Thrombosis or avulsion of the main renal artery or completely shattered kidney.

Grade I and II injuries can be managed conservatively but a close eye needs to be kept on development of infection and sepsis. Grade III injuries are more serious and although one can manage a patient conservatively with antibiotics, repeated imaging is necessary to rule out development of complications; however, a cardiovascularly unstable patient should be explored. Grade IV and V injuries are a urological emergency. All penetrating injuries need to be explored.

X-ray changes that are a clue to renal injury are:

- Loss of a psoas shadow.
- Fractured 11th or 12th rib.
- Fractured transverse processes of L1, L2 or L3.
- Scoliosis to the injured side.

Investigations

- Plain X-ray - findings as outlined above.
- IVU - non-opacification of the kidney suggests pedicle injury or renal artery thrombosis. An IVU is rarely performed as the initial investigation in the evaluation of renal trauma.

- A USS KUB may be able to identify the injury to the kidney but cannot be used to grade the severity.
- A CT scan is the gold-standard investigation of choice and is useful in evaluating other intra-abdominal injuries too.

Treatment

- ABC of resuscitation and ATLS® protocol.
- Rule out life-threatening intra-abdominal injuries.
- Minor renal trauma (85% of cases) are managed conservatively, but vital signs should be monitored.
- Major renal trauma (15% of cases) may be blunt or penetrating. Most of them require exploration. Renorrhaphy (surgical repair of damage to the kidney, eg. simple laceration), partial nephrectomy or simple nephrectomy is performed, depending on the severity of the condition.

Note

- In post-renal trauma, there may be hypertension, which, although transient, can be severe and intractable, occasionally requiring nephrectomy.
- Most renal trauma is managed conservatively.

Complications

There are similar complications as for nephrectomy, bearing in mind those patients who have suffered high energy trauma damaging a kidney sufficiently to require partial or total nephrectomy are unwell, and hence are more prone to complications.

Ureteric injuries

Ureteric injuries are either traumatic or iatrogenic, i.e endoscopic urological procedures or other surgical specialties accidentally lacerating the ureter. Management is by early repair if it is picked up within 24-36 hours. If late, benefit may be gained from using a stent and waiting until the patient is fitter. Stents are important in the early repair of ureters to prevent urine loss while the anastomosis heals.

Urethral injuries

Presentation

Most traumatic urethral injuries occur as a result of a high energy road traffic accident, and they are associated with a pelvic fracture. A high index of suspicion is required to make the diagnosis.

The main point to remember is that if urethral injury is suspected, do not catheterise per urethra; a suprapubic catheter is required. The signs of urethral injury are blood at the urethral meatus, perineal swelling and bruising in the scrotum.

Note

- 10% of pelvic fractures are associated with urethral rupture.
- Ruptures can be partial or complete.

The urethra is divided into four parts: prostatic, membranous, bulbar and penile. The prostatic part is the most dilatable; the membranous part is the least dilatable.

The prostate is held firmly by the puboprostatic ligaments, thus during a shearing injury, the membranous part can suffer rupture.

Investigations

An ascending urethrogram should be performed by injecting radiopaque dye (e.g. Omnipaque) per urethra whilst screening with an image intensifier. Any rupture will show up fairly obviously, at which point injection should cease and the image printed. A note of the level of rupture should be made.

Treatment

In the emergency setting, to prevent urinary retention or extravasation of urine on attempted micturition, a suprapubic catheter should be inserted. The on-call urologist should be contacted. The management options for a ruptured urethra include immediate exploration and direct repair, followed by two weeks' protection of the repair with a urethral catheter placed under direct vision at the time of the operation. This approach is shown to have a higher incidence of impotence and stricture formation. The preferred alternative is to leave the suprapubic catheter *in situ* and then perform a delayed surgical exploration and repair.

There are endoscopic techniques enabling realignment and visualisation of the passage of the urinary catheter. This visualisation helps to prevent conversion of a partial to a total rupture by an inadvertent pushing motion with the catheter when inserted 'blind'.

Note

— The most common cause of urethral damage is iatrogenic instrumentation.

Treatment modalities for urethral stricture include dilatation, optical urethrotomy (incision of scar), and excision of the stricture and end-to-end anastomosis.

Complications

- The complication of catheterisation of a partially ruptured urethra is the potential to convert a partial to a complete rupture.
- Untreated, a urethral rupture can form a urethral fistula.
- A healed partial rupture can go on to develop a urethral stricture in the future.
- In fact, a repaired urethral rupture is also at risk of future stricture formation.
- A risk of wound infection.

Infections of the kidney

Acute pyelonephritis

Presentation

The symptoms are fever, flank pain, systemic upset and dysuria. There are acute inflammatory changes in the parenchyma, which may develop into cortical abscesses, renal carbuncles (a carbuncle is simply a term meaning abscess, generally used to mean a large abscess, which is possibly multiloculated) or pyonephrosis (in the presence of obstruction).

What differentiates acute pyelonephritis from a simple UTI is an increase in the degree of systemic upset, and the flank pain previously mentioned. The patient requires IV antibiotics and hospital admission under the care of the acute medical team.

It is very important to differentiate between acute pyelonephritis from that of an infected obstructed system, as the latter requires urgent urological intervention.

Chronic pyelonephritis

A chronically shrunken kidney is susceptible to repeated infections. Most of the scarring is done to the kidney during childhood. There may be an element of reflux allowing infected urine to backtrack to the kidney.

Investigations

- Routine bloods including inflammatory markers, i.e. FBC, U+Es, CRP and ESR.
- Ultrasound examination of the urinary tract, looking for hydronephrosis (a distended renal pelvis and kidney) and any abscesses/ carbuncles.
- Urine sample for dipstick and MC+S.

Treatment

The treatment for pyelonephritis is with IV antibiotics, followed by two weeks of oral antibiotics. A carbuncle is treated by USS-guided drainage. Pyonephrosis is managed by relieving the obstruction (this is urgent, otherwise there is rapid irreversible damage done).

Complications

- If inadequately treated, pyelonephritis can be complicated by renal abscess formation, renal failure and permanent renal parenchymal damage.
- Side effects of antibiotic medication can include allergic reaction (ranging from simple rash to life-threatening angioedema), nausea, vomiting, as well as rarer more specific reactions depending on the specific antibiotic.

Xanthogranulomatous pyelonephritis (XGP)

Presentation

This is rare and presents as a mass in the kidney which macroscopically resembles renal cell carcinoma (or Wilms' tumour in children). It is caused by a recurrent UTI (Proteus infection being the commonest) in combination with stone disease. The resultant mass can invade local structures even beyond the renal capsule. Clinically it presents as fever, loin pain, dysuria and a mass palpable in the abdomen.

XGP can mimic a tumour in many ways. There is the chronically ill 'look' of the patient who has been suffering from weight loss, malaise and altered appetite for quite some time. There is also the ability for the granulomatous tissue around the kidney to actually infiltrate into/through local structures to the kidney, e.g. perinephric fat, bowel, spleen, etc. This is an unusual phenomenon in cases excepting of malignant tumours.

Investigations
- Routine bloods including inflammatory markers, i.e. FBC, U+Es, CRP and ESR.
- Urine sample for dipstick and MC+S.
- Urine microscopy may show xanthoma (lipid-laden macrophages) cells.
- Abdominal ultrasound will show the renal mass.
- Abdominal X-ray may show a staghorn calculus.
- CT will delineate the anatomy, showing any invasion of local structures.

Treatment

Antibiotics alone are insufficient to treat XGP. Surgical excision of the affected kidney (in entirety) is indicated, i.e. nephrectomy. No inflammatory (infected) tissue should be left behind, as it risks developing abdomino-cutaneous fistulae.

Complications

The complications are as for nephrectomy.

Additionally, there is the risk of incomplete excision of the inflammatory mass which can go on to cause further infective symptoms as well as abdomino-cutaneous fistulae.

Urachal abnormalities

The urachus is the fetal means of draining the bladder via the umbilicus.

The following represents a simple list of definitions to be aware of in the exam situation. The finer points of investigation and treatment of these (generally paediatric surgical) conditions is not expected of you.

Types of abnormalities

- Patent urachus requiring complete excision.
- Urachal sinus presents as umbilical discharge in a child or in adulthood, requiring imaging via a sinogram before surgical excision.
- Urachal cyst. Presents as a mass, which can become infected.
- Urachal diverticulum. The bladder has a diverticulum where the urachus was, but it does not usually cause problems.
- Urachal carcinoma. Rare, and usually an adenocarcinoma. This requires excision of the umbilicus, urachus and part of the bladder where the urachus attaches itself (omphalo-uracho-partial cystectomy).

Neurogenic bladder conditions

Presentation

A neurogenic bladder actually refers to any urinary malfunction symptoms secondary to a neurological cause. This can take the form of incontinence, urgency, urge incontinence or urinary retention. All these differing presentations of a neurogenic bladder depend on the exact cause, and neurological level of the lesion.

The list of key points to remember are:

- Voiding is the co-ordinated contraction of the detrusor muscle and relaxation of the distal urethral striated sphincter. The control of voiding is cortical, located in the pons.
- The detrusor muscle is a syncytium of smooth muscle cells, with cholinergic innervation, i.e. responds to anticholinergics.

- The bladder neck has smooth muscle with sympathetic innervation, i.e. responds to alpha-blockers.
- The urethra contains smooth muscle.
- The distal urethral striated sphincter (DUSS) contains voluntary muscle.
- The parasympathetic nerve supply to the bladder is from S2-S4.

Pathophysiology

The bladder has motor and sensory supply. The motor supply to the detrusor muscle is primarily parasympathetic from S2, 3 and 4. The sensory supply is both by parasympathetic (stretch, fullness, pain) and sympathetic nerves (pain, touch, temperature).

The urethral sphincter has two components: striated muscle also known as an intrinsic rhabdosphincter and a smooth muscle sphincter at the bladder neck. The striated sphincter is supplied by somatic nerves S2, 3 and 4. The smooth muscle fibres are innervated by sympathetic nerves derived from T10, 11 and 12.

Classification

The International Continence Society
Detrusor:

- Normal.
- Hyper-reflexic.
- Hyporeflexic.

Sphincter:

- Normal.
- Hyperactive.
- Incompetent.

Sensation:

- Normal.
- Hypersensitive.
- Insensitive.

Investigations

- Renal function. Measure serum creatinine.
- Imaging kidneys and bladder:
  - X-ray KUB. To rule out calculi which are quite common;
  - USS KUB. To look for the presence of hydronephrosis and also measuring the residual volume.
- Video cystometrogram (VCMG) assesses the following:
  - bladder capacity;
  - pressure changes during filling;
  - pressure at which voiding occurs;
  - ability for bladder to contract;
  - premature or unstable contractions;
  - presence of residual volume;
  - ability to perceive fullness;
  - ability to inhibit or initiate voiding.
  - incontinence.

Treatment

- Clean intermittent self-catheterisation (CISC).
- Palliative diversion (performed for patients who, for example, for reasons of quadriplegia, are unable to voluntarily self-catheterise, or for patients in whom renal function is deteriorating).

Complications

CISC, other than the obvious social and emotional difficulties, can result in an increased rate of UTI and haematuria.

Complications of permanent urinary diversion can be early or late.

Early:

- Urine leak.
- Ileus (transient).
- Wound haematoma.
- Wound infection.

Late:

- Problems of recurrent urinary tract infections.
- Urinary strictures.
- Parastomal herniation.
- Renal stones.
- Stoma retraction.
- Hydronephrosis.

Levels of neurological lesions

Suprapontine cord lesion

A suprapontine neurological lesion means a lesion occurring above the pons, i.e. after a CVA. As a result the ability is lost to voluntarily relax the DUSS, therefore suffering transient urinary retention. This is followed by the return of uninhibited detrusor muscle contraction, which results in urinary frequency and urgency. Patients also suffer from nocturia and urge incontinence.

Suprasacral cord lesion

If there is a partial traumatic lesion of the spinal nerve roots above the level of the sacrum, then spinal shock (inactivity, although transient, of the nerve roots distal to the lesion) can ensue. This results in an areflexic somatic paralysis of the portions of the lower limbs served by the affected nerve roots, including the bladder. This requires catheterisation (urethral or suprapubic), and when detrusor function returns it is hyper-reflexic (urgency, frequency, incomplete voiding). Also, the DUSS fails to relax at the time of detrusor contraction which is termed detrusor sphincter dyssynergia.

Conus/cauda equina lesions

Conus/cauda equina lesions result in complete interruption of innervation of the bladder, but it is not quite 'denervated'; it is more 'decentralised', meaning the patient can only void using abdominal straining or pressure. The DUSS is permanently relaxed and, therefore, this leads to genuine stress incontinence.

Note

- The cauda equina portion of the spinal cord begins at the level of L2.

Varicocoeles and epididymal cysts

Varicocoeles

Presentation

A collection of dilated tortuous veins of the pampiniform plexus of the spermatic cord. It is more common on the left. Fifteen percent of the adult male population have a left varicocoele. It may be associated with infertility (poor count and motility).

An untreated large varicocoele in children can cause testicular growth retardation and atrophy. A sudden formation of a varicocoele in a man over 50 years suggests the possibility of renal cell carcinoma obstructing the testicular vein due to its invasion into the renal vein.

Varicocoeles are often asymptomatic, but the patient can complain of ache. It is more often picked up as an incidental finding in investigation for infertility or during routine check-ups.

Examination findings include a sensation of a 'bag of worms' when the varicose vein plexus is rolled between the fingers. It is located above the testicle and is generally non-tender to palpation. It does not transilluminate (being blood-filled) and can be emptied of blood with simple compression, then watched to refill.

Investigations

- Colour flow Doppler identifies the varicocoele and can demonstrate reverse blood flow that is characteristic in this condition.
- In cases of clinical suspicion (e.g. new onset left-sided varicocoele in a patient over 50), abdominal USS can be used to exclude renal cell carcinoma.

Treatment

Treatment of a varicocoele in men with infertility may improve the semen parameters. However, the evidence that it increases the pregnancy rate is highly debatable. Therefore, men undergoing varicocoele repair should be thoroughly counselled on this fact. Options include surgical ligation (open, microscopic or laparoscopic) or embolisation of the varicocoele by an interventional radiologist.

Complications

♦ The recurrence rate of varicocoeles is approximately 10%, whatever technique is used.

♦ Due to the potential damage to the lymphatics, there is a risk of hydrocoele formation.

♦ Open techniques, of course, include wound infection and haematoma risks.

♦ Migration of the coils is a potential complication of embolisation technique.

Epididymal cysts

Presentation

The exact cause of epididymal cysts is not known. It is a cyst containing spermatozoa, located on the supero-lateral border of the testis. It is thought either to be a simple retention cyst or obstruction of some of the ducts along which the spermatozoa pass, resulting in a cystic collection.

They present either as an asymptomatic lump found incidentally or they can cause a minor ache or simply their size (some can be quite large) has caused the patient cosmetic embarrassment.

Clinical examination reveals a smooth mass, located on the supero-lateral border of the testis. They are usually non-tender on palpation and being cystic they transilluminate. The transillumination test is intended to help differentiate between a cystic or solid mass (solid is a concern for testicular tumour).

Investigations

Often the diagnosis of an epididymal cyst is clinical; however, in cases of doubt, a scrotal ultrasound can help exclude any solid masses (e.g. testicular tumour), and confirms the cystic nature of the lump.

Treatment

Treatment is conservative, unless they are symptomatic or very large. If they are, then the cyst can be excised surgically, although there exists a risk of postoperative fibrosis leading to infertility (if the opposite testis has compromised function) or postoperative scrotal pain. Aspiration of epididymal cysts is not recommended as they are almost certain to re-accumulate.

Complications

♦ Aspiration of epididymal cysts risks introducing infection and hence a scrotal abscess. Aspiration also carries with it a relatively high risk of recurrence/re-accumulation of the cyst.

♦ Surgical excision of the cyst, as previously mentioned, carries a risk of infertility secondary to epididymal fibrosis (if the opposite testis has compromised function).

♦ Surgical excision, as well as the risk of wound infection and scrotal haematoma, carries the risk of persistent scrotal pain.

Hydrocoele of the testis

A collection of fluid within the tunica or processus vaginalis.

Classification

♦ A. Primary:
  - congenital - the hydrocoele communicates between the peritoneal cavity and the tunica vaginalis;
  - encysted hydrocoele of the cord;
  - funicular, meaning the hydrocoele is open to the peritoneal cavity, but closed to the testis;
  - vaginal where the fluid is around the testis between the two layers of the tunica vaginalis and does not usually extend into the inguinal canal.

♦ B. Secondary:
  - inflammatory;
  - malignancy;
  - parasitic;
  - postoperative.

Note

– Vaginal hydrocoele does not mean that it occurs in women, but between the two layers of the tunica vaginalis of the testis. The female counterpart of this condition is known as a hydrocoele of canal of Nuck.

Presentation

Hydrocoeles are frequently asymptomatic and identified incidentally, e.g. during the course of a routine health check. The patient can present with an ache which is usually not severe, or with worries regarding the cause of the mass (i.e. worried about malignancy), or its cosmetic appearance.

Clinical examination can reveal the following:

- Smooth cystic swelling.
- Transillumination positive.
- Testis not felt separately.
- Can get above the swelling.
- Usually not tender.

Investigations

If suspicious clinically, a USS of the scrotum can be performed to rule out testicular neoplasms.

Treatment

Congenital hydrocoele

Requires a herniotomy as the hydrocoele is associated with a patent processus vaginalis.

Others

- Jaboulay's procedure. A trans-scrotal incision is performed exposing the testis with its tunica vaginalis layer. Then a circumferential incision of the tunica vaginalis is made, excising some of the redundant tissue so as not to leave too great a mass behind. The tunica is reflected, folding it upwards on itself and sutured. This preserves the tunica tissue and prevents re-accumulation of the cyst.
- Lord's plication. This is also a trans-scrotal incision, only this time the tunica vaginalis is not dissected, rather it is folded (plicated) with intermittently placed plicating sutures. This effectively occludes the parietal tunica vaginalis, providing its own haemostasis and preventing re-accumulation of the hydrocoele.
- Aspiration with or without injection of sclerosant. Different types of sclerosant have been tried, all with a relatively high incidence of recurrence. Examples include bismuth phosphate, talc and tetracycline. Aspiration is reserved for patients who are not fit for surgery as it carries a high risk of introducing infection, formation of haematoma and also a high risk of recurrence.

Complications

- Complications of aspiration include recurrence/re-accumulation of the hydrocoele and scrotal abscess.
- Complications of surgery on the hydrocoele also include recurrence/re-accumulation, although the incidence is considerably lower than for aspiration, at a rate of approximately 5%.
- Wound infection or scrotal haematoma.

Undescended testis (cryptorchidism)

Cryptorchidism is a Greek word meaning hidden testicle. As the term suggests the testicle has not fully descended from its position in the abdominal cavity into the scrotal sac. An undescended testis can be palpable or non-palpable: a palpable undescended testis is usually in the inguinal canal; a non-palpable testis is usually intra-abdominal. An undescended testis should be distinguished from a retractile testicle (the testicle moves intermittently from the scrotum to a position along the processus vaginalis, and back again). A retractile testis does not in most cases require any urological intervention.

The testis develops in the retroperitoneum and starts to descend into the scrotum. By the third month it is in the false pelvis and by the eighth month it is in the region of the deep inguinal ring, descending into the scrotum by the ninth month.

The concern with an undescended testis is that the testicle does not go on to develop properly, affecting its endocrine function, spermatogenesis, as well as having a risk of progressing to testicular cancer in the future. For these reasons, undescended testes are treated when identified.

Factors affecting the descent are:

◆ Testosterone.
◆ Gubernaculum testis (a specially adapted fold of tissue that precedes the descent of the testis).
◆ Intrinsic testicular defect.

Incidence:

◆ Premature infants: 30%.
◆ At term: 4%.
◆ At one year: 1%.

Presentation

The scrotal sac when palpated can be completely empty in the case of bilateral undescended testicles or contain only the one, in unilateral undescended testicles. In cases of bilateral undescended testes and a suspicion of ambiguous genitalia, it is necessary to involve the paediatric urologist to confirm the sex of the child.

Further palpation may reveal a palpable soft spherical mass in the groin (in the inguinal canal), or nothing at all in the case of a testicle that has remained entirely intra-abdominal. This examination, classically described, should be on a warm and relaxed patient in a warm room performed by a surgeon with warm hands to prevent cremasteric contraction and hence retraction of the testis.

An undescended testis has to be differentiated from a retractile testis, which can be brought down to the scrotum and is usually fully developed.

Investigations

When the testis is not palpable in the inguinal canal:

◆ USS. Useful in identifying testes in up to 15% of impalpable testes.
◆ MRI. Useful in 60-80% of cases.
◆ Laparoscopy. This is the modality of choice as it can be used to both detect and repair at the same time.

Treatment

Watchful waiting
After the first six months, spontaneous descent is rare, so it is reasonable to watch and wait for this length of time before considering surgery.

Hormone therapy
In physiologic cryptorchidism, treat with HCG 1500 units/week intramuscularly every other day or three times a week for a total of nine injections.

Surgery
◆ Orchidopexy (one-stage procedure). Identify the testicle by making an incision just above the inguinal ligament (take care to identify the rare subcutaneous testicles that lie outside of the inguinal ligament). Free up the cord structures and identify the patent processus vaginalis (an undescended testis almost always has a patent processus vaginalis). Place a stitch in the patent processus vaginalis, closing it (herniotomy). Pull down the testicle into the scrotal sac and place it in a subdartos pouch (which does not require a stitch).
◆ A two-stage procedure is usually done for a high-lying testis in the retroperitoneum where the cord cannot be mobilised sufficiently in one go without compromising the blood supply.

Complications

Complications of HCG injections include penile growth, increased scrotal rugae, pigmentation of the scrotum and pubic hair growth. These all regress after the course of injections.

Complications of orchidopexy include:

◆ Poor position of the testicle.
◆ Testicular atrophy (vascular injury due to surgical mobilisation of cord structures).
◆ Infection (wound or epididymo-orchitis).
◆ Scrotal haematoma or excessive oedema.
◆ Damage to the vas deferens and future infertility.

Normal   Bell clapper

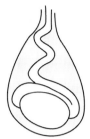

Normal level of
investment of
tunica vaginalis
from which testis
hangs.

Unusually high
investment of
tunica vaginalis
allowing testis
to hang
horizontally.

Figure 12.1. Torsion of the testes, showing bell clapper testicle.

Complications of undescended testicles carries a six-fold increase in infertility and a risk of malignant change (testicular cancer) in the affected testicle.

Torsion of the testis (Figure 12.1)

Presentation

Technically speaking, torsion of the testis is a misnomer, as it is the spermatic cord and its testicular artery and vein that are torted. It is the testis that becomes ischaemic (and eventually necrotic) as a result. This is commonly due to an unusually high lie of the tunica vaginalis, resulting in a horizontal lying and excessively mobile testis (bell-clapper testicle), therefore causing an increased predisposition to torsion (bilateral risk). This kind of torsion, known as intravaginal torsion, should be distinguished from extravaginal torsion that occurs in the perinatal and neonatal period.

It presents characteristically in the 14-20-year-old age group, with a sudden onset of pain and swelling in the testicle, and nausea/vomiting, although it can present as abdominal pain alone (rare, although this is a reason to examine the testicles in men presenting with severe abdominal pain, even though the diagnosis of torsion of the testicle is not usually the first thing that comes to mind when a patient presents with abdominal pain). Testicular torsion is a urological emergency and should be immediately explored. It is postulated that after eight hours, it is very unlikely to

salvage the testis, as there is irreversible damage to the seminiferous tubules.

The major differential diagnosis of testicular torsion in young men presenting with acute severe sudden onset testicular pain is epididymo-orchitis. It can be difficult to tell the two diagnoses apart on clinical grounds. One important difference (when present) is longer duration of symptoms in epididymo-orchitis and clinically the patient may be pyrexial. They may also give a history of urinary symptoms which can sometimes be evident on urine dipstick analysis. It is very important to ask for recent sexual contact, as STDs are a cause of epididymo-orchitis in younger men. A recent urinary tract infection or instrumentation may be the cause of epididymo-orchitis in older men.

Another differential diagnosis is that of torsion of the so called appendix of the testicle (a small structure attached to the testis itself known as the hydatid of Morgagni). It also causes sudden onset pain of the testicle, characteristically in younger adolescents, and can be difficult to tell apart from testicular torsion. The tenderness can be more highly localised, and (quite rarely) a dark dot can be seen through the scrotal skin of fair-skinned boys, representing the ischaemic appendix of the testis.

Investigations

Immediate surgical exploration is mandatory in patients with suspected testicular torsion. Time is of the essence, as delay in exploration will lead to more ischaemic damage to the testis and if delayed long enough, death of the testis. The decision to explore is based purely on clinical history and examination findings. Therefore, the role of imaging in suspected cases of torsion is minimal as this is time-consuming and none are 100% sensitive and specific.

Investigations are:

♦ Colour Doppler ultrasound shows vascularisation of the testes. A poorly vascularised testis indicates torsion. However, colour flow around the testis can sometimes give a false impression that the testis is vascularised. Therefore, there is a limited role for this investigation.
♦ Nuclear scintigraphy has been used in the past to demonstrate lack of blood flow to the testis in cases of torsion. However, as alluded to before, these investigations are time-consuming, of limited availability and are prone to variable false positive and false negative results.
♦ Blood tests, including inflammatory markers (i.e. FBC, U+Es, ESR and CRP), are useful in considering the differential diagnosis of epididymo-orchitis.
♦ MSU is also of use in patients with epididymo-orchitis, which can occur in cases of UTIs. A urethral swab should be taken in suspected cases of STDs.

Treatment

Testicular torsion is a urological emergency. The urology team should be involved immediately as the patient may need an immediate exploration. Exploration of the ipsilateral (affected) side is through a midline raphe incision. A torted testicle is dusky and hypovascular in appearance. The spermatic cord must be untwisted, and the testicle observed to return to its normal pink colour. A decision must be made at this point, if the testicle does not 'pink-up' whether it has necrosed, and hence requires orchidectomy (this takes both patience and experience, and administration of 100% oxygen by the anaesthetist and warm damp swabs). The untorted testicle should then be fixed to the scrotal sac to prevent recurrence. Because the risk of torsion is bilateral, especially in

the case of a bell-clapper testicle, one should (through the same incision) proceed to fix the contralateral testicle to the scrotal sac at the time of surgery.

Patients who have had orchidectomy (excision of the necrosed testicle) may wish to have a prosthetic replacement. This is generally advised to be placed anywhere between three and six months post-operation, when the scrotal oedema and other symptoms have settled down.

Complications

♦ Retention of a necrosed testicle carries with it the risk of antibody formation against testicular structures and hence may cause infertility. Thus, all necrosed testicles must be removed at the time of surgical exploration.
♦ There is an increasing risk of losing fertility of the torted testis the greater the delay between onset of symptoms and time of surgery. Delay of more than eight hours significantly reduces the chances of salvaging the testis.
♦ There is a risk of wound infection and scrotal haematoma.

Testicular tumours

Teratomas occur in younger men (age 20-30 years); seminomas occur in the age group of 30-40.

Note

– Lymphomas can also occur in testicles, e.g. non-Hodgkin's lymphoma (NHL).
– A choriocarcinoma in the testicles may secrete hormones.

Teratomas are germ cell tumours; therefore, the endoderm, ectoderm and mesoderm can all be part of the tumour.

Seminomas are also germ cell tumours. There are three subtypes:

♦ Classical seminoma.
♦ Spermocytic seminoma.
♦ Anaplastic seminoma.

Useful tumour markers

Useful tumour markers are beta-HCG and alpha-fetoprotein. These should be taken both before and after orchidectomy. LDH is also useful as it gives an estimation of the tumour burden.

Presentation

The tumour can present as a painless lump or as a painful testicle. There is often a history of recent trauma which brought attention to the lump (but did not cause it). It can also present as abdominal/back pain from para-aortic lymph nodes, or as chest symptoms from lung metastases.

On examination there is a smooth, hard lump in the body of the testis, loss of testicular sensation (quite early) and a thickened cord (if involved).

Investigations

- FBC, U+Es, CRP, ESR, alpha-fetoprotein, beta-HCG, LDH.
- Ultrasound examination of the testes.
- CT scan of the pelvis, abdomen and chest (shows presence of lymphadenopathy in the chest and abdomen or pulmonary metastases).

Treatment

Management is by a high inguinal (radical) orchidectomy. This is for both treatment and accurate staging of the disease.

Royal Marsden Hospital Staging
- I. Confined to testis.
- II. Abdominal LNs (A, B, C depending on size of the nodes).
- III. LNs above the diaphragm.
- IV. Extralymphatic metastases.

In recent times, the TNM classification of testicular tumours is gaining popularity as it has been shown to correlate with the disease outcome.

Treatment after orchidectomy

Treatment depends upon staging with the help of histology, tumour markers and CT staging:

- Watchful waiting in stage I disease with a six-monthly CT scan.
- Radiotherapy (seminomas are radiosensitive, but radiotherapy is not generally used in teratomas, which are better treated with chemotherapy).
- Chemotherapy.
- Surgery for para-aortic nodes in residual disease.
- Beta-HCG and alpha-fetoprotein levels can be used during follow-up, to screen for recurrence of the disease.

Complications

- Wound infection.
- Scrotal haematoma.
- Excision of abdominal lymph nodes, if performed, can result in ileus, damage to sympathetic nerves, resulting in loss of emission and ejaculation during orgasm and, rarely, damage to hollow or solid organs in the abdomen.
- Recurrence (or non-cure) of the disease. This risk increases with increasingly advanced stage at the time of presentation.
- Infertility. This can be either due to the orchidectomy itself, or radiotherapy scatter affecting the retained (normal) testicle.

Prognosis

The prognosis is excellent in stages 1 and 2, and even in stages 3 and 4, the long-term prognosis is approaching 70% disease-free survival.

Pearce's Surgical Companion *Essential notes for postgraduate exams*

Chapter 13

Examination techniques

Examination of the cranial nerves

This is particularly relevant for patient examination after a significant head injury. Remember, nerve palsies are often permanent and, hence, these cases can be brought into clinical exams for testing. You should, therefore, be comfortable with a neurological examination, and be able to answer questions on your findings.

Choose your own mnemonic for remembering these 12 nerves in order. Mine is unprintable, but the initial letters are OOOTTAFAGVAH!

◆ I. Olfactory:
  • test smell.
◆ II. Optic:
  • test visual fields with contralateral eye obscured;
  • test visual acuity with Snellen charts;
  • test colour vision with Ishihara charts;
  • fundoscopy.
◆ III. Oculomotor:
  • supplies all but two of the extrinsic muscles of the eye (exceptions are the superior oblique and lateral rectus). It also supplies levator palpabrae superioris and sphincter pupillae;
  • therefore, a III palsy results in a 'down and out' eye, with ptosis (droop of eyelid) and a fixed, dilated pupil.

◆ IV. Trochlear:
  • supplies superior oblique which turns the eye down and in, i.e. medially;
  • in IV palsy, the eye will look laterally on a downwards gaze and the patient will have a horizontal diplopia.
◆ V. Trigeminal:
  • sensory to the face, palate, teeth, conjunctiva and nasal mucous membrane;
  • three divisions of the trigeminal nerve:
    - ophthalmic;
    - maxillary;
    - mandibular.
  • the trigeminal nerve is the motor supply to the muscles of mastication (masseter, temporalis, pterygoids via the mandibular division of V;
  • test sensation on the face and conjunctiva (cotton wool bud). Test the motor function by clenching teeth.
◆ VI. Abducens:
  • supplies the lateral rectus muscle, which turns the eye outwards;
  • VI nerve palsy reveals an inability to turn the eye outwards, resulting in horizontal diplopia.
◆ VII. Facial:
  • supplies motor innervation to the muscles of facial expression;

- VII palsy results in hemifacial paresis and loss of taste, as the anterior two thirds of the tongue are also supplied by the VII nerve;

Note

— An upper motor neurone palsy results in sparing of the forehead frown as the occipitofrontal muscle is bilaterally represented in the cerebral cortex.

- test VII by screwing up eyes, baring the teeth, and frowning.
- VIII. Vestibulocochlear (auditory nerve):
  - test hearing by whispering and asking the patient to repeat.

Note

— Rinnie's and Weber's tests differentiate between nerve and conduction deafness.

Rinnie's test

In this test a tuning fork is held on the mastoid process which is heard. But, it is not heard, when held in air near the ear, i.e. this is conduction deafness because the nerve is intact.

Weber's test

A tuning fork on the vertex of the skull is heard loudest in the ear when conduction deafness is present.

Note

— With nerve deafness, the noise of the tuning fork will not be heard in the affected ear under any circumstances.

- IX. Glossopharyngeal:
  - supplies sensation to the posterior third of the pharynx, and posterior third of the tongue including taste. Tested by eliciting the gag reflex (swab at the back of the pharynx).

- X. Vagus:
  - supplies motor innervation to the soft palate, pharynx, larynx and the parasympathetic supply of the gut;
  - tested by opening the mouth and asking the patient to say 'Aah'. The uvula will deviate towards the functioning side, i.e. contralateral to the side of the lesion.

Note

— Recurrent laryngeal nerve palsy results in a hoarse voice; a paralyzed vocal cord can be seen on laryngoscopy.

- XI. Accessory:
  - supplies motor innervation to trapezius and the SCM. Tested by shrugging the shoulders and forcing the chin to the contralateral side of the SCM being tested.
- XII. Hypoglossal:
  - supplies motor innervation to the muscles of the tongue;
  - tested by asking the patient to push out their tongue. It will deviate to the affected side, which may also be wasted.

Foramina and their cranial nerves

- I. Olfactory. Through the cribriform plate of the ethmoid bone.
- II. Optic. Through the orbit to the retina (optic canal).
- III. Oculomotor. Through the superior orbital fissure to the extra-ocular muscles.
- IV. Trochlear. Through the superior orbital fissure to the superior oblique muscle.
- V. Trigeminal:
  - V1. Ophthalmic division. Through the superior orbital fisssure;
  - V2. Maxillary division. Through the foramen rotundum;
  - V3. Mandibular division. Through the foramen ovale.
- VI. Abducens. Through the superior orbital fissure to the lateral rectus muscle.
- VII. Facial. Through the stylomastoid foramen to the muscles of facial expression.

- VIII. Vestibulocochlear. Through the internal auditory meatus to the ear.
- IX. Glossopharyngeal. Through the jugular foramen posterior palate and the posterior third of the tongue.
- X. Vagus. Through the jugular foramen to the pharyngeal muscles, external auditory meatus, lung, heart, carotid sinus, liver, stomach, spleen, kidney, pancreas, and the small and large bowel to the level of the transverse colon.
- XI. Accessory. Through the jugular foramen to SCM and trapezius.
- XII. Hypoglossal. Through the hypoglossal (anterior condylar) canal to the muscles of the tongue and upper strap muscles.

Nerve and root supply of muscle groups

The table below may appear to be a dry list, but it is a very useful reference for examining the upper and lower limbs. The list is also helpful in answering common questions relating to the nerve root being tested in, for example, eliciting a knee jerk reflex. Another example would be testing the power of biceps brachii as part of your neurological examination of the upper limb.

Reflexes and their nerve root levels:

- Biceps brachii: C5-6.
- Triceps: C7.
- Ankle: S1.
- Knee: L3-4.

Nerve and root supply of muscle groups in the upper and lower limbs.

Cervical flexors:	C1-4
Cervical extensors:	C1-4
Trapezius:	Cranial nerve XI (accessory nerve)
Sternocleidomastoid:	Cranial nerve XI (accessory nerve)
Arm abduction:	0-15° supraspinatus C4-6 (suprascapular nerve)
	15-90° deltoid C5-6 (axillary nerve)
	>90° trapezius and serratus anterior C5-7 (long thoracic nerve)
Biceps brachii:	C5-6 (musculocutaneous nerve)
Forearm supination:	C5-6 (musculocutaneous nerve)
Forearm pronation:	C6-7 (median nerve)
Wrist flexors:	C7-8, T1 (median nerve)
Wrist extensors:	C6-8 (radial nerve)
Hand intrinsics:	C7-T1 (median and ulnar nerve)
Hip flexion:	L1-3 (femoral nerve)
Hip extension:	L4-S1 (sciatic nerve)
Thigh abduction:	L4-S2 (superior gluteal nerve)
Thigh adduction:	L2-4 (obturator nerve)
Leg flexion:	L4-S2 (sciatic nerve)
Leg extension:	L2-4 (femoral nerve)
Foot plantar flexion:	L5-S1 (superficial peroneal and tibial nerves)
Foot dorsiflexion:	L4-5 (deep peroneal nerve)
Great toe extension:	L4-5, S1 (deep peroneal nerve)
Foot inversion:	L4-5 (deep peroneal nerve)
Foot eversion:	L5-S1 (superficial peroneal nerve)
Rectal sphincters:	S2-4 (pudendal nerve)

Note

— There is no specific reflex to test for L5 function.

Peripheral vascular system

Classically, it is the legs that are more likely to be examined, as peripheral vascular disease is overwhelmingly more common there than in the upper limbs.

Ask about pain and cold extremities in the history. Inspect the legs for hair loss and smooth skin, which are common in chronic arterial insufficiency.

Feet

- ◆ Feel for temperature and colour.
- ◆ Look for oedema.
- ◆ Feel the pedal pulses, dorsalis pedis and posterior tibial (if absent, proceed to use a Doppler probe; one will be available in clinical exams).
- ◆ Look for the presence of ulcers. Arterial ulcers, remember, have punched out edges, not the sloping edges of venous or mixed ulcers, and tend to be located over the medial calf.

For varicose veins and venous ulcers, see the next section.

Other pulses

Palpate the popliteal pulse. Lie the patient down flat, relax the leg and gently place your index and middle finger pads behind the knee. Then feel slightly to the lateral side of the midline for any pulsation. Remember to use the Doppler if you cannot feel any pulse.

Palpate the femoral pulse. It is located at the mid-inguinal point, exactly half the distance between the anterior superior iliac spine and the pubic symphysis. Use the Doppler if impalpable.

Listen for a femoral bruit, sometimes known as a pistol shot femoral.

Examine for radiofemoral delay. This is present in coarctation of the aorta (a narrowing of the descending arch of the aorta). It slows down the blood flow after some has already travelled into the upper limbs, hence a delay in the time it takes for blood to reach the lower limb.

Buerger's test

Raise the leg (straight, flexing at the hip) to see if the limb goes pale. Record the angle at which this occurs. Then hang the leg over the side of the bed to look for reflex hyperaemia. The leg goes pale at this angle which results in a hydrostatic pressure that overcomes the pressure of arterial blood in the nearly critically stenosed artery of a patient with chronically ischaemic limbs. This would not happen in a patient with normal blood supply as the systolic pressure would be more than enough to compensate for raising the leg, even to the vertical.

Measure the ABPI

This is the Ankle Brachial Pressure Index. The patient lies supine, ideally rested for 10-20 minutes. Place an appropriately sized cuff around the arm and locate the brachial pulse with the Doppler probe, inflating the cuff until no signal is heard. Deflate the cuff and note the pressure at which the signal returns (brachial systolic). Repeat with the contralateral arm and record the highest of two readings. Place an appropriately sized cuff around the lower leg immediately above the malleoli. Repeat as for the upper limb using the posterior tibial pulse.

The actual ABPI is the highest ankle pressure (for each leg) divided by the highest brachial pressure. The normal value should be 1, in ischaemia it will be <1 and in critical ischaemia it is <0.6.

Clinical examination of varicose veins

This is very likely to come up in clinical exams, so it is advisable to become expert at the practice of examining varicose veins.

Ask the patient to stand first. Look for skin pigmentation, oedema, eczema, lipodermatosclerosis (also known as varicose eczema), and venous ulceration.

Look at both the front and back of the legs separately to see the distribution of varicose veins. Basically, the medial calf covers the great saphenous distribution, the lateral calf covers the small saphenous distribution.

Feel for short saphenopopliteal incompetence in the popliteal fossa. To do this the patient should be lying flat, raise the leg to drain the veins, press into the popliteal fossa and let the leg hang off the side of the bed. If the lateral varicose veins fill retrogradely when you release your pressure on the saphenopopliteal junction there is incompetence.

Tap distally on a varicose vein while palpating more proximally (on the same vein), testing for valvular incompetence. The normal presence of competent valves would prevent transmission of this impulse proximally, but if an impulse is felt, the valves must therefore be incompetent.

The same can be done for saphenofemoral (SF) incompetence. The SF junction is located one fingerbreadth medial to the femoral pulsation in the groin skin crease. It is an important definition, as it is frequently asked.

Trendelenberg's test for valvular incompetence

Raise the patient's leg, thus draining the veins, apply a tourniquet high around the leg and ask the patient to stand. If the varicose veins do not fill on standing (with the tourniquet on), this represents SF incompetence. If, however, they do fill (despite the tourniquet) then the site of incompetence must be distal to the tourniquet. Releasing the tourniquet, in SF incompetence, results in the veins rapidly filling from above (the opposite of what would happen normally).

You can narrow down the exact location of the incompetent valve by repeating the test with incrementally lower tourniquet applications.

Note

— A Doppler probe can be used to listen for biphasic flow in veins (after squeezing the calf muscles), which signifies reflux, as venous flow is supposed to be monophasic due to the presence of competent valves.

— Anatomy of the *deep* veins of the lower limb mirrors that of the arterial supply, i.e. the posterior tibial and peroneal join, as does the anterior tibial, becoming the popliteal. This becomes the femoral, receiving tributaries from the deep femoral (profunda femoris artery equivalent) and continues to become the external iliac before supplying the IVC.

— Do not forget the presence of the venae commitantes, paired veins on either side of arteries that benefit from pulsation of the artery to promote flow along the vein in one direction only due to the presence of the valve system.

— The concept of the muscle pump is similar to the above description, and is frequently asked in clinical exams. Muscle contraction promotes the flow of blood up the veins, because valves prevent backflow when competent.

Neck examination

When examining the neck, it should be inspected from the front, looking for any obvious swellings or scars.

The actual palpation of the neck, however, is supposed to be performed from behind the patient. If the patient is sitting on a chair, and the wall behind them prevents you from examining properly, you should ask the patient to stand, and move the chair accordingly. This position enables you to get the most sensitive parts of your fingers (the tips and pads) into contact with the patient's neck with little awkwardness.

During exams you are permitted, on occasion, to briefly question the patient. It is always wise to obtain some information, even if it is whilst performing the examination of the patient:

- Duration of symptoms?
- Presence of pain?
- Change in size?
- TB symptoms (night sweats, fevers, productive cough)?
- Hyper- or hypothyroid symptoms?
- Stridor?
- Difficulty swallowing?

Palpation

You should have a technique for logically including all relevant anatomical regions of the neck in your examination. The patient must be adequately exposed. You must be able to see as far as the tips of both clavicles and everything from that point upwards must be exposed.

You should palpate along the clavicle from lateral to medial, then track up the sternocleidomastoid (SCM) to the angle of the jaw (when doing so you should make a point to feel deep to its anterior border which enables you to feel the jugular chain of lymph nodes). This delineates the boundaries of the posterior triangle. You should then palpate inside the posterior triangle.

Thereafter, you should palpate along the ramus of the mandible to the midpoint and down the midline. This delineates the boundaries of the anterior triangle. You should then palpate inside the anterior triangle.

Any lumps felt within the neck must be examined for the following characteristics:

- Size.
- Firmness.
- Fluctuance.
- Regularity of border.
- Relation to underlying structures and skin, i.e. whether tethered or not.
- Transilluminability (if appears cystic).
- Tenderness.

You should decide which region of the neck the lump appears to be within (midline, anterior triangle, posterior triangle or supraclavicular). You must then be prepared to postulate as to the source of the lump.

For this see the section on 'Swellings in the neck' in Chapter 9.

Note

— If you identify a midline neck lump, you will note the examiner has kindly set out a glass of water by the patient's side. You should ask the patient to swallow, and stand by their side to observe (in profile) whether the lump rises on swallowing. This is said to be characteristic of a thyroglossal cyst, as the remnant of the thyroglossal tract connects the cyst to the tongue. It is wise to assess the position of the trachea with respect to any lumps identified, as it is possible for the trachea to be displaced by a lump.

Examination of the back

Examination

The patient needs to be quite exposed for adequate examination of the back. Ideally, they should only be in underwear, as you need to see the back, legs and feet. Inspect while standing, initially looking for scoliosis, chest wall deformity, surgical scars and café au lait patches (indicative of neurofibromatosis, which is associated with scoliosis). Then ask the patient to lean forwards to look for a 'rib hump', into lateral flexion (both sides) and extension. Ask the patient to put both hands on their hips and, keeping the hips still, to rotate left and right. Palpate the vertebral bodies looking for tenderness, as well as the paravertebral musculature looking for muscle spasm and tenderness. If you identify muscle spasm with the patient standing, you should go on to repeat your palpation of the paravertebral musculature with the patient relaxed, lying on their front on the examination couch. Then, with the patient recumbent on the examination couch, you should perform a full neurological examination of the lower limbs. This must include reflexes, as their absence is relevant in disc disease and other nerve compressive lesions. Also, straight leg raises should be performed, noting the angle at which the patient complains of leg pain. If they are prevented from going further, by back pain, and not leg pain, this renders the test useless from the point of view of any neurological implications.

Note

— Crossover pain is a very useful sign in a prolapsed disc, as it is suggestive of a large prolapsing central disc. Crossover pain, in this context, means pain felt down the opposite leg to that which is being raised.

— Also, the dermatome in which the patient has sensory loss, as well as where their pain is felt, can be correlated to the level at which they have nerve root compression.

Dermatomes

A useful mnemonic, if like the author, you have difficulty retaining this particular set of information, is:

2, 3, 4, 5, stand on S1, sit on S3.

This is accompanied by slapping thighs (lateral then medial) (L2, L3), then slapping the lower legs (medial then lateral) (L4, L5), stand on S1 (sole of feet) and sit on S3 (buttocks). (Figure 13.1. N.B. This is a teaching diagram and represents a simplified version of the dermatomes as an aide memoire).

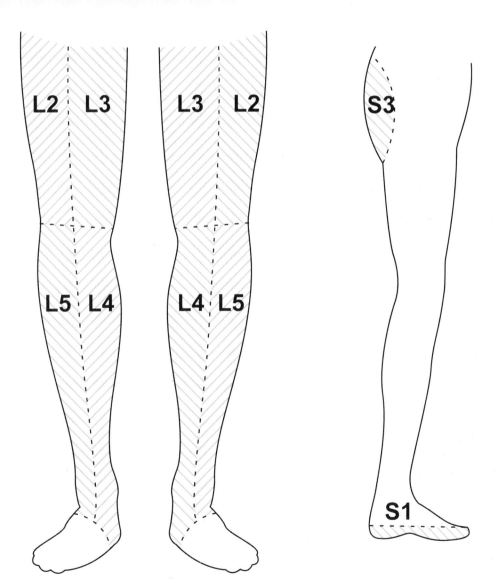

Figure 13.1. Examination of the back: dermatomes.

The more anatomically correct extent of the dermatomes is displayed in the section on 'Overall organisation of the nervous system' in Chapter 3.

Inguinoscrotal examination

Hernias are common, inguinal hernias moreso than femoral. They are on every general sugeon's waiting list in abundance. They form a regular source of patients for the clinical exam.

Strictly speaking, the patient should be exposed 'nipples to knees'. It is permissible to have loose underwear that can be drawn to the side to examine the groin in the exam situation.

If asked to examine the groin, then this is exactly what you should do. Do not look at the hands first, then the abdomen, and then the groin. If you are asked to examine the patient's abdominal system, then this is of course a different matter.

Being asked to examine a patient's groin is something of a clue that they are likely to have a hernia. The differential diagnoses here are: hydrocoele, ectopic testicle, lipoma of the spermatic cord, inguinal lymphadenopathy, femoral canal lipoma, saphena varix, psoas abscess and ileofemoral aneurysm.

Look for any scars, e.g. previous hernia repairs or a scar that is responsible for an incisional hernia.

Ask the patient to stand, if appropriate, as herniae are most likely to present themselves when standing.

Identify your landmarks:

◆ Pubic tubercle. Remember this lies immediately lateral to the pubic symphysis. They are not the same.
◆ Anterior superior iliac spine.
◆ The inguinal ligament is the line joining the previous two.
◆ The midpoint of the inguinal ligament is the internal inguinal ring. The external inguinal ring lies medial to the internal.

Once you are sure of your landmarks, feel for any masses. The location is your first clue to the diagnosis:

◆ Femoral herniae are below and lateral to the pubic tubercle.
◆ Inguinal herniae are above and medial to the pubic tubercle.
◆ Direct inguinal herniae are medial to the internal inguinal ring (as well as the inferior epigastric artery).
◆ Indirect inguinal herniae are also medial to the internal inguinal ring (as well as the inferior epigastric artery).

The usefulness of the inferior epigastric artery as an anatomical landmark is that it lies between the internal and external inguinal rings. So, when you identify the vessel, you know the rings lie on either side of it.

Herniae are reducible, and have a cough impulse. These differentiate them from other types of groin lumps.

The classical test you should be able to perform, to differentiate between indirect and direct inguinal herniae, is to reduce the hernia. Gently, with the patient on the couch, place your finger over the internal inguinal ring (midpoint of the inguinal ligament). Then ask the patient to stand. If this controls the hernia (prevents it from re-herniating), then the hernia is indirect. If, however, it re-herniates, medially to your finger, it is direct.

You can auscultate a hernia and would expect to hear bowel sounds. It is not the most sensitive of tests, as it is quite possible to hear normal bowel sounds when auscultating the groin of normal people.

You should also ensure that you palpate the femoral pulsation. In the case of males, you should state to the examiner that you would also examine the testicles as part of your normal abdominal examination. Herniae can extend into the scrotal sac, and testicles, quite apart from herniae, can have a separate pathology of their own.

Surgical lump examination

Lumps should be examined for the following criteria, to aid with your differential diagnosis:

- Site.
- Size.
- Shape.
- Colour and temperature.
- Consistency. Firm or soft. If firm, this has malignant implications.
- Surface. Smooth or irregular. If irregular, this has malignant implications.
- Relationship to surrounding tissues, i.e. tethered or free moving. If tethered, this has malignant implications.
- Margins. As for surface.
- Pulsatile. Then auscultate for a bruit.
- Fluctuant. If it is fluctuant, then you are expected to demonstrate if it transilluminates.
- Overlying skin changes. Ulceration and peau d'orange have malignant implications.

Abdominal examination

The patient should be exposed from 'nipple to knee', although for the purposes of clinical exams, it is permissible to retain the underwear. You should make judicious use of the sheet/blanket available to you to preserve modesty.

General observations

- State of nutrition and hydration of the patient.
- Presence of any peripheral oedema, which can imply hypoproteinaemia.
- Signs of liver disease, i.e. jaundiced sclerae or skin, liver flap, ascites, etc.
- Look at the flanks and back. Make a quick point of doing so; this way you will miss nothing.
- Examine the hands for nail changes, i.e. clubbing, splinter haemorrhages, leukoplakia, koilonychia.
- Eyes. Look for anaemia, and as previously mentioned, jaundice.

Inspection

- Ask the patient to lift their head off the bed, looking for herniae or divarication of the recti (a stretching of the linea alba, occurring in the obese, that results in a linear bulging of the abdomnal contents in the midline as the intra-abdominal pressure is raised by, for example, contracting the abdominal musculature, as you do when you raise your head in the lying position).
- Scars. You should recognise the varieties of abdominal scars (see the section on 'Abdominal wall incisions' in Chapter 3).
- Shape and symmetry.
- Abdominal wall veins. If distended, this signifies portal hypertension or IVC obstruction.
- Visible peristalsis, known as borborygmi.
- Presence of herniae.
- Spider naevi (>5 is significant, possibly indicating chronic liver disease or a liver tumour).

Palpation

Always remember to ask about pain before palpation. It is best to have a system of subdividing the abdomen into sections. The simplest is the 'quadrants' system, i.e. right and left upper quadrants, as well as right and left iliac fossae.

Use light palpation to assess tenderness and deep palpation to feel for masses. Palpate systematically for enlargement of the liver. Start in the right iliac fossa and palpate sequentially, asking the patient to inspire each time, up towards the right upper quadrant. Palpate the spleen, as for the liver, but from the right iliac fossa towards the left upper quadrant. Palpate the kidneys by ballotting them between left and right hands from anterior to posterior as the patient inspires.

Specifically feel for aortic pulsation, then assess to see if it is aneurysmal (a pulsatile, expansile mass).

Percussion

- Upper and lower liver margins.
- Shifting dullness (ascites).
- Suprapubic dullness.

Auscultation

- Bowel sounds.
- Aortic and renal bruits.
- Hepatic and splenic rubs.

Rectal examination

At the end of your abdominal examination you should state that you would complete your examination with a PR.

Look for:

- Presence of blood on the glove.
- Constipation.
- Prostate hypertrophy.
- Tenderness.
- Anal tone.
- Rectal masses.

Abdominal masses

You should have a system in your head when trying to identify the origin of an abdominal mass on examination. Perhaps the best system is to think of the organs in the abdominal cavity, their anatomical location, and the types of pathology that can cause them to be enlarged. The only exception to this system will be the generalised cause of abdominal distension: ascites.

Intestinal masses

Gastric

These will be located in the epigastric region of the abdomen; gastric carcinoma can sometimes be palpable as a firm deep mass.

Small bowel

These will be centrally abdominal; if the abdomen distends due to small bowel obstruction the small bowel loops will be palpable as a generalised mass. In complete obstruction there will be tinkling, or absent, bowel sounds, absolute constipation, and nausea with vomiting.

Large bowel

In volvulus of the caecum you would feel a mass extending up towards the left upper quadrant, from the right iliac fossa. There is a resonant note to percussion, tinkling or absent bowel sounds, absolute constipation, and possibly nausea and vomiting.

In sigmoid volvulus, there are similar findings as for caecal volvulus, except for the mass, which would be extending up towards the right upper quadrant, from the left iliac fossa. There is a resonant note to percussion.

In constipation you would feel indentable masses predominantly in the left half of the abdomen (the descending and sigmoid colon). PR would confirm a loaded rectum with a firm stool.

In carcinoma of the caecum and ascending colon, there is a firm, non-mobile mass in the right iliac fossa. You should be able to feel its irregular edge; it will be tender and you should be able to get beneath it as well as above it.

In carcinoma of the sigmoid and descending colon, there is a similar set of findings as for carcinoma of the caecum, but located instead in the left iliac fossa.

Rectal tumours tend to be impalpable on abdominal examination, unless they are extensive with local spread, in which case there would be a low abdominal mass you could not get below.

Appendix

It is unusual to be able to feel the appendix, except in the case of an appendix mass. This is a diffuse mass palpable in the right iliac fossa. The patient has a history of a number of days (possibly weeks) of abdominal upset, possible anorexia, fever and possible weight loss with tachycardia.

Hepatic

Hepatomegaly

Examine the liver as previously described. A palpable edge beneath the right costal margin is abnormal, indicating a degree of hepatomegaly. The edge can either be smooth or irregular; if irregular, this has malignant implications. Remember the causes of hepatomegaly are:

- Cirrhosis. Do not forget that the liver can also be shrunken in late cirrhosis.
- Tumours. A primary tumour is termed a hepatoma. Secondary tumours settle in the liver from other primaries, such as lung or colon cancers.
- Congestive cardiac failure.
- Hepatitis.
- Leukaemia/lymphoma.

Gallbladder

The gallbladder can be thought of as being in the hepatic section. Occasionally in gallstone disease, the gallbladder can distend so that it becomes palpable. It is a smooth, rounded, dull to percussion mass, and you cannot palpate it. It also moves with respiration.

Spleen

Splenomegaly

Examine the spleen as previously described. When enlarged it extends from the left upper quadrant (you cannot get above it) diagonally towards the umbilicus. It has a palpable notch, a dull note to percussion, and a firm and smooth edge. The causes of splenomegaly are:

- Infective. Leishmaniasis, CMV, HIV, malaria, etc.
- Haematological. Hereditary, spherocytosis, ITP, myelofibrosis, myelodysplasia.
- Malignant. Lymphoma/leukaemia.
- Portal hypertension.
- Rheumatoid arthritis (very rare).

Female pelvic organs

Uterus

The most common cause of a uterine mass is pregnancy (when characterising pregnancy as a mass, it is smooth-edged, a firm mass arising from the pelvis, and you cannot get below it).

Fibroids

When fibroids are multiple, or large, you will find them as a mass arising from the pelvis, possibly with an irregular edge. You cannot get beneath the mass.

Uterine carcinoma

Again this is a pelvic mass. It is either smooth-edged or irregular, you cannot get beneath it, it may be tender, and it is dull to percussion. Bimanual (per vaginum and abdominal examination) palpation may confirm the uterine nature of the mass.

Ovaries

Ovarian cysts, only when really very large, can be palpated as a mass arising from either the left or right pelvis. You cannot get beneath the mass, it is smooth, has curved edges, and is dull to percussion. You may feel a fluid thrill (this is difficult in this context though). Carcinoma is generally impalpable unless it is an extensive local invasion and is spread through the peritoneal cavity.

Aorta

An aneurysmal abdominal aorta is a pulsatile and expansile mass in the upper half of the central abdomen. You should be able to estimate the width by palpation, although this is a notoriously unreliable measure in inexperienced hands. You should remember to look for other aneurysms if you find an aortic aneurysm, e.g. femoral or popliteal.

Renal system

Distended bladder

Smooth-edged, spherical, dull to percussion and pressure on it causes a desire on the patient's behalf to micturate.

Enlarged kidney

Unilateral (in the loin) and felt by bimanual ballotting as the patient inspires fully. You can only feel the inferior pole, as the upper pole is behind the costal margin. If you think about it, the percussion note is irrelevant as it is a retroperitoneal structure with overlying bowel. The causes of an enlarged kidney are:

- Hydronephrosis.
- Carcinoma.
- Polycystic kidney disease, which tends to be bilateral.

Lymph nodes

Multiple enlarged lymph nodes (e.g. the para-aortic nodes) are palpable as a diffuse, deep, possibly tender mass in the central abdomen. You can usually get both above, as well as below, the abdominal mass caused by them. There is no change in the percussion note.

Generalised abdominal distension

Ascites

This is a collection of intra-peritoneal fluid. The abdomen can appear tensely distended (the umbilicus often everts). Ascites has a characteristic pattern of shifting dullness, i.e. the percussion note is dull over fluid (ascites), but it is more resonant over bowel, hence changing the position of the patient on the bed changes the relative position of the bowel within the ascitic fluid and the dullness thus shifts. You can also feel a fluid thrill by putting your fingertips on one side of the abdomen, and flicking the other side (after warning the patient), and feeling for a thrill with your first hand.

The causes of ascites are:

- Liver disease. Cirrhosis and resulting hypoproteinaemia.
- Cardiac. Right heart failure.
- Renal. Glomerulonephritis and resulting protein loss.
- Intestinal. Protein-losing enteropathy.
- Malignancy. Disseminated intraperitoneal secondaries.

Occasionally you may be asked which types of medical conditions can cause the ascites to be either a transudate or an exudate.

Transudate
- Hydrostatic. Cirrhosis, right heart failure.
- Plasma oncotic pressure (relating to decreased vascular oncotic pressure). Hypoproteinaemia, nephrotic syndrome.
- Metabolic. Hypothyroidism, hyperaldosteronism.

Exudate
- Inflammatory. Peritonitis, cancer.
- Iatrogenic. Operation, continuous ambulatory peritoneal dialysis.

Groin masses

See the earlier 'Inguinoscrotal examination' section for the technique of examination. You should be aware of the following differential diagnoses for a groin mass:

- Hydrocoele.
- Ectopic testicle.
- Lipoma of the spermatic cord.
- Inguinal lymphadenopathy.
- Femoral canal lipoma.
- Saphena varix.
- Psoas abscess.
- Ileofemoral aneurysm.

Breast examination

History

- Age.
- Presenting complaint:
  - pain (take a 'SOCRATES' history, i.e. site, onset, character, radiation, alleviating factors, timing, exacerbating factors, symptoms associated with it. Note whether the pain is cyclical);
  - lump/swelling (first noticed, change in size, related to cycle);
  - nipple discharge (amount, bilateral/ unilateral, related to cycle).
- Past breast history.
- Family history (FHx).
- Menarche, last menstrual period (LMP), pregnancies.
- Contraception/hormone replacement therapy.

Examination

Expose the patient and inspect the following with their arms by their sides.

- Symmetry.
- Volume.
- Scars.
- Nipple inversion.
- Pigmentation.
- Tethering/skin changes.

Lie the patient down and inspect with their arms behind their head. Lift the breast up with the thumb on the nipple and look in the axilla. Palpate the breast and axilla. Sit the patient up and examine the axilla with the arm lifted up and relaxed. Palpate the anterior and posterior fold as well as the mid-axillary line. Palpate the supraclavicular fossa. Advise that you would like to palpate the liver and percuss the lung fields.

Hip examination

Observation of gait

Antalgic gait

Means a painful gait, characterised by a short stance phase, i.e. spending a reduced amount of time bearing any weight through this leg.

Stiff hip gait

When you look analytically at the hip during its gait cycle you will note that the stiff hip gait involves no actual movement between the pelvis and femur (no hip flexion or extension in this context). Instead, the patient compensates by swinging their entire pelvis round before putting that foot to the ground. When well practised, this can be quite subtle, and hence difficult to spot.

Trendelenberg gait

This is a gait pattern resulting from unilateral weak hip abductors, the most common cause of which is hip replacement surgery to that side. If you stand on the leg with the weak abductors, the opposite hip sags downwards. Therefore, to be able to take a step the patient leans their body to the side of the weak abductors (away from the sagging 'good' side) to compensate for this, and thus their opposite foot does not scuff the floor as they step (which it otherwise would).

The corollary to this is the Trendelenburg test. Ask the patient to stand in front of you and put both their hands on yours. Ask them to stand on one leg, their good one to start with; they should be able to do so without putting undue pressure on your hands. But when you ask them to stand on their weak abductor leg side you will feel them rest heavily on your hand with their hand from the opposite side hip. This is to compensate for the opposite side of the pelvis dropping.

If it helps, remember this as 'the sound side sags'.

Expose and lie flat

Look

Check the position of the pelvis, i.e. ensure the patient is lying straight. Measure apparent leg length (e.g. xiphisternum to medial malleolus). Measure the true leg length, i.e. the anterior superior iliac spine (ASIS) to the medial malleolus. If there is shortening, ask the patient to bend their knees to 90° with the heels together on the bed to assess whether it is femoral or tibial shortening, by looking at the legs from the lateral side. Look for any soft tissue abnormality, scarring or obvious deformity.

Feel/move

Always ask about pain, first. Palpate the obvious bony landmarks, e.g. pubic rami, symphysis, greater trochanter (GT), ASIS, for pain. Thomas's test is performed by asking the patient to maximally flex one hip up and keep the other leg flat on the bed. Whilst they do this you must rest your hand under their lumbar spine to ensure the lumbar lordosis is not lost, indicating that the pelvis (and not the hip joint) is now flexing. If they cannot keep their leg flat on the bed with the other side maximally flexed, this is because there is actually a fixed flexion deformity of that hip.

The following represents a good system for examination of the hip joint:

- Flex hip (maximum 140°).
- Internal rotation (maximum 40°).
- External rotation (maximum 50°).
- Test abduction (maximum 45°) and adduction (maximum 30°) using either:
  - opposite leg locking. Examine the leg movements while the contralateral leg is left hanging off the side of the bed to prevent pelvic tilt; or
  - by feeling both ASISs with one forearm, whilst moving the leg. This ensures the movement is at the hip joint, and not a compensatory movement of the whole pelvis.

- With all these movements you are looking for a decreased range of movement or associated pain.
- Feel for pain over the GT, which is suggestive of trochanteric bursitis.
- Remember the pain of hip arthritis is felt in the groin, not over the GT. But it is possible for hip pain to radiate down to the knee (not vice versa).

Advise that you would also like to perform a neurovascular examination testing the tone, power, reflexes and peripheral pulses.

Knee examination

Look

Observe the gait, usually looking for an antalgic gait, characterised by a short stance phase and signs of discomfort on the face. Look for scarring, deformities or swellings. Look for quadriceps wasting. You may use a tape measure to measure girth at a fixed distance from a bony landmark. Look for the normal 5-7° valgus at the knee. N.B. Remember a valgus deformity means the apex points towards the midline (e.g. 'knock knees') and varus is the apex away from the midline (e.g. 'bow legged').

Feel

Always ask about pain first and feel for skin temperature and points of tenderness. Have a system: palpate the medial joint line, lateral joint line, patellar tendon, patella, quadriceps tendon and then feel the back of the knee.

Test for an effusion:

- Sweep your hand up the lateral side then down the medial side, looking for a brisk bulge of fluid on the contralateral side of the knee, indicative of a minor effusion.
- Force fluid down from the suprapatellar pouch and grip the patella, then tap the patella with the index finger of the other hand. A patellar tap indicates the presence of a moderate sized effusion if you have had to squeeze the

suprapatellar pouch to achieve it, and a large one if you have not had to squeeze the suprapatellar pouch.
- Examine behind the knee for a popliteal cyst.

Move

Check active and passive flexion. The maximum range of flexion varies markedly with age and flexibility, but usually 120-140° should be achieved. Check extension by lying the leg flat against the couch. Note that some are able to hyperextend 5°; this lifts the heel off the couch while the knee is still against the couch.

Test the collateral ligaments for laxity or pain. The lower leg is held under the arm whilst applying valgus or varus force above the knee joint. If this is done with the knee in extension, the tight posterior capsule contributes to stability, but in 20° of flexion this is negated, isolating the lateral cruciate ligament (LCL) and medial cruciate ligament (MCL).

Special tests

Anterior drawer test
With the knee bent to 90°, sit on the toes and pull the proximal tibia towards you. This will not work if the patient is tense, as the hamstrings can compensate, so you must ensure they are relaxed first.

Posterior drawer test
As above, but push the proximal tibia posteriorly. Do not be fooled by a pseudo-anterior drawer. This is caused by a posterior sag being present (posterior cruciate ligament [PCL] rupture) and you are then able to pull the knee anteriorly back to the normal anatomical position. You must flex both knees to 90° with the heels together on the couch, then look from the lateral side to see if one tibia is sagging posteriorly compared with the other knee.

Lachman's test
This is best performed by placing your flexed knee under their distal thigh on the couch, holding their thigh still with firm downward pressure with one hand and pulling the proximal tibia anteriorly with your other hand. The knee is necessarily flexed to about 20° in this test.

McMurray's test

This is only relevant if you are querying a meniscal tear. It is the forced internal and external rotation of the tibia (the foot is held with one hand) against a knee that is put through a full range of flexion and extension. The other hand supports under the knee to put it through the range of movement. A positive test is a sharp pain felt by the patient, as their torn meniscus is caught between one femoral condyle and the tibial plateau.

Pivot-shift test

With the patient's leg in full extension, rotate the foot into internal rotation, place a mild valgus strain across the knee (by pushing with your hand on their lateral calf towards the patient's opposite knee), and whilst doing this push the knee up into flexion. Watch for the tibial plateau to suddenly sublux anteriorly as you go from the extended position to flexed. This is because the absence of an anterior cruciate ligament (ACL) enables the knee in this position to shift around the pivot of the MCL, and this would normally be prevented by an intact ACL.

Advise that you would like to complete the examination by examining the hips (because hip pain can refer to the knee), as well as the neurovascular system of the lower limb.

Shoulder examination

The shoulder is a joint with a very large range of movement.

The planes in which movement takes place are:

- Forward flexion.
- Extension.
- Abduction.
- Adduction.
- Internal rotation.
- External rotation.

Occasionally the point might be raised in exams, that the scapula lies in a plane 45° anterior to the true lateral of the trunk, and hence abduction in the plane of the scapula only occurs when the arm is also 45° anterior, and then abducted. This is a semantic point, and more relevant to specialist shoulder surgeons than it is to the clinical exam. It is as well to be aware of this, however.

Look

Inspect the acromioclavicular joint (ACJ), clavicle, supraclavicular fossa, deltoid, biceps, both scapulae, and the muscle bulk of the supraspinatus and infraspinatus. You are looking for deformity, wasting or scars.

Feel

Palpate, specifically, the posterior shoulder for the C-spine, the paravertebral musculature, along the medial scapula down as far as the inferior angle, the posterior acromion, and trace your fingers around laterally to the acromion until you reach the anterior shoulder.

Palpate, specifically, the anterior shoulder for the biceps tendon, the anterior acromion and the coracoid process.

Palpate, specifically, the superior shoulder for the ACJ, clavicle, sternoclavicular joint and the supraclavicular fossa.

You are looking to identify points of tenderness or any masses.

Move

The range of movement should be assessed actively in:

- Forward flexion, whilst observing the scapulothoracic rhythm from behind. This is the smoothness of movement of the scapula with respect to the posterior chest wall; a disruption generally means a painful stimulus.
- Abduction, whilst observing the scapulothoracic rhythm.
- External rotation, and compare it with the other side.
- Internal rotation. This can be tested in one of two ways:
  - first, abduct the arm (with the elbow already bent to a right angle) to 90° at the shoulder, and rotate the forearm until it is pointing downwards; this is 90° of internal rotation;

* second, ask the patient how high they can get their thumb up their back, and make a note of the vertebral level.

The power can be assessed as follows:

◆ Trapezius. Ask the patient to shrug the shoulder against your hand.
◆ Rhomboids. Ask the patient to approximate their scapulae towards the midline.
◆ Winging of the scapula can be tested by asking the patient to push against a wall with their arm in the 90° forward flexed position, then, by observing the scapula to see if it lifts off the posterior chest wall; this is termed 'winging'.
◆ Latissimus dorsi. Ask the patient to abduct their arm to 90° and then try to adduct their arm downwards against your resistance.
◆ Biceps brachii. Ask the patient to flex their elbow against your downward resistance.
◆ Pectoralis major. Ask the patient to rotate their arm from the 90° abducted position towards forward flexion against your posterior resistance.

Special tests

In no other joint of the body are there more special tests, than in the shoulder. These tests attempt to identify shoulder impingement, instability, rotator cuff pathology and ACJ pathology.

You should certainly be aware of Jobe's test, Neer's sign, and the anterior apprehension test.

Jobe's test

Abduct the shoulder to 90°, with the arm straight and ask the patient to rotate their forearm such that the thumb is pointing to the ground. Then ask them to abduct upwards against the downward resistance of your hand on their arm. This tests for supraspinatus power and function, and (if painful) for impingement.

Hornblower's sign

Abduct the shoulder to 90° and flex the elbow to 90° with the forearm pointing upwards. Now ask the patient to try to internally rotate the shoulder (try to rotate the forearm to point downwards) against your

resistance posteriorly on their forearm. It is called the hornblower sign because hornblowers need to raise their arms into this position to blow the horn. This tests the power of infraspinatus.

Gerber's lift-off sign

Place the back of the patient's hand on their lumbar spine and ask them to push off their back posteriorly against the anterior resistance of your hand. This tests the power of subscapularis.

Hawkin's sign

Abduct the shoulder to 90°, support the patient's forearm and passively bring it through a range of internal rotation. At maximal internal rotation, the greater tuberosity of the humerus has been brought to its closest approach to the inferior surface of the acromion, and if they have impingement, this will result in a sharp pain.

Neer's sign

As for Hawkin's sign (same manoeuvre), but repeat the test 30 minutes after infiltrating local anaesthetic into the subacromial bursa. If this abolishes the pain, it is positive for impingement.

Acromioclavicular joint test

Palpate the ACJ for pain. Keep your hand over the ACJ and bring the arm around into maximal flexion across the chest horizontally. This is positive in ACJ pathology.

Sulcus sign

When the patient is relaxed with the arm hanging by their side, gently tug the arm down along its own axis, looking for the formation of a sulcus (an indentation) just inferior to the lateral border of the acromion. This demonstrates a trend to hypermobility, a risk factor for recurrent shoulder dislocations.

Anterior and posterior drawer signs

The humeral head in the relaxed patient should not be able to be pushed anteriorly (or posteriorly) by more than 50% of its own diameter. If it does, the shoulder is said to be hyperlax (or hypermobile).

Anterior apprehension test and Jobe's relocation test

With the arm hanging by the side, the elbow flexed up to 90°, place one hand on top of the shoulder (to stabilise the patient, not the shoulder) and gently force the shoulder into external rotation by the action of your hand on the patient's forearm. The Jobe's relocation test version of this is to perform the same manoeuvre with the patient supine on a couch, with the additional element of placing a posterior force with your other hand onto the anterior shoulder. The anterior apprehension test is positive if the patient becomes apprehensive (of dislocation), or if it hurts. The Jobe's relocation test is only positive if your stabilising force on the shoulder abolishes that apprehension (or pain). These are tests of anterior instability.

Wrist examination

Look

In rheumatoid arthritis you might see a prominent ulnar head and dorsal wrist swelling. Also, look for a ganglion, any relevant surgical scars or any associated forearm swellings.

Feel

Palpate the radial styloid, ulnar styloid, Lister's tubercle (on the dorsal distal radius), scaphoid tubercle (anterior radial border of the wrist), and the pisiform (anterior ulnar border of the wrist).

Palpate along both the anterior and posterior wrist joint lines. Compression between the scaphoid and the lunate anteriorly indicates scapholunate ligament instability. Tenderness between the distal radius and ulna, dorsally, can represent triangular fibrocartilage injury. Tenderness at the insertion of the extensor carpi ulnaris tendon at the wrist occurs in injury as well as in rheumatoid wrists. Tenderness over the thumb extensor tendons (dorsal radial wrist) may represent de Quervain's tenosynovitis.

Move

Stabilise the elbow (e.g. rest it on the table), hold the wrist (not the hand, as the carpal joints of the hand can mimic some pronation and supination, masking wrist pathology), and passively move the wrist through pronation and supination; also flexion, extension, radial and ulnar deviation. Compare with the other side.

Special tests

Finkelstein's test

This tests for de Quervain's tenosynovitis (inflammation of the tendon sheaths of extensor pollicis brevis and abductor pollicis longus). Ask the patient to make a fist over their thumb, then force the wrist into ulnar deviation. This is positive if the patient complains of dorsoradial pain.

Allen's test

This tests for vascular competence of both radial and ulnar arteries. Occlude both radial and ulnar arteries with your fingers. Ask the patient to repeatedly pump their fist as you maintain occlusion; this pumps the venous blood out of the hand, which goes white. Release your pressure over the ulnar artery; if the hand 'pinks-up' the patient's ulnar artery is competent to the hand.

Hand examination

This can usefully be divided up into two sections: the thumb and the fingers, although there is some overlap.

Examination of the thumb

Look

Inspect for deformities such as:

- Swan neck. Hyperextended MCPJ, flexed IPJ.
- Boutonniere. Flexed MCPJ, hyperextended IPJ.
- Gamekeeper's thumb. Excessive radial deviation at the MCPJ when gently forced.
- Swelling of either MCPJ or IPJ (arthritis).
- Subluxation of the thumb base at the CMCJ (osteoarthritis).

Feel

Palpate the thumb from the base to the tip for tenderness at the joints or over its bony surfaces. Feel for wasting of the thenar eminence, seen in carpal tunnel syndrome. Feel for swelling at the MCPJ or IPJ (arthritis).

Move

The movements of the thumb are more complex than for the fingers. Remember everything is 90° to the plane of the fingers. The thumb can flex across the plane of the palm and extend. It can abduct (if the palm is facing upwards and the back of the hand is resting on a table, then abduction is the action of raising the thumb vertically away from the table) and adduct. It can also oppose, which is a movement similar to flexion, but in opposition; the thumb is brought across the face of the palm into a form of two-digit-pinch-grip with the little finger.

You can formally test the action of flexor pollicis longus (FPL) by holding the proximal phalanx and asking the patient to flex the thumb at the IPJ. This neutralises the effect of flexor pollicis brevis (FPB), which flexes at the MCPJ only.

Special tests

Gamekeeper's thumb
Also known as skiier's thumb, nowadays, as the mechanism of the injury is to fall onto the thumb in forced abduction. The ulnar collateral ligament of the thumb MCPJ is torn in this condition, meaning that forced radial deviation at the MCPJ, with the metacarpal held fixed, results in excessive movement, radially, compared with the normal side.

Anterior interosseous nerve (AIN) palsy (the 'OK' sign)
Make a circle by bringing the tips of the thumb and index fingers together in a tip-pinch. Because the anterior interosseous nerve, which is a branch of the median nerve at the level of the elbow, supplies the FPL and flexor digitorum profundus (FDP) to the index finger, these are both used in this action. If the AIN has been damaged, the patient is unable to make the circular pinch grip and compensates by hyperextending the index DIPJ and the thumb IPJ, pinching with the pads of thumb and index, i.e. they cannot make the 'OK' sign.

Examination of the fingers

Look

Inspect the finger pads and look for wasting of the interossei, seen dorsally, as concavities between the metacarpals. Inspect the fingernails for psoriatic changes, e.g. pitting. Look for wasting of the thenar and hypothenar eminences (median and ulnar nerve lesions, respectively). Look for deformities of the fingers (ulnar deviation at the MCPJs is characteristic of rheumatoid arthritis), Heberden's nodes (bony swelling at the DIPJs, characteristic of osteoarthritis), Bouchard's nodes (bony swelling of the PIPJs, which are less common than Heberden's nodes and associated with osteoarthritis), and swelling of the MCPJs (characteristic of rheumatoid arthritis).

Feel

Palpate (gently, if the patient obviously has rheumatoid hands) the MCPJs, PIPJs and DIPJs, looking for tenderness.

Feel for soft tissue swelling in the region of the flexor tendons, indicative of flexor tenosynovitis, found in rheumatoid arthritis, most especially palpable at the level of the A1 pulley (level of the distal palmar crease).

Move

Testing movements of the hand is known as testing 'function' amongst hand surgeons.

Roll-up
Flexing all fingers together, gently, from an extended position to just about touching the distal crease of the palm. You should see a cascade, i.e. the little finger flexes ahead of the ring, followed by the middle and then index. Stiffness in any digit will disturb the cascade pattern of the roll-up.

Appositional grip
This is exactly as you would hold a key between your thumb pad and the lateral border of your index finger pad. Often tested by actually giving the patient a key to grip.

Power grip

Ask the patient to squeeze your hand. Remember, most of the power of grip comes from the little finger's side of the hand.

Tripod pinch

As you would hold a pen to write, involving the thumb pad, and both index and middle finger pads. Again, tested by giving the patient a pen to grip.

Precision grasp

As you would hold a screwdriver, i.e. power grip with the middle, ring and little fingers, combined with appositional grip of the thumb and index fingers.

Tip-pinch

As you would pick up a small object, i.e. between the tips of thumb and index fingers, often using the tips of the nails too.

Special tests

Isolating flexor digitorum superficialis (FDS)

Hold the other three fingers (other than the one you wish to test) in extension, and ask the patient to flex the remaining finger. You will note that it flexes at the PIPJ only, and that the DIPJ is 'floppy' if gently flicked to and fro. The reason for this is that holding the other fingers out straight prevents the action of FDP, which would normally flex the DIPJ. This is useful in looking for which tendon (FDS or FDP) has been ruptured or lacerated, e.g. a FDS laceration results in an inability to flex at the PIPJ.

Isolating flexor digitorum profundus (FDP)

Hold the middle phalanx of the finger with the finger extended. Then ask the patient to flex at the DIPJ. Keeping the PIPJ in extension negates the action of FDS, leaving only the FDP to flex the DIPJ. This is useful in looking for which tendon (FDS or FDP) has been ruptured or lacerated.

Testing median nerve motor function

Test thumb abduction (abductor pollicis brevis is supplied exclusively by the median nerve). To do this place the hand on a table, palm up, and ask the patient to raise the thumb so that it points to the ceiling.

Tinnel's test

Tap on the volar wrist crease to see if it reproduces tingling in the median nerve distribution (thumb, index, middle and radial border of the ring finger). If positive, this suggests carpal tunnel compression.

Phalen's test

Forcibly flex the wrist for one minute. If this reproduces the tingling in the distribution of the median nerve, it is positive for carpal tunnel compression.

Testing ulnar nerve motor function

Look for hypothenar eminence wasting.

Test the intrinsics of the hand. Ask the patient to spread their fingers (abduction, dorsal interossei) and test the power by resisting the movement. Then bring all the fingers together (adduction, palmar interossei) and test the power by asking them to trap your finger. Remember that the median nerve actually supplies the interossei to the index and middle fingers, so testing abduction and adduction specifically between these fingers would not be exclusively testing the ulnar nerve. To do so you can ask the patient to trap a sheet of paper between the sides of little and ring fingers, and ask them to resist you pulling the paper.

Froment's sign

This tests appositional grip of the thumb, by asking the patient to trap a piece of paper between the thumb's proximal phalanx and the index metacarpal's radial border, and hence function of the FPB muscle (the FPB flexes the MCPJ of the thumb). The test is positive for an ulnar nerve lesion if the patient tries to compensate for lack of FPB function by using FPL, i.e. flexes the thumb at the IPJ, rather than being able to keep it straight, when normal.

Ulnar paradox

This is the observation that clawing of the ring and little fingers occurring in ulnar nerve lesions only happens when the site of the lesion is said to be low. In this context it means distal to the elbow. The reason for this is that FDP needs to have some function to flex the fingers into the clawed position and if the lesion is above the level of the elbow, this interrupts the supply to FDP, hence abolishing clawing in a high lesion.

Testing radial nerve function

The radial nerve supplies sensation to a patch of skin on the dorsum of the thenar eminence. It supplies power to wrist extension and finger extension at the MCPJs. Thus, a high lesion, above the elbow, results in both wrist and finger drop, whereas a low lesion, below the elbow, results in finger and thumb drop only. This is because in the low lesion extensor carpi radialis and ulnaris are preserved, but extensor digiti communis and extensor pollicis longus are affected.

Testing dermatomes

The C6 dermatome includes the whole of the thumb and index finger. The C7 dermatome includes the whole of the middle finger and ring finger. The C8 dermatome includes the little finger and the ulnar border of the forearm. The T1 dermatome does not supply sensation to any skin on the forearm, only as far as the elbow along the inferior surface of the arm.

Elbow examination

Look

Inspect the carrying angle with the patient's arms down by their side, in supination and facing you, and look at the angle between the arm and forearm. It is normally valgus; this is the carrying angle. Inspect the anterior elbow and antecubital fossa, both posterior and medial aspects. Look for scars and deformity, etc.

Feel

Posteriorly

The olecranon and both humeral epicondyles.

Anteriorly

The cubital fossa, within which you should be able to feel the biceps tendon.

Medially

The medial epicondyle, looking for any tenderness of the ulnar nerve. A Tinnel's test can also be performed at this level, looking for tingling in the distribution of the ulnar nerve if it is entrapped at this level.

Laterally

The radial head and lateral humeral epicondyle.

Move

Range of movement

Move the elbow through flexion and extension, and compare with the other side. Also, test pronation and supination which occurs at the radiocapitellar joint, again comparing with the other side.

Power

Test grip strength. Resist elbow flexion (testing biceps brachii), and resist elbow extension (testing triceps).

Collateral ligaments

Place varus and valgus forces across the elbow with it held in extension, but also with it held in some flexion. This unlocks the olecranon from the olecranon fossa of the distal humerus, and hence tests the collateral ligaments more reliably.

Special tests

Tennis elbow

Also known as lateral epicondylitis. Place your finger on the common extensor origin (lateral humeral epicondylar region), then resist wrist extension of the patient. If this reproduces their pain they have an inflamed tendinous origin to their common extensors - tennis elbow.

Golfer's elbow

Also known as medial epicondylitis. It is similar to the above test, except you must place your finger on the common flexor origin (medial humeral epicondylar region), then resist wrist flexion of the patient. If this reproduces their pain they have an inflamed tendinous origin to their common flexors - golfer's elbow.

Foot and ankle examination

First, look at the hands for deformity, rheumatoid arthritis, psoriatic nail changes, Dupuytren's contracture, etc. Then look at the exposed lower limbs for deformity, muscle wasting, surgical scars, etc. Inspect the shoes for abnormal signs of wear, and look for any walking aids or callipers. Only then should you progress to examining the actual feet.

Look

In the first instance you should look at the feet with the patient standing. You are looking for clawing of the toes, any deformity, the medial arch (normal height, fallen as in pes planus, or high as in pes cavus), and abnormal prominence of either malleolus (as in varus or valgus hindfoot), scarring, and skin changes (e.g. trophic ulcers of neuropathy). Ask the patient to turn their back to you and stand with their feet together, so that you can then inspect their heels. You are looking for a varus or valgus calcaneum. The calcaneum is valgus in pes planus (fallen medial arch), and you can also identify the 'too many toes' sign. You should not normally be able to see more then the lateral two toes of the foot from behind, therefore three or more is 'too many', indicative of pes planus. If you identify pes planus, you should follow-up with observing tip-toeing to see if it corrects, indicating a flexible flat foot, e.g. tibialis posterior tendon dysfunction, as opposed to the fixed flat foot which is often due to tarsal coalitions in children.

Gait

Observe the sequence of the heel strike, stance phase, toe off and swing phase, and look for symmetry between sides.

Perform heel walking. This demonstrates the power of dorsiflexion (i.e. no foot-drop), and flexibility of the ankle (i.e. no stiffness).

Perform tip-toe walking. This demonstrates the arches of the foot, normal inversion of the heel, and good muscle power. Now, with the patient seated, you can inspect the soles of the feet. You are looking for callosities on the toe tips (in claw toes), metatarsal heads (in pes cavus), the lateral border of the foot (calcaneovarus), and the medial border of the foot (severe calcaneovalgus).

You should also make a point of inspecting between the toes (athlete's foot).

Feel

You should palpate the peroneal tendons, posterior to the lateral malleolus and along their course to the lateral foot for tenderness, the fifth metatarsal head, extensor tendons, the ankle joint medially, anteriorly and laterally, and both medial and lateral malleoli. Also palpate the tibialis posterior tendon, posterior to the medial malleolus and along its course to the medial foot, and the tendo achilles to its insertion to the superior border of the calcaneum. You are particularly feeling for tenderness and/or swelling.

Move

Test dosiflexion and plantar flexion of the ankle, comparing with the other side. Also, test eversion and inversion of the sub-talar joint, again comparing with the other side.

Stabilise the tarsal neck by gripping anterior to the ankle its medial and lateral eminences, and assess movement at the talonavicular and midtarsal joint, comparing with the other side.

Stabilise the heel by gripping the calcaneum medially and laterally, and assess abduction and adduction movements of the foot, comparing with the other side.

Assess the range of movement of the great and lesser toes, comparing with the other side.

You must always examine the back (including neurological examination of the lower limbs) at the end of a foot examination as there is considerable crossover of pathology between the back and the foot, e.g. spina bifida, spinal injury, neurological pes cavus and toe clawing, etc.

Special tests

Tibialis posterior

Perform resisted inversion. Remember that with tibialis posterior dysfunction, the patient is unable to tiptoe.

Peroneal tendons
Perform resisted eversion.

Tibialis anterior
Perform resisted dorsiflexion and inversion.

Drawer test
This tests for instability of the ankle, i.e. whether the talus is capable of anterior subluxation, which is not normal. Anterior subluxatory instability is most commonly caused by rupture of the anterior talofibular ligament (ATFL). Grip the ankle, and push the talus anteriorly with your hand on the posterior calcaneum.

Morton's neuroma
This is a neuroma in the common digital nerve between the metatarsal heads. In this condition there is tenderness on palpation between the metatarsal heads either side of the neuroma (pinch in the vertical plane).

You can also perform Mulder's click. Squeeze the foot's metatarsal heads together, with your other hand resting on the region of the metatarsal heads to feel for the click.

Grind test
This tests for hallux rigidis. Fix the metatarsal and rotate the great toe at the MTPJ. This is painful in hallux rigidis (OA of the first MTPJ).

Plantar fasciitis
This is tenderness on the sole of the foot at the level of the insertion of the plantar fascia with the inferior aspect of the calcaneum, as well as possible tenderness along the undersurface of the plantar fascia.

Simmond's test
Squeeze the calf when the patient is lying on their front on the couch with their foot hanging off the end. You should normally see the foot plantarflex as you squeeze. The test is considered positive (for a ruptured tendo achilles) if the foot does not plantarflex.

Coleman block test
This tests the flexibility (or rigidity) of the hindfoot in pes cavus. The foot is placed on a wooden block 3-4cm thick. The heel must be on the block. The 1st, 2nd and 3rd metatarsals must overhang off medially, leaving the 4th and 5th metatarsals on the block. In flexible pes cavus the heel varus corrects by this manoeuvre, and in rigid pes cavus, it does not. This has implications for the type of surgery that can be performed (as a rough guide: soft tissue surgery for flexible, and bony surgery for rigid).

Index